Pion and Heavy Ion Radiotherapy:

Pre-Clinical and Clinical Studies

Pion and Heavy Ion Radiotherapy:

Pre-Clinical and Clinical Studies

Proceedings of the International Workshop on Pion and Heavy Ion Radiotherapy:
Pre-Clinical and Clinical Studies, held in Vancouver, British Columbia, Canada,
July 29–31, 1981

Editor:

L. D. Skarsgard

Head, Medical Biophysics Unit
British Columbia Cancer Research Centre
Vancouver, B.C., Canada

Elsevier Biomedical
New York · Amsterdam · Oxford

The International Workshop on Pion and Heavy Ion Radiotherapy was sponsored by the British Columbia Cancer Foundation and by the National Health Research and Development Program of the Ministry of Health and Welfare Canada.

Published by:

Elsevier Science Publishing Co., Inc.
52 Vanderbilt Avenue, New York, New York 10017

Sole distributors outside the USA and Canada:

Elsevier Science Publishers B.V.
P.O. Box 211, 1000 AE, Amsterdam, The Netherlands

Library of Congress Cataloging in Publication Data

International Workshop on Pion and Heavy Ion Radio-therapy: Pre-Clinical and Clinical
    Studies (1981: Vancouver, B.C.)
    Pion and heavy ion radiotherapy.

    Includes index.
    1. Cancer—Radiotherapy—Congresses. 2. Pions—Therapeutic use—
    Congresses. 3. Heavy ions—Therapeutic use—Congresses. I. Skarsgard, L. D.
    II. Title.
RC271.R3I57 1981   616.99'4064   82-20956
ISBN 0-444-00765-2

Manufactured in the United States of America

Contents

RADIATION BIOLOGY IN VITRO

RADIATION BIOLOGY IN VIVO

Preface

The concept of using beams of pions and heavy ions in the radiation treatment of cancer arises logically from the physical properties of these particles: both particles are able to deliver maximum biological effect at a prescribed depth. When the depth is matched to the location of a tumour it allows the radiation effect to be concentrated in the tumour volume.

It is difficult to pinpoint the origin of the idea to use heavy charged particle beams for radiotherapy, though the names Robert Wilson, Chaim Richman, Raymond Zirkle, Cornelius Tobias, John Lawrence, Fowler and Perkins and others are certainly associated with this suggestion. Lawrence Berkeley Laboratory dominated the early development of heavy ion beams for radiobiological application and one of our contributors, Cornelius Tobias, has been involved with those developments since the 1940's. Another of our contributors, Carl von Essen, was a resident in radiotherapy in Chicago in 1953 when physicists Enrico Fermi and Herbert Anderson extolled to him the virtues of negative pi-mesons (pions) for radiotherapy. They suggested that within 20 years, pion beams appropriate for radiotherapy would be available. They were not far wrong.

Some of the intervening years were spent persuading the powers that be that facilities should be built to test these ideas and many more years were spent designing and building such facilities. For pions and the heavier ions, it is only in the last few years that actual clinical application of these beams has been possible and we are still at the early stages of such testing.

This monograph contains thirty-seven contributions from investigators who are actively involved in the development and testing of charged particle beam facilities. It provides an up-to-date review of the three major aspects of this field: the physics of charged particle beams, their biological effects in a variety of pre-clinical test systems and the clinical results obtained to date. Three contributions outline some of the recent technological advances in facilities to produce these beams, advances which promise more economic delivery of such beams. As well, two contributions review clinical results obtained with neutron beams which give ionization densities comparable to those of the heavier charged particles, though the depth doses are very different.

The numbers of patients treated to date with pions and heavy ions are far too small to allow us to draw conclusions as to the effectiveness of these new modalities for the treatment of cancer, though there are some encouraging signs as well as some disappointments. A continued and expanded program of clinical evaluation is essential if this question is to be answered.

It is a pleasure to acknowledge the support of the British
Columbia Cancer Foundation and the Ministry of Health and Welfare
Canada, whose sponsorship made this workshop possible.
We also wish to thank the authors who contributed to these procee-
dings and the publishers, Elsevier Science Publishing Company,
for their expert technical assistance. Special thanks are due to
Beverley Ersoy, Denise Jackson and Isabel Harrison for their efforts
in co-ordinating the workshop and the preparation of manuscripts.

L. D. Skarsgard

NEW DEVELOPMENTS IN FACILITIES

Published 1982 by Elsevier Science Publishing Co., Inc.
PION AND HEAVY ION RADIOTHERAPY:
Pre-Clinical and Clinical Studies
L. D. Skarsgard

3

THE PIGMI LINEAR-ACCELERATOR TECHNOLOGY*

T. J. Boyd, K. R. Crandall, R. W. Hamm, L. D. Hansborough, R. F. Hoeberling,
R. A. Jameson, E. A. Knapp, D. W. Mueller, J. M. Potter, R. H. Stokes,
J. E. Stovall, R. G. Sturgess, D. A. Swenson, P. J. Tallerico, T. P. Wangler,
and L. C. Wilkerson
Accelerator Technology Division, MS-H811, Los Alamos National Laboratory,
Los Alamos, New Mexico 87545

INTRODUCTION

A new linear-accelerator technology has been developed that makes pi-meson (pion) generation possible for cancer therapy in the setting of a major hospital center. This technology uses several new major inventions in particle accelerator science--such as a new accelerator system called the radio-frequency quadrupole (RFQ), and permanent-magnet drift-tube focusing--to substantially reduce the size, cost, and complexity of a "meson factory" for this use. This paper describes this technology, discusses other possible uses for these new developments and possible costs for such installations.

Innovation in the application of several new radiation types to cancer therapy has been pursued actively during the last 10 years, in both the United States and overseas. At present, the potential of pions, heavy ions, protons, and neutrons is being investigated in clinical trials. The technology of producing beams of these radiations also is under study, and significant advances have been made in the accelerator science necessary to produce cost-effective sources of them. This paper concentrates on proton linear-accelerator technology--essential to the production of pion beams for cancer therapy but also applicable to proton- or neutron-beam machines.

The PIGMI program,[1-4] funded by the National Cancer Institute (NCI), began in 1976 and has developed an entire technology that is capable of producing proton linear accelerators for installation in hospitals. These accelerators are significantly less expensive, are more reliable, and are smaller than any available before this program.[5-7] The rationale for this development involved a series of thrusts in technology development based on the philosophy

*Work supported by the US Department of Energy and by the National Cancer Institute, Division of Research, Resources, and Centers, US Department of Health and Human Services.

that several parameters traditionally chosen for research linacs were super-fluous for a medically dedicated machine. The rationale chosen involved

- an intermediate current goal,
- a minimum energy consistent with pion production,
- a minimum size,
- a maximum simplicity in operation,
- a low "duty factor" to allow standard power sources,
- compatibility with all known or contemplated pion delivery systems, and
- optimum reliability.

These directions then defined the PIGMI parameters.

Starting with a pion dose rate of 50-100 R/min/$_\ell$ and an upper limit on the performance of a large acceptance pion channel of 3% $\Delta P/_p$ at 0.5 steradian, the accelerator parameters required are

E	650 MeV
I	100 μA
ε_n	0.05 π cm· rad
$\dfrac{\Delta E}{E}$	0.5%

Using the newly developed PIGMI technology, these parameters are relatively easy to achieve without exceptional measures; they yield desired performance and have convenient beam-handling characteristics.

THE PIGMI TECHNOLOGY

With the above parameters and rationale, the PIGMI program has developed an innovative design for the required hospital-based pion generator. Figure 1 shows the components of a PIGMI accelerator and indicates the innovations and design used in the final proposed solution.

A high-energy proton linac generally consists of a chain of separate accel-erators, each adding an increment to the energy of the final beam. In the cur-rent PIGMI design, the first of these accelerators is a 30 kV injector with an ion source, where protons are generated and accelerated to low energy for injection into the next acceleration stage. Because of the development of the RFQ structure,[8] which will be described next, the design of this injector has been simplified dramatically.

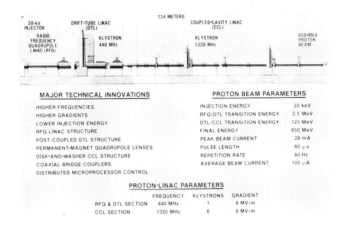

Fig. 1. Pion generator for medical irradiations.

The second accelerator in this chain is the RFQ accelerator, invented in the Soviet Union and first developed in the United States for the PIGMI program. This accelerator accepts the 30 keV proton beam from the injector and prepares this beam by bunching and further acceleration for injection again into the next acceleration stage, the drift-tube linac (DTL). The RFQ is unique in this function: it allows very efficient capture of the injector beam with extremely low degradation of beam parameters in this transfer process. We believe the RFQ represents a major advance in accelerator science and significantly improves the performance of a PIGMI system.

The third accelerator in this chain is the DTL; this is the classic, conventional ion linear accelerator. In the PIGMI design we have made an innovation, the permanent-magnet drift-tube focusing lens, that allows the design to be executed at a considerably higher frequency than is normally the case. This higher frequency (440 MHz) results in two major savings in the final system: high-power klystrons are available at this frequency, thus lowering costs substantially; and the higher frequency results in appreciably smaller component size.

The fourth and last accelerator system in this chain is the disk-and-washer (DAW) system,[9] also a newly developed technology, with possibilities for high acceleration rates. As in the DTL, permanent-magnet focusing may be used to ensure simple and reliable operation. The DAW accelerates the proton beam to the final output energy, then must couple into a beam transport system that carries the protons to a pion producing target, and a pion collection channel that gathers and focuses the pion beam on the tumor for treatment. A more detailed discussion of the individual accelerator systems is given below.

The Injector

The injector system into a conventional proton linac traditionally has been an extremely expensive and complex component. The advent of the RFQ system has simplified the PIGMI injector to the point where it is of minor cost and size in the PIGMI system. Figure 2 shows an artist's concept of the PIGMI injector system,[10,11] consisting of a duoplasmatron ion source and a single accelerating gap acceleration column, with all required power supplies, gas systems, etc., contained in a single rack of electronics contiguous to the source. The geometry of the source extraction region is designed to provide a converging focused beam that is then refocused to a second waist at the input to the RFQ. This refocusing is accomplished by an "einzel" or electrostatic focusing lens operated at the same polarity and slightly lower voltage than the main extraction gap. This injector system has been assembled and tested, and performs up to specification in all respects.

The RFQ Linac

The RFQ represents a revolutionary new focusing, bunching, and accelerating structure that promises to be an important part of many future proton, light ion, and heavy ion facilities.[12-15] The first RFQ structure outside the USSR was tested in the PIGMI laboratory in February 1980.[16] These tests were highly successful, confirming the general properties of the RFQ structure, and gave excellent agreement between the beam's measured properties and its predicted performance. The tests established that the RFQ operates in a stable manner that is remarkably insensitive to injection energy errors, rf excitation errors, and structural fabrication errors.

The RFQ represents a superb answer to one of the most difficult remaining questions of how to build simple, reliable, and inexpensive proton or ion linacs. The RFQ offers the lowest injection energy of any known linac structure, it is the best buncher ever conceived, and it bunches and accelerates the

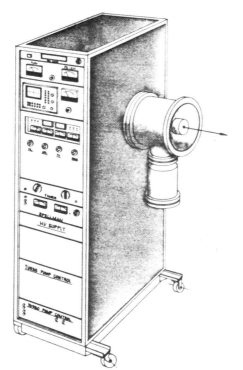

Fig. 2. Ion source and associated equipment.

beam with less emittance growth than any other known system.[17] It represents the best transformation ever seen between the continuous beams that come
from ion sources and the bunched and accelerated beams required by conventional
linacs. The RFQ eliminates the need for large and costly Cockcroft-Walton
power supplies, complex multicavity buncher systems, low-energy beam-transport
systems, and their associated controls and instrumentation.

The RFQ is essentially a vane-loaded cylinder (Fig. 3) excited in a modified TE_{210} cavity mode that produces a strong electric quadrupole field near the axis. This field's transverse components, which are uniform in space and alternating in time, give rise to strong, alternating-gradient, focusing effects that can focus beams of particles traveling along the axis of the structure. By scalloping the vane-tip geometry as shown in Fig. 3, a longitudinal component, which can bunch and accelerate the beam, is introduced into the rf electric field near the axis. Thus, the RFQ structure is capable of focusing, bunching, and accelerating beams of charged particles.

The structure is so simple that, for the first time, it is possible to configure the linac for adiabatic capture of continuous beams at low energy. This configuration introduces the scallops gradually, so that the structure acts primarily as a buncher at the beginning, transforming gradually to an accelerator at the end. A cutaway view of the RFQ structure is shown in Fig. 4 and a computer-generated picture of such a vane tip is shown in Fig. 5.

The RFQ contains four regions: the radial matching section, the shaper, the gentle buncher, and the accelerating section.[18] In the radial-matching section, the vane aperture is tapered to adjust the focusing strength from almost zero to its full value in a very short distance; this allows the dc injected beam to be matched into the time-dependent focusing. In the next two regions (shaper and gentle buncher), the beam is adiabatically bunched as it is accelerated. At the end of the gentle buncher, the beam's synchronous phase angle reaches its final value, and the bunched beam is then accelerated in the final region (accelerating section). In this region, the vane radius, vane modulation, and phase angle are held constant to obtain the maximum acceleration gradient.

The PIGMI RFQ was designed and its performance analyzed with PARMTEQ, the RFQ-linac design and simulation computer code. The RFQ's operating frequency is 440 MHz. It is designed to accept a 30 keV proton beam from the ion source,

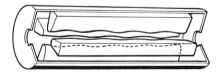

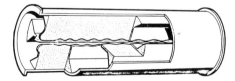

Fig. 3. General configuration of the RFQ.

Fig. 4. Cutaway view of the RFQ structure.

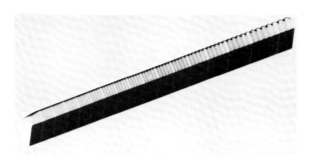

Fig. 5. Computer-generated view of the RFQ vane tip.

then to focus, bunch, and accelerate that beam to a 2.5 MeV energy in 1.78 m.
Each vane tip has a total of 200 scallops, varying in length from 0.27 cm at
the beginning to 2.47 cm at the end. The structure's minimum radial aperture
is 1.9 mm. The RFQ captures 92% of a 30 mA beam to yield the PIGMI 28 mA
design current. The transverse emittance growth (for the 90% contour) is
approximately a factor of 1.4, which is better than can be achieved by any
other buncher/linac combination.

A coaxial manifold has been developed that provides a symmetrical, multislot
driving arrangement for the RFQ cavity.[19] A coaxial cavity surrounding the
RFQ cavity is excited in a coaxial TEM mode. The magnetic fields in the TEM
mode are orthogonal to the magnetic fields in the RFQ mode. These fields can
be coupled by diagonal slots that have their angles determined by the magnitude
and direction of adjacent magnetic fields. We are investigating techniques for
resonating these slots to provide resonant coupling between the RFQ manifold
and the RFQ cavity.

A technique has been proposed for coupling the RFQ manifold to the DTL so
that the RFQ can derive its rf power from the DTL, thereby eliminating the
necessity for a separate rf power source and drive line.[8]

The Drift Tube Linac

The vast majority of proton linacs are of the DTL type. Most of the linacs
designed in the last 10 years use post couplers[20] (developed at Los Alamos
by the principal investigators of the PIGMI program) to stabilize the distribution of the electromagnetic fields within the structure. These structures'
properties and their performance are well known.

The PIGMI DTL differs from conventional DTLs primarily in scale, being more than twice the frequency, and hence, less than one-quarter the cross-sectional area of conventional linacs. The higher frequency and the low duty factor of PIGMI make its optimum accelerating gradient higher than normal for conventional linacs, thus making the PIGMI facility significantly shorter.

The small size of the PIGMI DTL precludes normal fabrication and assembly techniques, which require entry of personnel into the interior of the structure for assembly and alignment.[21,22] The PIGMI scheme is based on the preassembly of short (2.5 m) linac tank sections, into which the drift tubes can be introduced from the ends, or through slots in the top, into precision-bored holes along the bottom of the tank sections.

The PIGMI drift tubes also are considerably smaller than those in conventional DTLs, precluding the use of electromagnetic quadrupole lenses for focusing the beam. The PIGMI solution is to use permanent-magnet quadrupole lenses, made of modern materials in the best geometrical configuration (Fig. 6); this results in compact magnetic lenses of sufficient strength.[23,24] The design is further simplified by allowing all quadrupoles to have a common length and strength throughout the structure.

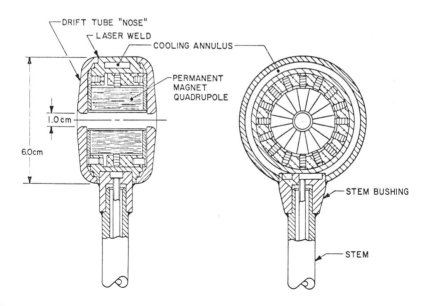

Fig. 6. DTL drift tube and quadrupole configuration.

The PIGMI DTL is conceived as a single-tank, post-coupled DTL that is ~30 m long and 0.4 m in diameter. The DTL operates at 440 MHz, the same as that of the RFQ, and accelerates the proton beam from 2.5 MeV to 125 MeV, with an average axial electric field of 6 MV/m. Its peak power dissipation is 14.2 MW and peak beam power is 3.4 MW, for a total peak-power requirement of 17.6 MW. The average power dissipated in the structure is only 51 kW or 1.7 kW/m.

The DTL structure has 150 drift tubes and 74 post couplers. All drift tubes have a 6 cm o.d., a 1 cm diameter bore hole, and are supported on a single stem from the bottom of the tank. Figure 7 shows a cutaway view of a portion of the DTL structure.

Each drift tube contains a permanent-magnet quadrupole lens to focus the beam. All 150 quadrupole magnets are identical in size and strength. They are made of samarium cobalt and are magnetized to produce a quadrupole gradient of 20 kG/cm over the 1 cm diameter bore.

The DTL structure is designed and analyzed with the aid of the linac design and simulation code, PARMILA. The structure accepts essentially 100% of the accelerated beam from the RFQ and accelerates it to 125 MeV.

The 30 m linac structure is fabricated as twelve tank sections, each about 2.5 m long. The tank sections' ends are located at points corresponding to the midplane of a drift-tube gap. The length, number of drift tubes, and maximum energy associated with each tank section are given in Table 1. The general mechanical features of the first and last tank sections are shown in Fig. 8.

The tank sections are stiffened along the bottom by a structural member that supports the drift tubes. The drift-tube mounting holes are precision bored through this structural member and tank wall. Post-coupler mounting holes are bored along the side of the tank at locations corresponding to the midplane of every other drift tube and alternating from side-to-side of the structure.

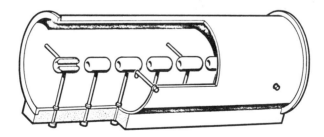

Fig. 7. Cutaway view of the DTL structure.

TABLE 1

PIGMI DTL TANK SECTIONS

Section	Length (m)	Number of Drift Tubes	Energy (MeV)
1	2.502	30	13.4
2	2.570	19	25.0
3	2.375	14	35.7
4	2.556	13	47.2
5	2.411	11	57.5
6	2.624	11	68.5
7	2.557	10	78.7
8	2.433	9	88.2
9	2.550	9	97.8
10	2.360	8	106.5
11	2.443	8	115.2
12	2.680	8	125.0
Total	30.061	150	125.0

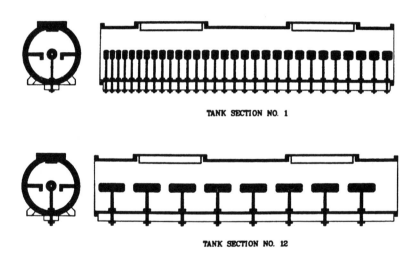

TANK SECTION NO. 1

TANK SECTION NO. 12

Fig. 8. First and last DTL tank sections.

Each tank section has two half-meter-long slots in the top surface for access to the interior and for mounting vacuum pumps, fixed tuners, variable tuners, etc.

The DAW Accelerator System

Significant discoveries made at Los Alamos during the development of LAMPF in the 1960s led the way to practical coupled-cavity linac structures for acceleration of protons at energies in excess of 200 MeV. The major advance made at that time was the recognition of the importance of using biperiodic standing-wave structures excited in the $\pi/2$ cavity mode.[25] The structure developed at that time is called the side-coupled structure[26] and, when properly tuned, offers high efficiency in the conversion of rf power to beam power, with exceptional stability in the distribution of the accelerating fields--a feature that is essential for reliable operation.

The Russians, in their interest in building a LAMPF-type machine, considered the LAMPF side-coupled structure and two other structures: the ring-coupled structure and a DAW structure. They selected the latter because of its large intercavity coupling constant and its potential for simple fabrication.

At the outset of the PIGMI program, it was assumed that the "high-beta" portion of PIGMI would use a scaled-down version of the LAMPF side-coupled structure. The only developments envisioned were methods for increasing the intercavity coupling and for simplifying the fabrication. It was quickly realized that the outstanding properties of the DAW structure satisfied both these goals.[27,28] A cutaway view of the DAW structure is shown in Fig. 9.

SUPERFISH,[28,29] a powerful rf-cavity calculational program developed at Los Alamos (partly in response to the needs of the PIGMI program), was used to analyze the DAW structure in detail. Exhaustive computer studies using this program, coupled with test-cavity experiments, led to a thorough understanding of this structure's performance and to an optimized set of parameters for the PIGMI application.[30]

In long linac structures such as PIGMI, there is a need to break the structure into shorter sections to allow the introduction of auxiliary apparatus such as beam-focusing quadrupoles, beam-diagnostic equipment, vacuum isolation valves, etc. In many cases it is also desirable to couple these sections into longer resonant units to reduce the required number of rf-power drive points and to lock the relative phase and amplitude of the fields in adjacent sections. To take optimum advantage of the structure's superior properties, any required rf couplers also should be of the resonantly coupled type with large

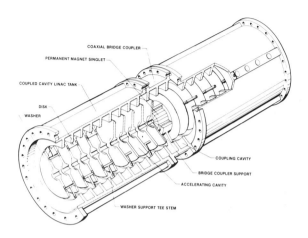

COAXIAL BRIDGE COUPLER

PERMANENT MAGNET SINGLET

COUPLED CAVITY LINAC TANK

DISK

WASHER

COUPLING CAVITY

BRIDGE COUPLER SUPPORT

ACCELERATING CAVITY

WASHER SUPPORT TEE STEM

Fig. 9. Cutaway view of the DAW structure.

coupling constants and, for the practical reasons of structure tuning, the linac structures' rf coupling should represent a minimum distortion of the field patterns in either element. Such couplers at LAMPF have been called "bridge couplers" because they bridge the resonant properties of the linac structure around the auxiliary apparatus.

For the PIGMI application, single-cell bridge couplers have been developed that are adequate to house the required apparatus within the linac struc-ture.[31] Figure 10 shows the general geometry of these bridge couplers for the values of ß equal to 0.5, 0.6, 0.7, and 0.8. In each bridge coupler's center there is a region of high magnetic field and zero electric field. In this plane, conducting radial supports have a negligible effect on the accel-erating mode and a tolerable effect on the coupling mode. Hollow conducting radial supports provide suitable channels for the services required by the auxiliary apparatus housed within the bridge couplers, such as cooling water for the bridge-coupler parts, signal leads for beam-diagnostic devices, and control rods for mechanical devices. Practical designs incorporating a variety of these features have been made for bridge couplers.

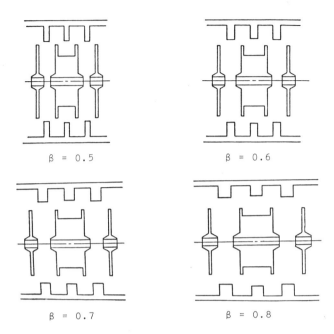

β = 0.5   β = 0.6

β = 0.7   β = 0.8

Fig. 10. Single-cell bridge coupler geometries.

The PIGMI DAW is ∿100 m long and 0.34 m in diameter, with a 1320 MHz operating frequency, three times that of the DTL. The DAW accelerates the proton beam from 125 MeV to 650 MeV with an 8 MV/m average axial electric field. The structure's peak-power dissipation is 69 MW and its peak beam power is 14.6 MW, for a total peak-power requirement of 81.4 MW. The average power dissipated in the structure is only 250 kW, or about 2.5 kW/m.

The PIGMI DAW comprises 108 tanks of 11 cells each, whose lengths vary from 0.6 m to 1.0 m. The cell geometries are uniform throughout each tank, but differ from tank to tank. The tanks are resonantly coupled by 107 single-cell bridge couplers, each containing a permanent-magnet quadrupole singlet for focusing the beam. All 107 quadrupole singlets are identical; they are made of a ceramic material magnetized to produce a 5 kG/cm quadrupole gradient over the 2 cm diameter bore. The bore-hole diameter of the structure and of the bridge coupler is 2 cm.

The structure accepts essentially 100% of the accelerated beam from the DTL and accelerates it to 650 MeV; apparently the beam suffers no emittance growth in this portion of the PIGMI facility.

For facility organization, the DAW is subdivided into 6 modules of 18 tanks each. A high degree of similarity is imposed on the organization of each module with regard to the distribution of the necessary auxiliary features such as rf drive points, beam and accelerator diagnostic instrumentation, and vacuum equipment. Each module's center bridge coupler accommodates one of the six 1320 MHz rf power systems. Each module's end bridge coupler is outfitted with a coaxial ceramic window and a compact beamline valve to provide vacuum isolation between modules for maintenance purposes. The remaining bridge couplers accommodate an array of vacuum pumps and diagnostic gear. Figure 11 shows a typical module, and Table 2 gives the length and maximum energy associated with each module.

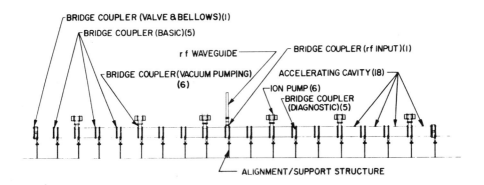

Fig. 11. Typical module of the DAW.

TABLE 2

PIGMI DAW MODULES

Modules	Length (m)	Number of Tanks	Energy (MeV)
1	12.60	18	193
2	14.61	18	271
3	16.22	18	357
4	17.52	18	450
5	18.56	18	548
6	19.42	18	650
Total	98.93	108	650

The rf Power Systems

The PIGMI frequencies of 440 MHz and 1320 MHz were chosen partly on beam-dynamics considerations and partly on the availability of suitable klystrons. Many military radar klystrons have been designed to operate in the 400 to 450 MHz band and the next higher frequency band of 1250 to 1350 MHz. The PIGMI frequencies, which must be harmonically related, were chosen to fall in these ranges.

The costs of the rf systems were compared for three different beam-pulse patterns with identical duty factor: 10 μs beam pulses at a 360 Hz repetition rate, 30 μs beam pulses at a 120 Hz repetition rate, and 60 μs beam pulses at a 60 Hz repetition rate. The shorter beam pulse and higher repetition rate reduce the cost of the pulse-forming network (PFN) modulator but consume more average power because of the larger number of cavity fill times. The longer beam pulse and lower repetition rate result in a 100 kW power saving over the medium-pulse alternative and a 240 kW power saving over the short pulse alternative. The 60 μs, 60 Hz option has been adopted for PIGMI on the basis that the power savings resulting from the lower repetition rate will override the additional cost of the PFN modulators associated with the longer pulse length.

The cavity power dissipation for the 440 MHz portions of PIGMI (RFQ and DTL) are estimated to be 16.2 MW, and the beam loading for this same region corresponds to 3.5 MW. The rf pulse length must exceed the beam pulse length by the cavity fill time of $\sim$15.6 μs. The rf duty factor is 60 x 75.6 x 10^{-6}, or 0.004536. The total peak-power requirement at 440 MHz is 19.7 MW and the average-power requirement is 89.4 kW. A single Varian VA-812E klystron can satisfy both the peak- and average-power requirements of the 440 MHz portion of PIGMI.

The cavity power dissipation for the 1320 MHz portion of PIGMI is estimated to be 66.8 MW; the beam loading for this same region corresponds to 14.6 MW. The cavity fill time of the 1320 MHz structure is only 3.6 μs, and the rf duty factor is 0.003816. The total peak-power requirement at 1320 MHz is 81.4 MW and the average-power requirement is 310.6 kW. Five Litton L-5081 klystrons are capable of satisfying both the peak- and average-power requirements of the 1320 MHz portion of PIGMI. The PIGMI design is based on six such klystrons operating at a reduced level, providing the possibility, in emergencies, to continue operation if there is failure of a single klystron.

An appropriate PFN modulator has been designed and is being fabricated for the PIGMI component test program.

Computer Control and Instrumentation System

The PIGMI control and instrumentation system will provide the operator with a three-state control: OFF, STANDBY, and ON. The STANDBY and ON states are identical in that all equipment is on and running within tolerance, with the exception that the beam is inhibited at the ion source and certain beam stops are inserted in the STANDBY state.

In either of these states, the operator can monitor the detailed performance of each system in the facility. All of the set points designed to influence the machine's performance are available to the operator through the control system and can be set up, monitored, and/or recorded for future setup purposes by convenient parameter-management procedures.

In the ON state, the operator can monitor the properties of the beam, the evidence of beam loss (if any), and the effects of beam loading on the accelerator equipment systems. Certain tuning procedures will be available to the operator for fine-tuning of the performance.

If there is equipment failure, the control and diagnostic system will identify the faulty equipment and will notify the operator. In some cases, further diagnostics may be available to pinpoint the faulty unit; most repairs will be accomplished by unit replacement.

All critical parameters will be monitored periodically and will be compared to their current set-point values and tolerance limits. The operator will be notified of out-of-tolerance conditions, and in some cases, corrective action will be automated. Selected data will be collected on a regular basis for general and specialized logs to support machine records and statistical studies of machine performance.

The control system comprises a minicomputer, a control console, and a distributed array of small, modular, and intelligent control stations. The design is based on an advanced architecture developed and demonstrated at the Fermi National Accelerator Laboratory (FNAL). The design benefits from state-of-the-art engineering and from years of experience in controlling an operating linac. Soon this general configuration will control several new accelerator facilities, including the injector linac of FNAL and the antiproton accumulator ring at FNAL. The PIGMI system will benefit from these related applications.

The equipment systems under the surveillance of the control system include injector parameters, cavity field parameters, temperature-control systems, forward and reflected powers, PFN modulator parameters, beam diagnostics, beam-spill radiation monitors, and a few electromagnetic quadrupoles and steering magnets. A few protection systems, such as the personnel-safety system, the run-permit system, and the fast-protect system, are implemented independently of the control system, and provide their status, but no control, to the computer control system.

PIGMI FACILITY COSTS AND INSTALLATION

A PIGMI facility clearly is suitable only for a large hospital complex. Siting at such a center might be configured as shown in Fig. 12 where the adjacent parking lot provides open space in which to bury a tunnel; this tunnel would house the accelerator and provide radiation shielding if inadvertant beam loss occurs along the accelerator's length. It is essential that a hospital be involved that is large enough to provide the engineering and medical backup required for operating such a complex device. In this context, then, the cost figures for a PIGMI facility can be estimated. We estimate that such an accelerator would cost between $10 M and $12 M for the technical component costs, with a $5-6 M construction project for housing the accelerator. In addition, a $10 M treatment facility would be required for providing pion beam channels,

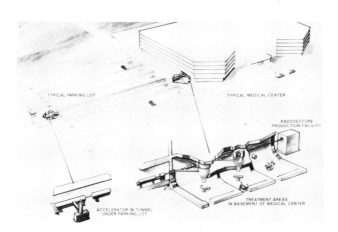

Fig. 12. Typical PIGMI-facility layout.

patient handling, and so on. Therefore, the current estimate is a total cost of $25-30 M for a clinical pion installation to be established in a hospital environment. In contrast, a LAMPF accelerator system would certainly be in the $100 M category if built today.

Such a facility, however, would have a large treatment capacity, if operated in a manner that recognizes the high capital costs involved and makes suitable provision for optimum use of the equipment. At the assumed dose rate we would have an irradiation time per fraction (125 rads) of 2-3 min; setup time would dominate, as in conventional radiotherapy. With three channels accepting beam from the PIGMI accelerator, and automated patient positioning as used in the Los Alamos clinical trial, it would seem possible to treat 10-15 patients/hour. Using a 16 h day for treatment yields a 160-200 patient/day throughput; or with a 5 wk cycle, gives the capability of 2000 new patients/year. Thus the cost per patient will be high, but not excessively so, if pion radiotherapy is seen to be extremely effective at the conclusion of the clinical trials.

CONCLUSIONS

The NCI-funded PIGMI program has resulted in several revolutionary accelerator science innovations, making possible the design and fabrication of a pion-producing linear accelerator for use in a hospital environment. The resulting accelerator complex would be compact enough to be located in many regional hospital centers, would be reliable and easy to operate, and would be compatible with reasonable patient cost if pion therapy turns out to be extremely effective.

REFERENCES

1. Knapp EA, Bradbury JN (1975) Medical Linac Design Possibilities. Springfield, Virginia: National Technical Information Services, CONF-741040:304.

2. Bradbury JN, Knapp EA, Nagle DE (1975) Light Ion Linacs for Medical Application. IEEE Trans Nucl Sci 22:1755.

3. Knapp EA, Bradbury JN (1975) Proposal for Development of a Pion Generator for Medical Application. Los Alamos National Laboratory proposal P-540.

4. Knapp EA, Swenson DA (1977) The PIGMI Program at LASL. Chalk River Nuclear Laboratory report AECL-5677:230.

5. Hansborough LD, Compiler (1981) PIGMI: A Design Report for a Pion Generator for Medical Irradiations. Los Alamos National Laboratory report LA-8880.

6. Hansborough LD, Hamm RW, Stovall JE, Swenson DA (1981) An Optimized Design for PIGMI. IEEE Trans Nucl Sci 28:1511.

7. Swenson DA (1980) Low-Beta Linac Structures. Brookhaven National Laboratory report BNL-51134:129.

8. Swenson DA (1980) Resonant Coupling of an RFQ Manifold to a Drift-Tube Linac Cavity. Los Alamos National Laboratory, Accelerator Technology Division, Group AT-1 memorandum AT-1-197.

9. Schriber SO (1980) High-Beta Linac Structures. Brookhaven National Laboratory report BNL-51134:164.

10. Hamm RW, Lederer HM, Mueller DW, Stevens RR (1979) A Compact 250-kV Injector System for PIGMI. IEEE Trans Nucl Sci 26:1493.

11. Hamm RW (1980) Los Alamos National Laboratory, Accelerator Technology Division, Group AT-1 memorandum AT-1-270.

12. Wangler TP, Stokes RH (1981) The Radio-Frequency Quadrupole Linear Accelerator. IEEE Trans Nucl Sci 28:1484.

13. Stokes RH, Crandall KR, Hamm RW, Humphry FJ, Jameson RA, Knapp EA, Potter JM, Rodenz GW, Stovall JE, Swenson DA, Wangler TP (1981) The Radio-Frequency Quadrupole: General Properties and Specific Applications. Experimentia: Supplement 40:399.

14. Hamm RW, Crandall KR, Fuller CW, Hansborough LD, Jameson RA, Knapp EA, Machalek MD, Potter JM, Rodenz GW, Stokes RH, Stovall JE, Swenson DA, Wangler TP, Williams SW (1981) The RF Quadrupole Linac: A New Low-Energy Accelerator. Inst Phys, Bristol: Conf. Ser. 54:54.

15. Potter JM, Humphry FJ, Rodenz GW, Williams SW (1979) Radio-Frequency Quadrupole Accelerating Structure Research at Los Alamos. IEEE Trans Nucl Sci 26:3745.

16. Stovall JE, Crandall KR, Hamm RW (1981) Performance Characteristics of a 425-MHz RFQ Linac. IEEE Trans Nucl Sci 28:1508.

17. Jameson RA, Mills RS (1980) On Emittance Growth in Linear Accelerators. Brookhaven National Laboratory report BNL-51134:231.

18. Crandall KR, Stokes RH, Wangler TP (1980) RF Quadrupole Beam-Dynamics Design Studies. Brookhaven National Laboratory report BNL-51134:205.

19. Potter JM (1980) An RF Power Manifold for the Radio-Frequency Quadrupole Linear Accelerator. Brookhaven National Laboratory report BNL-51134:205.

20. Swenson DA, Knapp EA, Potter JM, Schneider EJ (1967) Stabilization of the Drift-Tube Linac by Operation in the $\pi/2$ Cavity Mode. Cambridge Electron Accelerator Laboratory report CEAL-2000:167.

21. Hart VE (1976) PIGMI Mechanical Fabrication. Chalk River Nuclear Laboratory report AECL-5677:358.

22. Hansborough LD, Bush ED, Hart VE (1979) Mechanical Description of Pigmi. IEEE Trans Nucl Sci 26:1464.

23. Holsinger RF (1980) The Drift-Tube and Beam-Line Quadrupole Permanent Magnets for the New Proton Linac. Brookhaven National Laboratory report BNL-51134:373:230.

24. Lazarev NV, Skachkov VS (1980) Tipless Permanent-Magnet Quadrupole Lenses. Brookhaven National Laboratory report BNL-51134:380.

25. Nagle DE, Knapp BC, Knapp EA (1967) Coupled Resonator Model for Standing-Wave Accelerator Tanks. Rev Sci Instrum 38(11):1583.

26. Knapp EA, Knapp BC, Potter JM (1968) Standing-Wave High-Energy Linear Accelerator Structures. Rev Sci Instrum 39:979.

27. Manca JJ, Knapp EA, Swenson DA (1977) High-Energy Accelerating Structures for High-Gradient Proton Linac Applications. IEEE Trans Nucl Sci 24:1087.

28. Halbach K, Holsinger RF (1976) SUPERFISH - A Computer Program for Evaluation of RF Cavities with Cylindrical Symmetry. Particle Accelerators 7:213.

29. Halbach K, Holsinger RF, Jule WE, Swenson DA (1977) Properties of the Cylindrical RF Cavity Evaluation Code SUPERFISH. Chalk River National Laboratory report AECL-5677:122.

30. Schriber SO (1979) Room-Temperature Cavities for High-Beta Accelerating Structures. Proc Conf on Future Possibilities for Electron Accelerators, University of Virginia, Charlottesville, Virginia: L-1.

31. Swenson DA, Potter JM (1980) Resonantly Coupled Bridge Couplers for the Disk-and Washer Linac Structure. Los Alamos National Laboratory, Accelerator Technology Division, Group AT-1 memorandum AT-10186.

THE PIOTRON

GEORG VECSEY
Swiss Institute for Nuclear Research, 5234 Villigen, Switzerland

INTRODUCTION

In many cases positive results fully justify the use of γ rays
for radiotherapy, but their wide spread application is mainly based
on their relatively simple availability. In still many other cases
of cancer, where local failure of treatment remains the cause of
high mortality, significant changes of the cure rate should hopefully be achieved by new methods in radiotherapy using particle
beams. For reasons given below, negative pi mesons were identified
as most promising candidates by Fowler and Perkins[1] as early as
1961. It is only recently, however, that pion beams of sufficient
intensity can be generated at the meson factories, LAMPF, TRIUMF
and SIN.

Ideally, the irradiation method should guarantee the deposition
of a highly homogeneous dose distribution inside an arbitrary but
well defined 3 dimensional boundary in the body. A selective effect
such as repair enhancement of healthy tissue by fractionation of
the dose, or at least no negative selectivity with respect to the
healthy tissue is required.

The absorption of a monoenergetic parallel beam of pions shows
a characteristic momentum-dependent range in matter with a flat,
weakly ionizing entrance dose region. As stopped π^- are captured
and subsequently the nuclei decay into heavy fragments with small
range and high linear energy transfer (LET), a strongly pronounced
peak appears at a definite momentum-dependent depth (star region),
(Fig. 1). Clearly, this peculiar characteristic should be reason
enough to give π^- a chance in radiotherapy. Fortunately, there are
two more potential advantages to be mentioned: the high LET contribution in the star region results in a higher biological effectiveness (RBE) leading to an enhancement of the peak to plateau ratio
on the effective or biological dose scale and this higher effectiveness is expected to be less dependent on the oxygen tension

TABLE 1

CHARACTERISTIC DATA OF MEDICAL PION FACILITIES

Laboratory	Range in H_2O (cm)	Ω (msr)	ΔP (%)	Decay.corr. (220 MeV/c)	$\dfrac{d}{d\Omega}$	Ip (µA)	P.
SIN	30	.75	10	.5	1.0	20	1.0 (75)
LOS ALAMOS	25	.16	20	.41	.6	500	.49
TRIUMF (M8)	30	.08	13	.52	1.0	100	.07

Note: 1. $P = \Omega\ \Delta P\ (Decay)\ \dfrac{d\rho}{d\Omega}$ Ip/same for SIN Torus

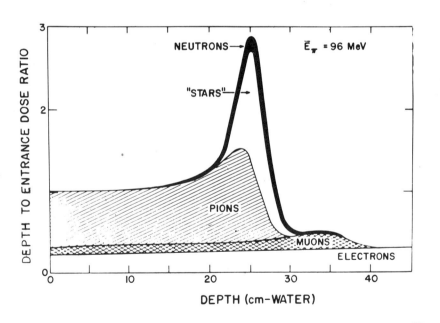

Fig. 1. Depth-dose distribution of a monoenergetic pion beam[22]

The first of these advantages is clearly demonstrated in a single
beam pion experiment on a cell culture. In Figure 2 the physical
depth-dose distribution is compared with the corresponding cell
survival rates.

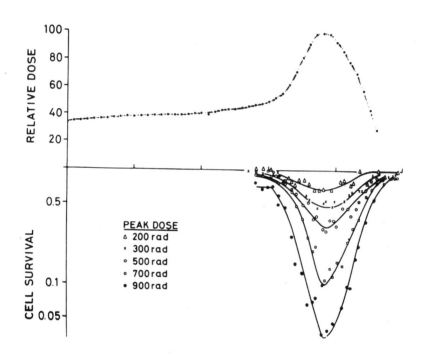

Fig. 2. In-vitro demonstration of enhanced radiobiological
         effectiveness in the star region[23]

BASIC CONSIDERATIONS

Negative pi mesons are generated above the threshold of about
400 MeV in a target hit by a proton beam. In order to obtain pions
of sufficient energy to penetrate tissue or water of adequate depth
for treatment purposes (120 MeV for 30 cm typical) protons of
500-800 MeV are required. High intensity accelerators working in
this energy range with a proton current of 100-1000 µA (called

meson factories for obvious reasons) are operating at Los Alamos
(LAMPF), Vancouver (TRIUMF) and Villigen (SIN).

Negative pi mesons are relatively rare particles even at a meson
factory. Their production cross section at 600 MeV proton energy
is in the order of 10 µb/St MeV for heavy target materials and
60^0 production angle[3]. Rising forward production preference is
observed for higher pion momentum, coupled however, with extremely
high contamination by protons and electrons. Spontaneous decay of
the particles is limiting the available path length for the optical
system to about 8 m for high intensity purposes. The limited system
length practically excludes the use of decontaminating separation-
methods for forward production. Properly designed clean, high intensity systems therefore are oriented slightly forward or perpendicular to the primary beam.

The useful target length cannot exceed 4 to 5 cm for heavy materials at the given proton energies without significant loss in
production intensity along the target.

Keeping all these limitations in mind, for a pion channel of
classical design with solid angle acceptance of perhaps 20 msr at
best, several hundred to 1000 µA of protons is needed in order to
achieve a desired irradiation dose rate of at least 10 rad l/min,
representing a lower limit for the work of the therapist.

CLASSICAL CHANNELS

The first generation of biomedical channels were built in all
three meson factories on a classical basis i.e. using dipole and
quadrupole magnets of conventional design. They were all useful in
operation at least for the preliminary biological experiments.
However, only the beam line at LAMPF has been effectively used for
therapeutic trials, where up to 500 µA of protons were available
for pion production. As a typical example the LAMPF biomedical
facility is based on a beamline with 8 quadrupoles and 3 bending
magnets. A beryllium wedge degrader is used to compress the accepted
20% momentum band by a factor of 6 in order to achieve favourably
narrow depth-dose distributions. For arbitrary 3 dimensional shaping of the homogenous dose distribution zone dynamical treatment
is required for all facilities. At the LAMPF beam the basic distribution is a slab of variable length, (the fan type beam is collimated
at both edges). The depth of the slab in the body is changed by a
rapidly actuated liquid degrader, in the third direction relative
movement of the patient is needed. First treatments at LAMPF using

static spots were started as early as 1975 and since that time over 200 patients were treated[2]. Despite the available high proton current, dose rate limitation caused by the relatively low acceptance is felt to be critical on the long term. The TRIUMF facility is suffering even more from its low acceptance because of its limitation to 100-200 μA in proton current.

THE PIOTRON AT SIN

The former single beam facility at SIN was recently replaced by a new powerful device.

Based on a reevaluation of medical needs in 1975 it was decided at SIN to build a high solid angle acceptance pion beam line facility dedicated specifically to medical purposes.[4,5,6]. It was envisaged to follow a brilliant idea of the Stanford team[7] and to develop a large superconducting ring spectrometer similar to their experimental prototype device[8] but highly upgraded and fully equipped for hospital - like operation.

Corresponding to the entirely different pion production conditions (the Stanford device was designed to be operated by an electron linac injector) and according to the ambitious plans regarding clinical trials, and last but not least, based on technical considerations related to the existing experience in the superconducting field at SIN, a complete redesign was started in 1976.

SYSTEM DESIGN

The SIN double stage proton cyclotron operates at present at 600 MeV with a maximum current of 100 μA. In order to make medical operations independent of the basic high energy physics activities, a fraction of the order of 20% is split off from the main beam and is guided to the medical area outside the experimental hall (Fig. 3). The production target unit is an integral but removable part of the spectrometer assembly (Fig. 4).

The remotely controlled target changer offers a choice of 11 different targets. Molybdenium targets are used if high intensity is required. Be is taken if lower electron contamination is crucial.

28

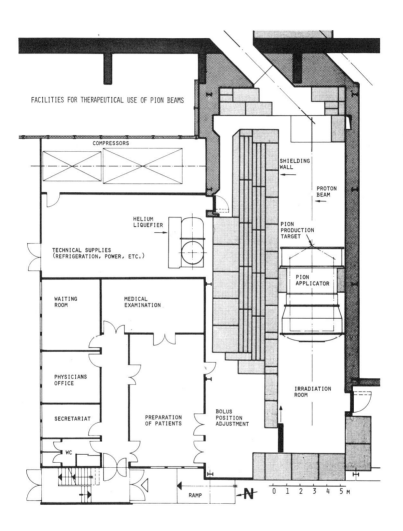

Fig. 3. Medical area

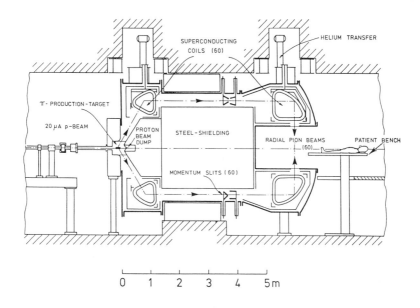

Fig. 4.   Simplified section of the medical facility

The length of the targets (25 - 70 mm) defines the axial size of
the pion spot. The automatic target change takes about 1 minute.

The large acceptance optical system is essentially an assymetric
but dispersionfree double wheel orange spectrometer doubly focusing
because of its axial symmetry. A slightly forward production angle
(60°) was chosen for higher intensity, 90° extraction is needed for
simplified treatment symmetry.

Overall dimensions were defined by 0 order analytical calculations
optimizing with respect to available space for treatment inside the
second ring, adequate shielding between beam dump and treatment
area weigthed against intensity losses by pion decay.

Exact coil contour locations, curvatures, tilt, effects of fringe
field and coil precision, momentum slit position and characteristics
were covered by extensive first and second order optical calculations
using two different models [9,10].

It has to be noticed that the pions do not always reach the focal
region at the axis after the second bend. In the high resolution

30

mode they are preferably stopped at a given distance from the axis
producing a ringlike absorption pattern. Special attention therefore
had to be paid also to the beam convergence, including corrections
due to scattering in windows, bolus, and patient in order to achieve
azimuthal ring homogeneity by multiple overlap at large radii
(see below Fig. 5).

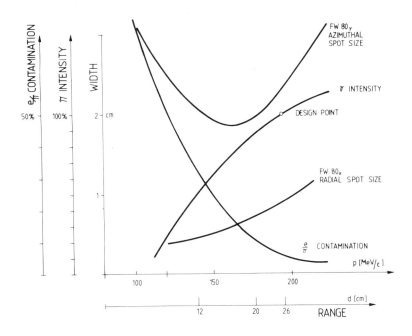

Fig. 5.   Pion intensity, electron contamination and characteristic
          width (full width at 80%) as function of π-momentum or
          range (design range 14-30 cm)

The maximum final design flux of $2 \cdot 10^9$ π/sec (30 mm Mo target)
corresponds to a maximum available rate of 50 rad 1/min for large
cylindrical target volumes.

OPERATING MODES

The use of toroidal coils results in a simultaneous momentum
equality for all radial beams. Nevertheless, the device is still
extremely flexible due to the fact that all 60 beams (separated by
the pancakes of the toroidal magnets) can be individually modulated
by 60 independent, rapidly activated slits. (on - off 0.2 sec). In
fact, early criticism was focussed on the expected complexity of
therapy planning if such a large number of beams is used simultaneously.
It could be proven, however, that matching the symmetry of the
device - by choosing unconventional but simple treatment modes and
corresponding auxiliary equipment such as a solid cylindrical bolus
-can in fact significantly simplify the procedure. A certain effort
is naturally unavoidable if we want to realize the extreme potential
of generating an arbitrary 3 dimensional homogenous dose distribution.

Surrounding the region of the body near the treatment area by a
cylindrical bolus of tissue equivalent material and positioning the
patient with the cylinder co-axial to the optical system, the dose
will be deposited in a region of a form similar to a donut (Fig.6).

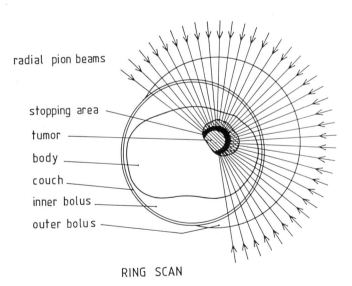

RING SCAN

Fig. 6.   Dose ring segment produced by a limited number of beams
          with overlapping peak regions.

By appropriate change of the magnetic field (momentum-scan) and corresponding slit actuation, the required homogenous distribution can be produced with sufficient precision (5%) and good contour definition. Only stepwise axial motion of the patient is needed for this treatment mode[11,12].

Alternatively, spot or raster type scan by properly programmed 3-dimensional movement of the patient with respect to the central stopping region (hot spot) could in principle be used[13] with similar results. For this method therapy planning efforts are considerably higher. Complexity of required bolus equipment and inconvenience and precision limitation of 3 dimensional patient movement are on the long term for routine operation hardly justifiable. Nevertheless, the SIN piotron is equipped for both operational modes.

OPERATIONAL EXPERIENCE

During the very first operation trial June 21, 1980 satisfactory performance of the complex system could be roughly demonstrated by the impressive photographic picture of a ring-shaped dose distribution (Fig.7). Since then, all the optical and dosimetric data, as far as available, have confirmed the proper functioning of the system[18,19]

Despite some corrections to the control system in progress and a provisional intensity limitation at 76% of the maximum design value patient treatments were started at the end of 1980.

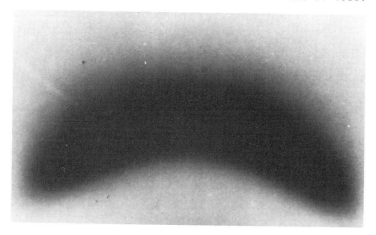

Fig. 7. Stopping region of 15 pion beams

FUTURE TRENDS IN PION FACILITIES

A comparison of proven efficiencies in terms of available pion dose per required proton current results for Piotron to LAMPF channel in a dramatic ratio of 50. Clearly the general urgent interest in typical annular type channels such as the Piotron is reawakened at the meson factories. Related but slightly different approaches using the relatively simple double co-axial solenoid geometry[20] or the more complex combination of a piotron ring with several solenoids[21] demonstrate a peculiar trend towards conversion of the cylindrical symmetry at the channel entrance into a single-beam-like operation at the output, and a certain preference for three-dimensional scanning of the treatment area. In the opinion of the author a more courageous integration of the optical system symmetry in the choice of dynamic treatment modality leads to better or at least technically simpler results. As an example the obvious advantage of the multiport-effect using the radial beams of the Piotron should be noted. Another remarkable example is the simple one dimensional patient movement in connection with the fan-scan of the LAMPF beam or the ring scan at the Piotron. According to our technical experience proper 3-dimensional motion could become a noteworthy difficulty in dynamic treatment if much higher intensities than present could be achieved. This is certainly not expected for single beam facilities. For the usual superconducting annular devices serious investigations of the nuclear heat load have to be carried out before significantly higher intensity gains (>2) can be envisaged.

REFERENCES

1. Fowler P.H., Perkins D.H. Nature (1961) 189,524
   Possibility of therapeutic applications of beams of negative
   π mesons.
2. Kligerman M.M. et al., Cancer (1979) 43, 1043
   Experience with pion radiotherapy.
3. Frosch R. et al., SIN PR 79-010 (1979)
   Measurement of cross sections and asymmetry parameters for
   the production of charged pions from various nuclei by
   585 MeV protons.
4. Blaser J.P., Krebsinformation (Schweiz.Krebsliga) (1976) Vol.11
   Medizinisches und biologisches Forschungsprogramm mit Pionen-
   strahlen am SIN.
5. Vécsey G., SIN-Newsletter No 6 (1976)
   The new medical pion beam.
6. Vécsey G., SIN TM-62-01 (1976)
   Status Report of the Pion-Therapy Program at SIN,
   Report delivered at the IAE Conference on Radiotherapy, Vienna
   November 1976.
7. Boyd D., Schwettman H.A., Nuclear Instruments & Methods (1973)
   111, 315, A large acceptance pion channel for cancer therapy.
8. Stekly J.J.J. et al., MT5 (1975) 419, a large toroidal coil
   system for the Stanford medical pion generator, Paper delivered
   at the Fifth International Conference on Magnet Technology
   Roma 1975.
9. Frosch R., Culloch Mc., SIN-TM 37-03 (1975), First order beam
   transport matrices for the "double wheel" medical pion channel,
   SIN-TM-37-04 (1975), Effect of curved magnet boundaries for
   the "double wheel" medical pion facility, SIN-TM-37-05 (1977)
   Second order beam optics of the double wheel medical pion
   applicator, SIN-TM-37-07 (1977) Particle distributions in the
   pion applicator.
10. Crawford J., SIN-TM-37-08 (1977), Calculation of the properties
    of the new pion therapy channel, SIN-TM-37-09 (1977), further
    calculations on the new pion therapy channel
11. Vécsey G., SIN-internal Note 6-15-1977
12. Crawford J., SIN-TM-37-10 (1978), DOSER; a simple therapy
    planing program.
13. Zellweger J., SIN-TM-65-01 (1978) Dynamic machine parameter
    design and basic ideas for an optimum three dimensional treat-
    ment.
14. Besse L., SIN-Annual Report (1978) 1.3, therapy control system
15. Horvath I. Vécsey G. Zellweger J., EC-12, The piotron at SIN -
    A large superconducting double torus spectrometer, Paper
    delivered at the Seventh International Conference on Magnet
    Technology, Karlsruhe March-April 1981.
16. Maix R.K. et al., GA-9,The superconducting coils for the pion
    therapy facility of the Swiss Institute for Nuclear Research,
    Paper delivered at the Seventh International Conference on
    Magnet Technology, Karlsruhe March-April 1981.

17. Zellweger J. Vécsey G. Horvath I, Superconducting magnets of the biomedical facility at SIN, Advances in Cryogenic Engineering, (1979) 25, 232.
18. Kluge W. Matthäy H. Biological and Medical applications, SIN-Newsletter No 13, (1980) 13,46.
19. Vécsey G, SIN Superconducting facility for medical applications, HB-1, Paper delivered at the Seventh International Conference on Magnet Technology, Karlsruhe March-April 1981.
20. Lobb D.E., Beam-Optical properties of the Magnetic field produced by two co-axial coils to be published Nuclear Instruments Methods 1981.
21. Sugimitou, Swenson D.A., Investigation of a large solid angle pion channel for medical applications utilizing current sheets and solenoid elements, LA-8356-MS, Los Alamos, May 1980.
22. Curtis, S.B. et al., UCRL-17606, A calculation of the physical characteristics of negative pion beams - Energy-loss distribution and bragg curves, Lawrence radiation Laboratory University of California, Berkeley, and Southwest Center for Advanced Studies, Dallas, Texas, (1968)
23. Tremp J. Blattmann H. Fritz-Niggli H., Cell survival over the depth profile after irradiation with a negative pion beam, Radiation and Environmental Biophysics, 16, 267 (1979)

Copyright 1982 by Elsevier Science Publishing Co., Inc.
PION AND HEAVY ION RADIOTHERAPY:
Pre-Clinical and Clinical Studies
L. D. Skarsgard

MEDICAL ACCELERATOR RESEARCH INSTITUTE IN ALBERTA (MARIA)

J.D. CHAPMAN
Department of Radiation Oncology, Cross Cancer Institute and Department
of Radiology, University of Alberta, Edmonton, Canada, T6G 1Z2

INTRODUCTION

The Medical Accelerator Research Institute in Alberta (MARIA) is a
"world-ciass" research facility built around an array of interactive
particle accelerators. It was conceived and proposed by a few basic and
applied scientists at the University of Alberta (U.A.), Edmonton who
believed that existing strengths in several scientific fields would serve
as a superb foundation upon which to launch such a major research
endeavour in Canada. A large component of support and justification for
MARIA comes from areas of basic and applied medical research. One
unique feature of this proposed facility is its primary commitment to
medical research. We strongly believe that such a commitment does not
preclude the use of the MARIA facility for superb research in the basic
physical sciences.

The Government of Alberta through its Provincial Cancer Hospitals
Board has commissioned an advanced study of this project which we
have called Phase IIA. It was to include work on the conceptual design,
the anticipated location, construction and operating costs, and the
anticipated scientific and economic benefits of such a "world-class"
accelerator facility. In this paper I have summarized several details of
that Phase IIA study which was carried out by the Scientific Advisory
Committee – MARIA and the MARIA Phase IIA Design Team. I have had
the privilege to serve as Chairman of this Committee and Design Team
during this phase of the project.

BRIEF HISTORY OF PROJECT

The Medical Accelerator Research Institute in Alberta (MARIA) is the
title given to a multi-disciplinary, multi-user research facility defined
for the U.A. in Edmonton. Proposals from at least five independent
research groups were merged in the fall of 1977 and have formed the
basis for MARIA planning to date. These U.A. based research groups
are now listed.

I. Radiopharmacists and Nuclear Physicians had identified the need for a hospital-based cyclotron for production of medical radionuclides. The short-, intermediate- and long-lived radioisotopes which could be produced by such an accelerator were envisioned as the resource material for a strongly interactive research program covering fundamental and basic, developmental, and applied medical research.

2. Radiation Oncologists and Radiobiologists had evaluated various types of radiation beams for the treatment of cancer and determined that charged-particle beams offered considerable potential, as yet inadequately investigated, for an improved local treatment of some human cancers. Several centers were currently evaluating or installing equipment to evaluate the use of neutrons in radiotherapy. At least three centers around the world, including TRIUMF in Vancouver, Canada, were evaluating negative pi-mesons as a potential new modality in cancer therapy. The Lawrence Berkeley Laboratory is the only accelerator facility today with a medical program which includes the evaluation of charged-particle beams in cancer therapy. The need for a hospital-based research program with charged-particle beams was apparent. As well, the potential for novel contributions to applied medical research was judged to be greatest with accelerator produced charged-particle beams.

3. Scientists at the Nuclear Research Centre (U.A) in looking beyond the usefulness of the Van de Graaff accelerator on-site and their involvement in the TRIUMF project in Vancouver recognized the unique opportunity for performing both atomic and nuclear physics research with charged-particle beams required for the proposed medical applications. The MARIA philosophy, from the beginning, has consequently included a component of basic physics research which we believe to be essential for the innovation and vitality of the more applied medical programs on site.

4. A large group of individual investigators in several fields of basic physical, chemical and biological sciences (radiation biology, genetics, radiology, endocrinology, surgery, biochemistry, biophysics, chemistry, geology and anthropology) defined basic research projects which could effectively utilize various charged-particle beams. Some of these projects would constitute an extension of existing studies with low-LET radiations to particle beams which deposit their energy at high-LETs. Other basic research projects would constitute new programs for this University, several of which are on-going at the Lawrence Berkeley Laboratory.

5. Various medical physicists and researchers within the Faculty of Medicine had recognized the need for an imaging research center with computerized-tomographic-scanning, gamma-imaging, positron-emission-tomography and nuclear-magnetic-resonance (NMR) – imaging represented. The development of charged-particle imaging techniques at the MARIA facility is proposed as a major research activity and could provide the focus and possibly space for a more broadly-based imaging research group.

This evolving interest led to the formation of a Scientific Advisory Committee to define the specifications of the MARIA accelerator(s) and the research programs to be conducted at the facility. At the same time a Steering Committee was formed to seek funding for initial studies and to advance the project. The outcome of these activities was the commissioning of DSMA ATCON Ltd. to carry out the preliminary feasibility study. This study showed that the various research activities could be effectively carried out in one facility which housed various accelerators. The favourable findings contained in their report led the Government of Alberta to fund scientific workshops and a more comprehensive design study (Phase IIA).

The Phase IIA MARIA study compiled information from several studies performed by local members of the MARIA design team as well as local, national and international accelerator and engineering experts who had been contracted by the MARIA project during Phase IIA. Increased user expectations in MARIA as a major national research facility resulted in more than a doubling of the design specifications for the proposed accelerators, the space required for accelerator operations and for on-site research, and the operating and research staff at MARIA than had been included in the preliminary feasibility study completed in 1979. The research facility which has now been defined and costed represents the largest and most technically advanced accelerator laboratory in the world to be justified primarily on the basis of medical research. As well we believe MARIA offers to Canadian physicists a unique facility in which to perform intermediate energy charged-particle physics which is not available elsewhere in Canada.

The schematic shown in Figure I emphasizes the fact that MARIA has been proposed as a research facility to be sited in Alberta as a national research resource. It furthermore indicates that a unique balance between basic and applied research has been defined with a dominant emphasis on biological and medical research. It is our opinion that such a facility will complement existing activities in Canada and have a useful lifetime of from 20 to 50 years.

MARIA CONCEPT - RESEARCH FACILITY

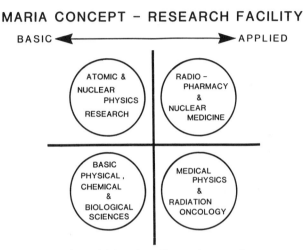

Fig. 1. A schematic which describes the various research activities proposed for MARIA.

CHARGED-PARTICLE REQUIREMENTS OF VARIOUS USERS

Charged-particle beam requirements for various research applications were defined by a series of three MARIA Design Symposia held in the fall of 1980.[3,1,4] The beam requirements of the diverse research groups could not be met by constructing a single accelerator. The first MARIA Design Symposium[3] which dealt with medical radionuclide production concluded that the requirements for high current beams of protons, deuterons, and possibly other particles for the production of radio-nuclides could best be met by two cyclotrons. The lower energy cyclotron of the K-16 class would be dedicated to the production of short-lived clinical gases for the University of Alberta and Cross Cancer Hospital in addition to those radioactive gases required for the in-house research program at MARIA. A higher energy cyclotron of the K-90 class will produce longer-lived radionuclides for medical research, clinical use and possibly commercial sales. This higher energy cyclotron could also be designed to provide back-up heavy-ion injection into the synchrotron accelerator.

The heavy-ion requirements for the field of radiation oncology research (including radiobiology and diagnostic radiography) were defined by the second MARIA Design Symposium[1]. Table 1 summarizes particle specifications required for this research.

TABLE 1

PARTICLE-BEAM REQUIREMENTS OF RADIATION ONCOLOGY
(INCLUDING RADIOBIOLOGY AND RADIOGRAPHY)

    Particles – Protons to Argon/including radioactive beams
                Interchange between any two particles in $\leq$ 2 min.
    Energy – $\sim$250 MeV for protons
           – I GeV/nucleon for other particles
                Variable energy: patient to patient and continuously for
                range modulation.
    Intensity – $\geq$ 1000 rad/min into I liter of tissue

P^{1+}	1.3×10^{11} particles/sec	
He^{2+}	3×10^{10} "	"
C^{6+}	7×10^{9} "	"
Ne^{10+}	3×10^{9} "	"
Si^{14+}	2×10^{9} "	"
Ar^{18+}	1×10^{9} "	"

    Time Structure – Microdose not to exceed 10^{6} rad/sec

                   – Mean dose rate $\sim 10^{3}$ rad/min/liter
                   – Long, uniform beams with macroduty cycle $\geq 25\%$
    Physical Beam Size – $\leq$ 1 cm FWHM

    Energy Spread – $dE/E \leq 10^{-3}$

A third MARIA Design Symposium[4] dealt with accelerator systems for relativistic heavy ions in medical and scientific research and also defined the particle specifications of interest to proposed researchers in the field of atomic and nuclear physics. Table 2 summarizes the specifications of the various particle beams required for this research.

It was recognized that the linac injector accelerator could be used as an ultra-sensitive mass spectrometer. The capability to accelerate ^{10}Be, ^{14}C, ^{26}Al, ^{32}Cl, and ^{41}Ca to an energy of 10MeV/nucleon would be of interest to basic researchers involved in dating samples from such diverse fields as geology, anthropology, and the fine arts.

The Phase IIA MARIA Design Study defined a configuration for an array of accelerators which was capable of meeting the requirements of the various users.

TABLE 2

PARTICLE BEAM REQUIREMENTS FOR BASIC PHYSICS

ATOMIC PHYSICS

Particles	— Zr, Nb, Mo $\sim$ .2MeV/amu
	— Cr, Fe, Ni $\sim$ .8MeV/amu
	— Zr, Nb, Mo 1–3MeV/amu
	— Ta, V, Re, Pt, Au 2MeV/amu
Intensity	— 10^{10} – 10^{12} particles/sec.
Beam Size	— $\sim$0.5 cm FWHM

NUCLEAR PHYSICS

Particles	— Initially protons through argon
	— polarized ions (p → Li)
	— Future acceleration of ions to A $\sim$ 130
Energy	— > 800 MeV/amu up to A=40
	— Continuously variable from 50MeV/amu
Particle Intensity	—>5x10^{10} nucleons/sec (polarized)
	—>5x10^{11} nucleons/sec (unpolarized)
Time Structure	— High duty factor, > 25%
Physical Beam Size	—≤0.5 cm (FWHM in two dimensions)
Energy Spread	— dE/E ≤ 3.5x10^{-4}

DESCRIPTION OF PROPOSED FACILITY

That MARIA should be a multi-disciplinary, multi-user research facility was the initial concept adopted by those researchers who merged interests in 1977 and this concept determined several principles used in the planning phase. Firstly, the accelerator(s) required to produce particle beams for the various research applications were to be designed into one research center. This approach provided the opportunity for assembling a large technical support staff, including accelerator physicists and engineers, to maintain and operate the accelerators. If independent research functions were housed in different facilities some duplication of technical support staff would be required and beneficial interaction amongst all of the staff would be lessened. Figure 2 shows a schematic of the layout of accelerators defined to meet the various research needs. MARIA consists of four different accelerators with varying degrees of interactivity. The low energy (K-16 cyclotron) is dedicated to the application of short-lived radioisotopes for pharmaceutical and medical research. The higher energy cyclotron (K-90) will be used primarily for the production of longer-lived radioisotopes for research, clinical use, and possibly commercial sale. This cyclotron might also be designed to serve as a back-up injector of various charged particles into the high energy synchrotron ring. A linear accelerator was chosen as the primary injector system for heavy ions into the synchrotron because of the high reliability required by the medical applications of energetic charged–particle beams. The linear accelerator designed for MARIA will consist of three different ion sources, a pre–accelerator of the RFQ type[2] and two drift tube linacs (DTL) in series. The energies of the particle beams emerging from the RFQ, the first–stage DTL and the second–stage DTL will be approximately 600 KeV/nucleon, 5 MeV/nucleon and 10 MeV/nucleon, respectively. Beam emerging from the second–stage DTL will inject into a synchrotron ring which is similar to the SATURNE II synchrotron at Saclay, France. Basic research such as atomic physics or radiation biophysics will be carried out in a low–energy particle laboratory with beams extracted at various energies from the injector linac. Two extraction ports for high–energy particle beams from the synchrotron are planned to facilitate both intermediate–energy particle physics as well as both basic biological and clinical research.

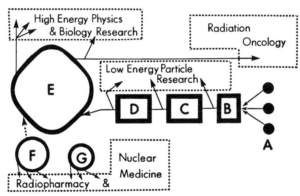

Fig. 2. A schematic of the layout of accelerators proposed for MARIA. Research functions with various particle beams are indicated. A=three ion sources, B=RFQ accelerator, C=first–stage drift tube linac, D=second–stage drift tube linac, E=synchrotron, F=K–90 cyclotron, G=K–16 cyclotron.

MARIA has been designed with three rooms in which cancer therapy research will be performed with beams from different directions. One room will have only a horizontal beam, a second room will have two beam ports emerging downwards and upwards into the room at 45° to the horizontal and intersecting at the isocenter of a treatment couch, and a third room will have one vertically downward beam and one horizontal beam intersecting at the isocenter of a treatment couch. This arrangement gives the radiotherapist and medical physicist the opportunity for treatment planning with parallel opposed beams in three directions as well as one beam directed vertically downward. Figures 3 shows the ports available for treating cancer patients in the supine position when the treatment couch is permitted to rotate 180° in the horizontal plane.

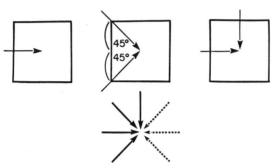

Fig. 3. A schematic of the three radiation oncology treatment rooms proposed for MARIA. The various treatment ports available for therapy planning are indicated below.

This first principle of planning for MARIA has defined a research facility housed on six different floors with a space of approximately 30,000 m². This includes space to house the various accelerators, particle beam lines, isotope handling, research areas, patient areas, office space for approximately 350 MARIA personnel, library, conference room, cafeteria and administrative offices.

The multi-user concept for MARIA has dictated a commitment to time-sharing. It is envisaged that the beam intensities from the various accelerators in the MARIA facility will be adequate so that all proposed research activities, both basic and applied, can be scheduled into any given week. The concept of ultimate time-sharing requires the capability for a rapid shifting of energetic particle beams to any one of several research areas in MARIA in a short time (about one minute). This flexibility of dumping high-energy particle beams into various beamlines with speed demands sophisticated switching magnets under the control of the most advanced computerized control systems.

The clinical research proposed for MARIA requires the highest level of beam reliability ever designed into a particle accelerator. This can be achieved, in part, by over-designing several accelerator components so that for specific medical applications the accelerator is not expected to operate at maximum design specifications and to have an adequate level of spare components capable of quick replacement in several systems.

It is known that many advances in science have occured because of developments at interfaces of scientific disciplines. The MARIA facility provides the unique opportunity for the co-existence of and cooperation between scientists of several basic disciplines around an array of accelerators producing particle beams of mutual interest. It is expected that such interdisiplinary activities will result in several discoveries of benefit to mankind which would not have resulted without such cross-fertilization of scientific thought.

ANTICIPATED IMPACT OF MARIA

The MARIA research facility as defined in the Phase IIA study represents the largest accelerator installation ever proposed for Canada. Furthermore with applied medical research as its primary objective and basic biological and physical research providing secondary justification, the MARIA concept is unique in the world. Such a high-technology research facility constructed in Alberta would positively impact on several facets of the business, manufacturing, engineering, research and educational components of the Albertan economy. The research program proposed for MARIA would complement several existing high-technology programs in Canada as well as provide a new setting for unique technology with which to perform research into areas, which at present, are unavailable in Canada. MARIA would rank as a research facility with a few of the best accelerators in the world today.

The construction of MARIA by the Government of Alberta would generate enthusiasm and good will amongst Canadian researchers and engineers, in particular, and amongst all Canadians by providing a research resource for this country which otherwise will not be realized. It indeed would serve to attract high technology and medical researchers to the province of Alberta. The scientific break-throughs and medical benefits generated by the MARIA research programs could presumably be made available to many. Such a large international research center would become a training ground for scientists and technologists from within Canada and from several other countries. It is expected that the construction of MARIA would spawn secondary industries in the fields of nucleonics, radiopharmaceuticals, accelerator components, engineering consultants (high-technology), biomedical engineering and diagnostics, etc. Such a large-scale high technology project would result in a significant upgrading of some Canadian manufacturing and fabricating industries. Proposals for heavy-ion accelerator facilities are being developed in several other countries and the MARIA expertise could be expected to interact strongly with other "world-class" projects. This project consti- tutes that type of an investment which undoubtedly will generate over its lifetime both direct and indirect benefits which could be costed at several times the initial investment.

The Government of Alberta has been asked to capitalize and imple- ment the construction of MARIA. Our request includes a commitment to a core operating budget for several years so that the ultimate research potential of such a national research resource can be realized.

ACKNOWLEDGEMENTS

The MARIA concept and the Phase IIA Proposal are both team efforts. I would like to acknowledge major input to each by members of the Scien- tific Advisory Committee – MARIA which over the past two years has in- cluded Drs. J.J. Battista, J.M. Cameron, R. Hooper, B.C. Lentle, A.A. Noujaim, T.R. Overton, J.G. Pearson, W.M. Saunders, J.W. Scrimger, D.M. Sheppard, R.C. Urtasun, and G.B. Walker. Mr. K. Lacey, as Phase IIA project coordinator, has made several major contributions. The skillful assistance of B. Gartner and K. Liesner in preparing this manuscript is appreciated.

REFERENCES

1. Battista, J.J., Scrimger, J.W., and Urtasun, R.C. editors (1981). MARIA Design Symposium – Volume II "Radiation Oncology". The University of Alberta Press.
2. Crandell, K.R., Stokes, R.H., and Wangler,T.P. "R.F. Quadrupole Beam Dynamics Design Studies". Proceedings of Linear Accelerator Conference. Brookhaven National Laboratory. Report No. 51134: 205.
3. Noujaim, A.A., McQuarrie, S.A., and Wiebe, L.I. editors (1981). MARIA Design Symposium – Volume I "Medical Radionuclide Produc- tion". The University of Alberta Press.
4. Sheppard, D.M., Cameron, J.M., and Neilson, G.C. editors (1981). MARIA Design Symposium – Volume III. "Accelerator Systems for Relativistic Heavy Ions in Medical and Scientific Research". The University of Alberta Press.

PHYSICS, DOSIMETRY AND TREATMENT PLANNING

DOSIMETRY INTERCOMPARISONS BETWEEN HEAVY CHARGED PARTICLE RADIOTHERAPY
FACILITIES

ALFRED SMITH[1], ROBERT HILCO[1], JOHN DICELLO[2], PETER FESSENDEN[3], MARK HENKELMAN[4],
KEN HOGSTROM[5], GABRIEL LAM[6], JOHN LYMAN[7], HANS BLATTMANN[8], MYRIAM SALZMANN[8],
DOUGLAS READING[9] AND LYNN VERHEY[10]

[1]Cancer Research and Treatment Center, c/o Los Alamos National Laboratory, Los
Alamos, N.M.; [2]Los Alamos National Laboratory; [3]Stanford University Medical
Centre; [4]Ontario Cancer Institute, Toronto; [5]M.D. Anderson Hospital and Tumor
Institute, Houston; [6]British Columbia Cancer Foundation, Vancouver; [7]Lawrence
Berkeley Laboratory, Berkeley; [8]SIN, Villigen; [9]Rutherford Laboratory, Oxford;
[10]Massachusetts General Hospital, Boston.

INTRODUCTION

Three facilities in the United States are using heavy charged particle
beams in clinical trials: (a) protons are being used at the 160 MeV Harvard
Cyclotron; (b) helium ions are being used at the Lawrence-Berkeley 184" Cyclotron and carbon ions are being used at the Lawrence Berkeley BEVALAC; and (c)
negative pi-mesons (pions) are being used at the Los Alamos Meson Physics Facility. Heavy charged particle therapy projects are also in progress or being
developed in other countries, notably pion facilities at TRIUMF, Canada, and at
SIN, Switzerland; a helium ion facility at SACLAY, France; and proton facilities in Sweden, Russia, and Japan. When the efficacy of a new radiation therapy modality is being investigated, it is important that the dosimetry is compatible among the various institutions involved in the clinical trials. It is
also important that the dosimetry be accurate so that the clinical and radiobiological data from the various facilities can be compared. These concerns
are especially acute when charged particle beams are being employed with no established guidelines or protocols available to standardize dosimetry practices.
The complicated nature of these beams and the differences in dosimetry practices at various institutions could lead to large differences in actual delivered
dose for the same stated nominal dose at different facilities. Adequate agreement in delivered dose is unlikely to be achieved without an extensive program

of experimental intercomparison of charged particle beam dosimetry. The Amer-
can Association of Physicists in Medicine (AAPM) has established a Task Group,
(#20), operating under its Radiation Therapy Committee, to address the problems
of heavy charged particle dosimetry. This task Group is composed of approximately 40 physicists from the USA, Canada, England, France, Switzerland, Germany, Sweden, and Japan who are directly involved in charged particle therapy
projects or who are experts in dosimetry related fields. The activities of the
Task group are funded by the National Cancer Institute through a Grant to the
AAPM.*

The Task Group has conducted intercomparisons of dosimetry methodologies at
the various charged particle facilities in order to provide some basis for dosimetry recommendations and to lay groundwork for the uniformity of patient dosimetry at all facilities. Members of the Task Group have designed and built a
calorimeter which measures the absolute absorbed dose in charged particle beams
and which will be used as a standard for all dose measurements. This instrument has been used in all of the charged particle therapy beams to calibrate
ionization chambers which are routinely used for dosimetry at each facility.
The Task Group is continuing the intercomparison of dosimetry at charged particle therapy facilities and is designing a protocol for charged particle beam
dosimetry which will standardize the instrumentation, methodologies, data, and
quality control at all facilities to insure that the results of the clinical
trials rest on a firm physical foundation.

This paper presents the results of Phase I intercomparisons which were
designed to establish techniques, procedures and instrumentation which would
form the basis for absolute dose intercomparisons in Phase II studies.

GOALS

Ionization chambers have become the principal instruments employed for routine measurement of the absorbed dose in tissue. Ionization methods require
conversion factors which rest on physical interpretation of the energy absorption processes and involve such considerations as secondary charged particle
spectra, relative stopping power ratios, the energy required of secondary
charged particles to produce ion pairs in various gases, and corrections for the
non-tissue equivalence of chamber walls. The use of ionization chambers requires a primary calibration of the response of the chamber in a standard beam
(usually cobalt-60) whose output calibration is traceable to the National Bureau

*PHS Grant CA22286 awarded by the National Cancer Institute DHHS.

of standards. This calibration is used to determine the volume of the chamber or the mass of the gas in the chamber under normal gassing conditions. Also, it is important that an accurate measurement of the collected charge in the chamber be made when the chamber is irradiated.

Phase I intercomparisons with ionization chambers were designed to determine the agreement among the physicists representing the various charged particle therapy facilities in the measurement of:

1) integrated charge with respective electrometers using a standard current source;

2) pion/X-ray chamber response ratios with respective electrometer and ion chamber systems;

3) response of ion chambers for helium ions using a common electrometer;

4) absorbed dose for cobalt-60 irradiation;

5) proton, helium ion, and carbon ion beam measurements.

Phase II intercomparisons were designed to directly compare measurements with ionization chambers and a calorimeter on pion, proton, helium ion and carbon ion beams. These measurements provide the conversion factors necessary to state the absorbed dose in the chamber walls since the ion chamber walls and the calorimeter are fabricated from the same material (Shonka A150 plastic). The results of Phase II intercomparisons are still being analyzed and will be presented at a later date.

RESULTS

The chronology of the Phase I measurements was:

1) Los Alamos National Laboratory - March 1978

    Integrated Charge

    Pion/X-ray chamber response

2) Massachusetts General Hospital/Harvard Cyclotron Laboratory-January, 1979

    Cobalt-60 absorbed dose

    Proton beam measurements

3) Lawrence Berkeley Laboratory-June 1979

    Cobalt-60 absorbed dose

    Helium ion chamber response

    Helium ion beam measurements

    Carbon ion beam measurements

Integrated charge measurements

Each group, using their respective electrometers, measured the integrated current from a calibrated picoampere source. Currents of 10^{-10}, 10^{-11}, and 10^{-12} coul/sec, were integrated on electrometers using the 10^{-8}, 10^{-9}, and 10^{-10} coulomb scales, respectively. Measurements were corrected for background and electrometer correction factors (when available). The data were analyzed by calculating the mean of all data from each group for each current scale then calculating the ratio of the mean and each datum. The results are shown in Table 1. The standard deviations of the means of these ratios are 2.8%, 1.8%, and 1.2% for the 10^{-10}, 10^{-11} and 10^{-12} ampere scales respectively. For the 10^{-10} ampere scale, if the institution (SIN) with the ratio differing the greatest from 1.0 is omitted, the standard deviation of the mean for that scale is reduced to 1.2 %. This group found that they had problems with their Cary electrometer during intercomparisons. With this correction, the standard deviation of the means for all scales is less than 2% and the maximum difference for all scales is 5%.

TABLE 1

INTEGRATED CHARGE MEASUREMENTS

Institution	Mean/Institution		
	10^{-10} amps	10^{-11} amps	10^{-12} amps
Berkeley	–	–	–
Harvard	0.9729	0.9784	1.0161
Rutherford	1.0009	0.9959	0.9985
SIN	1.0546*	1.0245*	0.9965*
Stanford	0.9904	0.9973	0.9990
TRIUMF	1.0007*	1.0187*	1.0081*
UNM/LANL	0.9839	0.9869	0.9822
SD =	2.8%	1.8%	1.2%

*not corrected for background

Pion/X-ray response ratios

The object of these experiments was to identify individual ionization chambers, or types of chambers, with deviant response ratios for pion and x-rays and to test how the different groups of physicists using their total measuring systems (ion chambers plus electrometers) would agree in their respective measurements of two beams of differing radiation qualities and experimental geometry.

Measurements were first performed on X-ray beams of two qualities--1.38 and 3.7 mm Cu HVL. Data were taken with ionization chambers placed in air using both air and tissue equivalent (TE)* gas and with the chambers positioned in a lucite phantom using TE gas.

Measurements were then performed on a pion beam of approximately 9.5 cm penetration in H_2O. The pion stopping region was spread to approximately 3 cm and was uniform over this dimension to within ±1.5%. The ionization chambers were placed in lucite phantoms at the focal point of the beam. Additional material was placed above the lucite phantom to cause the chamber centers to be placed at the center of the spread peak. TE gas was used in the chambers.

We report here only the pion and X-ray response ratios for data taken in the lucite phantom and using TE gas for both pions and X-rays. All data were corrected for temperature and pressure but not corrected for the differences in integrated current measurements since these cancel out in the ratios. The results of the pion/X-ray (1.38 mm Cu) and pion/X-ray (3.7 mm Cu) are shown in Tables 2 and 3, respectively.

The mean pion/X-ray ratio for pion vs 1.38 mm Cu X-rays is 0.1127±2.6% for EG&G chambers (excluding SIN) and 0.1157±7.6% for Spokas chambers. The difference in the means of the response ratios is only 3% which is probably not significant and cannot be explained by chamber volume effects. For pions vs 3.7 mm Cu X-rays the mean pion/X-ray ratio for EG&G chambers (excluding SIN) is 0.0946 ±2.4% and 0.0952 ± 7.5% for Spokas chambers. The difference in the means of the responses here is 1%. The larger standard deviations for the Spokas chambers are not considered significant because there were only two data for each case.

Helium ion chamber response

Ionization chambers were exposed to high-energy helium ions in the plateau region of a 10-cm spread peak therapy beam. The chambers were placed in a lucite phantom and were electrically connected to a common recycling integrator. This procedure eliminated possible differences due to electrometer calibrations. The measurements were performed only with a negative polarizing voltage and with air-filled chambers. Each chamber received the same exposure. The integrated counts for each chamber were corrected for temperature and pressure and multiplied by the chamber's cobalt-60 correction factor. The results are given in Table 4. The standard deviation of the mean for all chambers was 2% and the maximum difference was 7%. There was no significant difference in the means or standard deviations among the different types of chambers.

---

*Nominally 10.2% H, 45.6% C, 40.7% O, and 3.5% N by weight or 64.4% CH_4, 32.4% CO_2 and 3.2% N_2 by partial pressures.

TABLE 2

PION/X-RAY MEASUREMENTS IN PHANTOM (1.38 mm Cu HVL-TE GAS)

Chamber	Institution	Pion/X-ray
0.1cc EG&G	Harvard	0.1086
	SIN	0.1438
	Stanford	0.1155
	TRIUMF	0.1126
	UNM/LANL	0.1141
0.55cc Spokas	SIN	0.1263
	Stanford	0.1220
	TRIUMF	0.1095
0.2cc Farmer	Rutherford	0.0975*

*air filled

0.1cc EG&G(4 chambers excluding SIN)	mean =	0.1127
	SD =	2.6%
0.55cc Spokas (2 chambers excluding SIN)	mean =	0.1157
	SD =	7.6%

TABLE 3

PION/X-RAY MEASUREMENTS IN PHANTOM (3.7 mm Cu HVL-TE GAS)

Chamber	Institution	Pion/X-ray
0.1cc EG&G	Harvard	0.0928
	SIN	0.1273
	Stanford	0.0956
	TRIUMF	0.0927
	UNM/LANL	0.0973
0.55cc Spokas	SIN	0.1047
	Stanford	0.1003
	TRIUMF	0.0902
0.2cc Farmer	Rutherford	0.0876*
1.0cc Far West	Berkeley	0.0936

*air filled

0.1cc EG&G (4 chambers excluding SIN)	mean =	0.0946
	SD =	2.4%
0.55cc Spokas (2 Chambers excluding SIN)	mean =	0.0952
	SD =	7.5%

Cobalt-60 absorbed dose

Cobalt-60 measurements were first performed at Massachusetts General Hospital. Measurements were made with the chambers in air with a cobalt-60 build-up cap and in a standard lucite phantom. Each group used the gas of their preference (air or TE) and applied standard cobalt-60 correction factors to calculate the

TABLE 4

HELIUM ION CHAMBER RESPONSE

Chamber	Institution	Corrected Response x10-11
0.1ccEG&G	Berkeley	256.4
	Harvard	270.1
	SIN	260.5
	Stanford	259.1
	TRIUMF	270.0
	UNM/LANL	264.9
0.1cc Far West	Berkeley	258.6
0.55cc Spokas	Berkeley	255.7
	SIN	258.0
	Stanford	260.6
	TRIUMF	265.1
	TRIUMF	263.2
1.0cc EG&G	Berkeley	258.3
1.0cc Far West	Berkeley	252.8
		mean = 261.0
		SD = 2%
0.1cc Chambers (7)		mean = 262.8
		SD = 2%
0.55 cc Chambers (5)		mean = 260.5
		SD = 1.5%
1.0cc Chambers (2)		mean = 255.6
		SD = 1.5%

absorbed dose in H_2O. The results of the in-air measurements are given in Table 5 and the lucite phantom results are given in Table 6. The standard deviation of the mean for both the in-air and in-phantom measurements is 2% or less and the maximum difference is 5%. No significant differences were seen in either chamber type or gassing conditions.

The second set of cobalt-60 measurements were made at the Lawrence Berkeley Laboratory. Data were taken with chambers in a lucite phantom in standard geometry and standard cobalt-60 factors were used to calculate the absorbed dose in tissue. The mean of the calibrations with the TE gas filled ionization chambers was 1.5% higher than the mean obtained with the air-filled chambers. In order to determine the cause of the difference, the ratio of the chamber responses when filled with TE gas and air were calculated. The mean ratio (TE/air) was 1.171±0.010. If the chamber calibration factors are not in this ratio then the difference between the TE and air data can be explained by the fact that each physicist calibrated his chamber with a TE gas with slightly different composition than the gas used at Berkeley. The ratio of the calibration factors for TE and air by the physicists varied from 1.108 to 1.178. If the TE data

TABLE 5

COBALT 60 MEASUREMENTS IN AIR (Massachusetts General Hospital)

Chamber	Institution	Water rads/min air gas	TE gas
0.1cc EG&G	Berkeley	115.4	–
	Harvard	–	115.1
	SIN	–	115.3
	Stanford	–	113.0
	TRIUMF	113.4	–
	UNM/LANL	–	116.9
0.55cc Spokas	Berkeley	113.3	–
	SIN	–	116.0
	Stanford	–	111.8
0.1cc PTW	Harvard	116.1	–
0.6cc Farmer	UNM/LANL	116.0	–
1.0cc Far West	Berkeley	112.4	–
	mean =	114.4	114.7
	SD =	1.4%	1.7%

TABLE 6

COBALT 60 MEASUREMENTS IN PHANTOM (Massachusetts General Hospital)

Chamber	Institution	Water rads/min air gas	TE gas
0.1cc EG&G	Berkeley	113.9	–
	Harvard	–	112.4
	SIN	–	113.4
	Stanford	–	112.5
	TRIUMF	114.1	–
	UNM/LANL	–	116.7
0.55cc Spokas	Berkeley	114.4	–
	SIN	–	116.9
	Stanford	–	111.3
0.1cc PTW	Harvard	115.0	–
0.6cc Farmer	UNM/LANL	116.8	–
1.0cc Far West	Berkeley	113.1	–
	mean =	114.6	113.9
	SD =	1.1%	2.1%

are recalculated using a new calibration factor that is 1.171 times less than the air calibration factor, then the air and TE results are in excellent agreement for the individual ionization chambers as well as the mean values. The Berkeley cobalt-60 results with corrected TE data are shown in Table 7. The standard deviation of the mean of all data is less than 2% and the maximum difference is 4%.

TABLE 7

COBALT 60 MEASUREMENTS IN PHANTOM (Lawrence Berkeley Laboratory)

Chamber	Institution	Tissue rads/MU*	
		air gas	TE gas
0.1cc EG&G	Berkeley	1.198	1.206
	Harvard	1.227	1.229
	SIN	1.213	1.217
	Stanford	1.184	1.189
	TRIUMF	1.217	1.198
0.1cc Far West	Berkeley	1.208	1.205
	UNM/LANL	1.177	1.194
0.55cc Spokas	Berkeley	1.218	1.227
	SIN	1.205	1.203
	Stanford	1.191	1.189
	TRIUMF	1.187	1.197
1.0cc Far West	Berkeley	1.194	1.186
	mean =	1.202	1.203
	SD =	1.3%	1.2%
0.1cc Chambers (7)	mean =	1.203	1.205
	SD =	1.5%	1.1%
0.55cc Chambers (4)	mean =	1.200	1.204
	SD =	1.2%	1.4%

* MU: monitor unit

Proton beam measurements

Measurements were performed on the proton therapy beam at the Harvard Cyclotron Laboratory. The chambers were placed in a lucite phantom in the center of a 12-cm spread peak. The data were taken with both negative and positive bias voltage and corrected for temperature and pressure. Cobalt-60 calibration factors and dose conversion factors were applied to the data to calculate absorbed dose. The goal here was not to determine the absolute proton absorbed dose, but to determine how well the participants agreed in stating a dose by using their respective measurement systems and techniques and using common conversion factors. The absolute proton absorbed dose measurements were the object of a separate intercomparison to be reported elsewhere. The results of the proton beam measurements are given in Table 8.

TABLE 8

PROTON BEAM MEASUREMENTS

Chamber	Institution	Water rads/MU	
		air gas	TE gas
0.1cc EG&G	Berkeley	0.413	–
	Harvard	–	0.418
	SIN	–	0.450
	Stanford	–	0.430
	TRIUMF	0.406	–
	UNM/LANL	–	0.430
0.55cc Spokas	Berkeley	0.412	–
	SIN	–	0.444
	Stanford	–	0.427
0.1cc PTW	Harvard	0.411	–
0.6cc Farmer	UNM/LANL	0.410	–
1.0cc Far West	Berkeley	0.402	–
	mean =	0.409	0.433
	SD =	1.0%	2.7%

There are no significant differences between types of chambers (0.424±3.7% for 0.1 cc chambers (6) versus 0.428±3.8% for 0.55cc chambers (3)). However, there is a large and somewhat surprising difference of approximately 6% between the results using air and TE gas in the chambers, TE results being higher. Also, the spread in the data is greater when TE gas was used. One conclusion is that when the chambers are exposed to the proton beam the results are more sensitive, than for cobalt-60, to the variations in the TE gas compositions used by the participants to calibrate their chambers and to the difference in their respective gasses and that used at Harvard.

Helium ion beam measurements

Measurements were made in the proximal and distal peak of a 10 cm spread therapy beam. The spread peak was shaped to produce a uniform biological effect across the peak and therefore the physical dose at the proximal and distal positions had a ratio of approximately 0.79. The chambers were moved from one position to the other by the insertion or removal of a lucite absorber in the beam path. These measurements were generally made with air filled chambers. As was done for the proton beam measurements, cobalt-60 correction factors and dose conversion factors were applied to the collected charge after correction for temperature, pressure, and polarity effects. The results are shown in Table 9.

The standard deviations of the means for all measurements is less than 2% and the maximum difference is 6%. The chambers with the larger volumes are

TABLE 9

HELIUM ION BEAM MEASUREMENTS

Chamber	Institution	Tissue rads/MU	
		proximal peak	distal peak
0.1cc EG&G	Berkeley	0.983	0.779
	Harvard	0.997	0.776
	SIN	0.997	0.779
	Stanford	0.963	0.779
	TRIUMF	1.005	0.787
0.1cc Far West	UNM/LANL	0.968	0.754
0.55cc Spokas	Berkeley	0.990	0.794
	SIN	0.991	0.788
	Stanford	0.972	0.770
	TRIUMF	0.988	0.787
	TRIUMF	0.984	0.785
1.0cc Far West	Berkeley	0.969	0.784
		mean = 0.984	0.778
		SD = 1.4%	1.8%
0.1cc chambers (6)		mean = 0.986	0.771
		SD = 1.7%	2.0%
0.55cc chambers (5)		mean = 0.985	0.785
		SD = 0.8%	1.1%

effectively at a point slightly more upstream than the smaller chambers and are therefore expected to give a slightly larger response. The ratio of distal/ proximal for the 0.1, 0.55, and 1.0cc chambers are 0.782, 0.797, and 0.809, respectively, which bears out this expectation.

Carbon ion beam measurements

The carbon ion irradiations were performed in a fashion similar to the helium ion irradiations and the data were handled in the same fashion. The results are given in Table 10.

The standard deviations of the means for all measurements is less than 3% and the maximum difference is 8%. The ratio of distal/proximal for the 0.1, 0.55, and 1.0 cc chambers are 0.753, 0.760, and 0.766 respectively. The effect of volume size is smaller because the carbon ion peak had less slope than the helium ion peak between the proximal and distal measurement points.

CONCLUSIONS AND DISCUSSION

The agreement among the physicists for the various measurements is reasonable but steps can be taken which will improve the results of intercomparisons. The

TABLE 10

CARBON ION BEAM MEASUREMENTS

Chambers	Institution	Tissue rads/MU	
		proximal peak	distal peak
0.1cc EG&G	Berkeley	0.934	0.710
	Harvard	0.971	0.732
	SIN	0.922	0.692
	Stanford	0.900	0.673
0.1cc Far West	UNM/LANL	0.922	0.695
0.55cc Spokas	Berkeley	0.935	0.720
	SIN	0.947	0.720
	Stanford	0.912	0.684
	TRIUMF	0.941	0.719
	TRIUMF	0.944	0.714
1.0cc Far West	Berkeley	0.923	0.715
	Berkeley	0.942	0.715
		mean = 0.933	0.707
		SD = 2.0%	2.5%
0.1cc chambers (5)		mean = 0.930	0.700
		SD = 2.8%	3.1%
0.55cc chambers (5)		mean = 0.936	0.711
		SD = 1.5%	2.2%
1.0cc chambers (2)		mean = 0.933	0.715
		SD = 1.4%	0.0%

following recommendations are made on the basis of the Phase I studies reported here:

1) Institutional calibrations of electrometers should be done using a standard capacitor and bridge circuit. Most institutions use calibrations furnished by the electrometer manufacturer at the time of purchase and these calibrations are known to change with use and aging of components.

2) Physicists should have an analysis made of the TE gas used for their chamber calibrations and the TE gas used during intercomparisons. Corrections can be applied which account for different gas compositions.

3) Physicists should calibrate their own ionization chambers against a chamber whose calibration is traceable to NBS or send the chamber to a calibration laboratory. Manufacturers calibrations are known to be inconsistent and unreliable.

4) When possible, intercomparisons on cobalt-60 beams should be made using both air and TE gassing for chambers, being careful to flush chambers well when gasses are changed. The ratio of the cobalt-60 responses for air and TE will indicate a TE gas composition different than that used at the home institution.

5)   When chambers of different volumes are intercompared the volume differences must be accounted for when measurements are performed in a dose gradient.   Different volumes, in general, result in different effective points of
measurement.   Phase I intercomparisons failed to show any differences in types
of ionization chambers other than expected volume effects.

6)   All instruments should be calibrated at the home institution both
before and after they are taken to an intercomparison.

7)   Dosimetry protocols need to be written to establish guidelines, instrumentation, methodology, and to recommended data bases for heavy charged
particle dosimetry.

Phase I intercomparisons have laid the groundwork for intercomparisons of
the absorbed dose at the various charged particle therapy facilties.   Most
of the differences in the Phase I studies are a result of inappropriate
calibrations of electrometers and ionization chambers.   In particular, the
composition of TE gas at the various facilities needs better quality control.

Note:

Institutions are identified in Tables as follows:

Berkeley	=	Lawrence Berkeley Laboratory
Harvard	=	Massachusetts General Hospital/Harvard Cyclotron Laboratory
Rutherford	=	Rutherford Laboratory, England
SIN	=	Swiss Institute for Nuclear Research, Switzerland
Stanford	=	Stanford University
TRIUMF	=	Tri-University Meson Facility, Canada
UNM/LANL	=	University of New Mexico/Los Alamos National Laboratory

RADIATION QUALITY OF BEAMS OF NEGATIVE PIONS

J. F. DICELLO AND D. J. BRENNER

Los Alamos National Laboratory, Los Alamos, NM 87545 USA

INTRODUCTION

As a negative pion stops in tissue, it attaches itself to an adjacent atom to form a mesonic atom. Subsequently, the wave function of the pion interacts with that of the nucleus and the pion is absorbed. Because the energy associated with the rest mass of the pion is greater than the separation energy of the nuclear particles, the nucleus disintegrates (pion star). In tissue, approximately 40 MeV goes into overcoming the binding energies; 20 MeV goes into kinetic energy of charged particles; 80 MeV goes into kinetic energy of neutrons.

In cases where biological studies are performed with beams of negative pions, as much as 20% of the total absorbed dose in the treatment volume and about 50% of the high-LET dose (> 100 keV/μm) can result from neutrons.[1-3] The degree of biological response and the variation of that response throughout the treatment volume can be altered by the neutron dose.[4] A significant amount of work has been performed by several groups in order to quantify the effects of neutrons from pion stars.[3,5-9] It is frequently difficult to follow the underlying physics associated with pions because of the complexity of most calculations and experiments. It is the purpose of this paper to review some of the basic effects with a simplified but semiquantitative approach.

CALCULATIONAL RESULTS

By eliminating energy straggling, a second-order effect in terms of integral dose, one can simplify calculations of absorbed dose by pion beams in uniform media. Consider a parallel pion beam with a uniform fluence over a cross-sectional area of 2.7 x 2.7 cm^2. The momentum spread of the incident beam is chosen to obtain a uniform stopping distribution 2.7 cm in depth, as illustrated in Fig. 1. There are three primary sources of energy deposited by such a beam: atomic collisions (dE/dx), charged particles from stars, and neutrons from stars. Doses as a function of depth for these three components

64

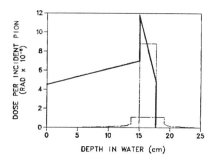

Fig. 1. Dose in water as a function of depth for a 76-MeV beam of negative pions. The heavy curve is the dose from atomic collisions of the pions, referenced as the pion dose throughout this article. The light curve is the dose deposited by charged particles from pion stars. The dashed curve is the dose deposited by neutrons from pion stars.

are plotted in Fig. 1. The energy deposited by atomic collisions will be called "pion dose." The maximum pion energy has been chosen to be 76 MeV. The total kinetic energy of charged particles from stars is chosen to be 20 MeV and is assumed to be locally deposited. The total kinetic energy of neutrons from stars is chosen to be 80 MeV. The distribution of dose per stopped pion from neutrons is assumed to be that calculated by Schillaci and Roeder[5] for a sphere, 2.7 cm diameter, as shown in Fig. 2. In order to examine the effects of neutron dose near and distant to the source (star), this dose has been divided into two components, that closer than 2.7 cm and that beyond 2.7 cm ("tails"). The dose closer than 2.7 cm is approximated by a uniform distribution with the same integral dose.

In addition to energy straggling, the dose from in-flight decay products and from secondary particles produced by in-flight interactions are neglected, along with any muon-electron contamination.

The simplified beam can be used to construct larger stopping volumes in order to examine changes in the four components (dose from pions, star dose from charged particles, star dose near the source from neutrons, and star dose distant to the source from neutrons). Remember that changes in the magnitude of the dose per incident pion change dose rate, but not necessarily radiation quality. The initial energy and dimensions were chosen specifically in order to compare with similar experimental results.

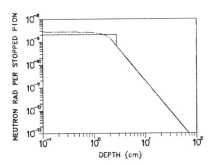

Fig. 2. Dose in water from star neutrons as a function of distance. The dashed curve is the result of a calculation for a uniform, spherical stopping distribution, 2.7 cm in diameter, by Schillaci and Roeder (Ref. 5). The heavy curve is the distribution used in the present calculation for a 2.7 x 2.7 x 2.7 cm^3 stopping volume. In the calculations the distribution has been normalized to a value of 80-MeV total neutron energy per stopped pion, rather than 60-MeV as originally used.

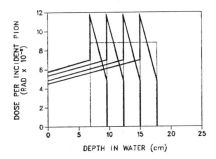

Fig. 3. An overlaying of four pion beams in order to produce a beam broadened in depth with a uniform stopping distribution. The four beams are obtained by shifting the range of the initial beam shown in Fig. 1 with an external range-shifter. The heavy curves are the pion dose. The light curves are the dose deposited by charged particles from stars.

Consider a case where the beam is broadened in depth (z) as shown in Fig. 3. The volume of the stopping region increases by a factor of four. The star dose from charged particles at any position in the stopping region remains unaltered.

However, the pion dose in the stopping region increases because more dose from energetic pions (plateau or entrance dose) is included in the stopping volume. Therefore, the dose of charged particles relative to that of pions has actually decreased as seen in Fig. 4. This can be seen more precisely if integral doses, i.e., the total energy deposited in the entire mass, rather than doses at a single position are compared. Percent integral doses are given in Table I.

The neutron dose near the source relative to the ionization dose is plotted in Fig. 5. Because the width of the neutron dose is larger than the width of the stopping distribution, there is an overlapping of neutron doses when the

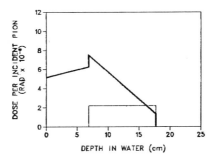

Fig. 4. Dose in water as a function of depth for the range-modulated beams shown in Fig. 3. The heavy curve is the pion dose. The light curve is the charged-particle dose.

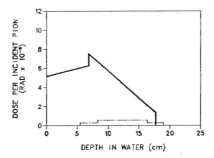

Fig. 5. Dose in water as a function of depth for the range-modulated beam shown in Fig. 4. The solid curve is the pion dose. The dashed curve is the dose deposited close to the source (star) by star neutrons.

TABLE 1

A COMPARISON OF THE PERCENTAGE CONTRIBUTIONS BY VARIOUS COMPONENTS OF A BEAM OF NEGATIVE PIONS TO THE TOTAL INTEGRAL DOSE IN THE STOPPING VOLUME. THESE VALUES ARE THE RESULT OF THE PRESENT CALCULATIONS FOR A UNIFORM STOPPING DISTRIBUTION IN WATER.

VOLUME (cm^3)	20	59	79	177	709	1260	5030
STOPPING WIDTHS (x,y,z)	(2.7,2.7,2.7)	(8.1,2.7,2.7)	(2.7,2.7,10.8)	(8.1,8.1,2.7)	(8.1,8.1,10.8)	(21.6,21.6,2.7)	(21.6,21.6,10.8)
DOSE FROM PIONS	54%	52%	61%	48%	54%	47%	51%
STAR DOSE	46%	48%	39%	52%	46%	53%	49%
STAR DOSE FROM CHARGED PARTICLES	41%	39%	31%	37%	27%	35%	26%
STAR DOSE CLOSE TO SOURCE FROM NEUTRONS	5%	8%	7%	13%	16%	16%	20%
STAR DOSE DISTANT TO SOURCE FROM NEUTRONS	0%	~ 1%	~ 1%	~ 2%	< 5%	< 3%	~ 3%
STAR DOSE FROM NEUTRONS	5%	9%	8%	15%	19%	18%	23%

TABLE II

PERCENTAGE INTEGRAL DOSE IN THE STOPPING REGION FROM STAR NEUTRONS FOR NEGATIVE PION BEAMS IN WATER. THESE VALUES WERE DERIVED FROM EXPERIMENTAL DATA FOR PION BEAMS IN C_2H_6. ALL OF THESE BEAMS HAVE TRANSVERSE STOPPING DISTRIBUTIONS WHICH ARE APPROXIMATELY GAUSSIAN AND HAVE BEEN INTEGRATED ONLY IN DEPTH. THE PRESENT RESULTS ARE FOR A UNIFORM STOPPING DISTRIBUTION IN DEPTH. THE BEAMS USED IN REF. 3 DID NOT HAVE A UNIFORM STOPPING DISTRIBUTION. SEE TEXT FOR DETAILS.

FWHM (x,y,z)	(7.5,7.5,2.5)	(20,20,9.4)
STAR DOSE FROM NEUTRONS	~ 10%	~ 20%
FWHM (x,y,z)	REF. 3 (7.5,7.5,9.4)	REF. 3 (20,20,9.4)
STAR DOSE FROM NEUTRONS	~ 11%	~ 15%

*THE MUON-ELECTRON CONTAMINATIONS HAVE BEEN SUBTRACTED FROM THE EXPERIMENTAL DATA.

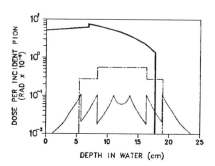

Fig. 6. Dose in water as a function of depth for the range—modulated beam shown in Fig. 4. The heavy and dashed curves are the pion and star neutron doses plotted in Fig. 5. The light curve is the dose deposited distant to the source (star) from star neutrons.

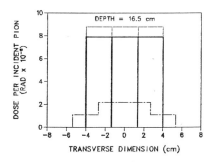

Fig. 7. Dose in water as a function of distance from the central beam axis in the plane perpendicular to the beam axis at a depth of 16.5 cm. The heavy curve is the pion dose. This beam is produced by abutting the initial beam in Fig. 1 against itself. The light curve is the charged—particle dose. The dashed curve is the dose near the source from star neutrons.

stopping distributions are abutted and their contribution increases relative to the total dose. The neutron dose from the tails is plotted in Fig. 6. This dose represents such a small fraction of the total dose ($\sim 1\%$), and must be compared on a logarithmic scale. (The sharp peaks in Fig. 5 are artifacts resulting from the separation of the neutron dose into two components. They do not alter the value of the integral dose.)

Consider another case where the initial beam is broadened in a transverse dimension (x or y) as shown in Fig. 7. Again, the doses from charged particles abut and this dose at any position remains unaltered. Again, the doses from neutrons overlap and their relative contribution increases. In contrast to the previous case, the pion doses remain unaltered at any position. Obviously, there is no change in the contribution of energetic pions (plateau) to the pion dose when the beam is broadened in x or y. Therefore, the relative contribution of stars increases more rapidly with changes in volume when the beam is broadened in the transverse dimensions as compared with broadening in depth.

Some additional examples are listed in Table I for comparison.

EXPERIMENTAL RESULTS

The experimental technique of Dicello et al.[2] has been used to directly measure that fraction of the total dose resulting from neutron-induced proton recoils in polyethylene (C_2H_4). Basically, the measured dose in polyethylene is compared with that in carbon, the difference being from proton recoils produced by neutrons. For more details, see Ref. (2).

Data have been obtained for an unmodulated pion beam having a stopping distribution with full-widths-half-maximum (FWHM) of about (7.5 cm, 7.5 cm, 2.5 cm) and for a beam with a uniform stopping distribution in depth[2] with FWHMs of about (20,20,9.4).

For the broad beam, stopping distributions in the transverse dimensions are approximately Gaussian. For the narrow beam, the distributions are Gaussian in all dimensions. Results are presented in Figs. 8 and 9. That fraction of the total dose resulting from proton-recoils is 9% for the narrow beam and 16% for the broad beam. This corresponds to a total dose in water from neutrons of approximately 10 and 20% respectively. (The ratio of proton-recoil dose in polyethylene to neutron dose in water as calculated in Ref. (2), was used to obtain these latter values.) Results are listed in Table II. Also listed are results obtained from the data of Dicello et al.[2] for a beam with constant total dose as a function of depth (20,20,9.4) and a beam having this same stopping distribution in depth but a narrower distribution in the transverse plane (7.5,7.5,9.4).

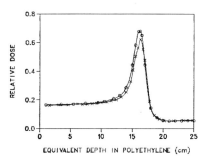

Fig. 8. Dose as a function of depth for a relatively narrow pion beam. The open circles are doses in polyethylene ($C_{2n}H_{4n}$) and the crosses are doses in carbon.

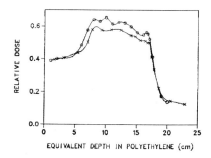

Fig. 9. Dose as a function of depth for a range-shifted pion beam. The open circles are doses in polyethylene ($C_{2n}H_{4n}$) and the crosses are doses in carbon.

DISCUSSION AND CONCLUSIONS

With the results in Tables I and II, we can arrive at some general conclusions with regard to variations in the integral dose in the treatment volume. These depend only on the assumption that the width of the neutron dose distribution is greater than that of either the pions or charged particles.

1. The fractional contribution of neutrons to the total dose increases with increasing field size (x,y).

2. The fractional contribution from neutrons increases with increasing width in

z of the stopping distribution; however, the change occurs more slowly than with changes in field size.

3. The percentage star dose (integral) always increases with increasing field size. However, the central-axis dose will slowly increase only as a result of the tails once the beam is wider than the width of the local neutron dose. Additionally, the percentage star dose can decrease with broadening with depth.

4. The increased (%) neutron dose with increasing volume is primarily a result of the greater width of the dose distribution of neutrons as compared with that of pions or charged particles. The dose from long-range interactions (the tails) represents only a small fraction of the neutron dose in the treatment volume.

5. Although the neutrons do contribute to a smearing of the dose at the edges of the field, it is a fairly local effect (within about a centimeter or so of the edge). Long-range interactions make only a small contribution to these effects.

6. The previous conclusions are consistent with available experimental data.

It is obvious that the above conclusions would still be valid even if the tails of the dose distributions from neutrons were negligible as long as the width is greater than that of pions or charged particles.

Another interesting conclusion can be inferred from a comparison of the calculated and experimental results. The calculated values of neutron dose are higher than the measured values, but closer for the wider distribution. A straightforward but lengthy calculation shows that the fractional contribution of neutrons to the total dose is greater for a Gaussian than for a uniform stopping distribution when integrated over the entire volume, but less for a Gaussian when integrated only along the central axis.

None of the previous conclusions are particularly new. Nevertheless, it seems appropriate to reiterate them in the context of a relatively simple model in order to review the relative contributions of neutrons in beams of negative pions.

ACKNOWLEDGMENTS

The authors wish to thank Drs. Peter Berardo, Stanley Curtis, Edward Knapp, and John Lyman for their useful discussions and comments.

REFERENCES

1. Dicello JF and Zaider M (1978) Investigation of the microdosimetric characteristics of broad, therapeutic beams of negative pions at LAMPF. Proceedings of the Sixth Symposium on Microdosimetry, J Booz and HG Ebert, eds. London: Harwood Academic Publishers Ltd.

2. Dicello JF, Zaider M., and Takai M (1979) Physical characteristics of range-modulated beams of pions, p. 221 High LET Radiations in Clinical Radiotherapy, GW Barendsen, J Broerse, and K Breur eds. Suppl to European J of Cancer. New York: Pergamon Press.

3. Dicello JF, Brenner DJ, Zink S, Berardo PA, and Rosen, II (1981) A method for the direct measurement in the treatment volume of neutron dose from pion stars. Los Alamos National Laboratory Report LA-UR 81-1683. Proceedings of the 4th Symposium on Neutron Dosimetry, Neuherberg, Germany. In press.

4. Brenner DJ, Dicello JF, and Zaider M (1981) An interpretation of some biological results obtained in range-modulated negative pion beams. Los Alamos National Laboratory Report LA-UR 80-3419, Int J Radiat Oncol Biol Phys. In press.

5. Schillaci ME and Roeder DL (1973) Dose distribution due to neutrons and photons resulting from negative pion capture in tissue. Phys Med Biol 18: 821-829.

6. Brenner DJ and Smith FA (1977) Dose and LET distributions due to neutrons and photons emitted from stopped negative pions. Phys Med Biol 22: 451-465.

7. Amols HI, Bradbury JN, Dicello JF, Helland JA, Kligerman MM, Lane, TF, Paciotti MA, Roeder DL, and Schillaci ME (1978) Dose outside of the treatment volume for irradiation with negative pions. Phys Med Biol 23: 385-369.

8. Klein U (1978) Measurement of neutron spectra from absorption of stopped negative pions in the biologically interesting nuclei ^{12}C, ^{14}N, and ^{16}O. Inst of Nucl Phys. Thesis. Karlsruhe University.

9. Wright HA, Hamm RN, Bishop BL, and Turner JE (1978) Neutron dose distributions in tissue irradiated by negative pion beams. Nucl Instr Meth 157: 405-414.

CRITERIA AND TECHNIQUES FOR THREE-DIMENSIONAL TREATMENT PLANNING WITH PIONS

PETER BERARDO, SANDRA ZINK, MICHAEL PACIOTTI, AND JAMES BRADBURY

Los Alamos National Laboratory, MS H809, Los Alamos, New Mexico 87545

INTRODUCTION

The ability to predict a pion dose distribution in a patient is a major objective of the clinical trials at LAMPF. Accurate predictions are essential for evaluation of pion therapy. But accuracy must be in the context of clinical utility. That is, reasonable approximations must be made in calculational methods so that treatment planning can proceed in a timely and efficient manner. We present here a few of the techniques and current developments used to achieve that objective.

METHOD OF DOSE CALCULATION

The treatment-planning program PIPLAN calculates a dose distribution by summing the contributions of individual pencil beams as they pass through various clinical appliances and patient anatomy. One-dimensional depth dose distributions for pencil beams of each type of incident particle and for each of their dose components are precalculated analytically in water and include the effects of inflight interactions, straggling, and decay. Additionally, a two-dimensional distribution is precalculated for long range neutrons that are emitted by inflight and stopping pion interactions. Secondary muons from pion decay are treated as a composite psuedo-particle with its own dose distribution. Primary electron dose is obtained from fits to high-energy electron depth-dose curves. Long-range electron dose from muon decay is obtained from a separate model during the dose accumulation process.

For a given pencil beam, dose is distributed in depth as a function of water-equivalent range along the incident trajectory and then further distributed radially as a function of multiple Coulomb scattering. A dose calculation then entails accumulating at each point of interest the amount of energy from each incident pencil beam and then dividing by the local mass density. To model the complex, non-analytic, phase space of treatment beams, measurements of individual trajectories or rays are used as input to the calculation. This introduces a Monte Carlo aspect into the calculation and associated statistical uncertainties. However, the otherwise analytic nature of the calculation and distributed dose for each pencil beam yields a result comparable to Monte Carlo in much less time.

PIPLAN calculations are initially verified with measurements of unmodulated beams in water. Figure 1 shows a typical comparison after slight adjustments in the beam momentum and background. However, these adjustments are within experimental uncertainties, are only beam-tune dependent, and are then constant for all subsequent calculations. PIPLAN verification then consists of comparing predicted and measured dose distributions for various beam-modulation functions and geometries. Predictions typically match measurements to better than four percent of maximum, as shown in Figure 2. An inability to measure the entire beam phase-space passing through the primary monitor chamber presently requires that normalized comparisons be made.

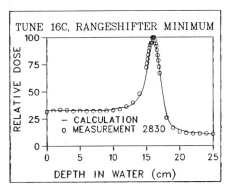

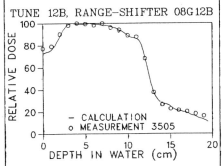

Fig. 1. Comparison of calculation and measurement of depth-dose curves for an unmodulated, medium-energy, large-field beam.

Fig. 2. Comparison of calculation and measurement of depth-dose curves for a modulated, low-energy, medium-field beam.

CT DATA

The value of CT data in radiotherapy in general is widely accepted. In particular, it is used for at least three different purposes: diagnosis, treatment planning calculations, and evaluation of dose distributions on a CT image background. For the latter two purposes it is possible to significantly reduce the bulk of CT data without significant loss of calculational accuracy or visual resolution. The corresponding reduction in processing time, data storage space, and data transfer time between machines can be substantial, especially for computers capable of 8-bit byte processing.

TABLE 1

RESULTS OF REDUCED CT NUMERICAL PRECISION AND SPATIAL RESOLUTION

SITE	TEST CASES	AVERAGE INTEGRAL CHANGES (mm)	AVERAGE INCREASE CHANGES (mm)
SINUSES	4/9	-0.14 (0.40)	0.0 (0.08)
	-1,+1	-0.07 (0.38)	0.0 (0.08)
	BOTH	-0.07 (0.37)	0.0 (0.08)
LUNG	4/9	0.0 (0.05)	0.0 (0.05)
	-1,+1	-0.02 (0.23)	0.0 (0.08)
	BOTH	-0.02 (0.23)	0.0 (0.08)
PELVIS	4/9	0.0 (0.06)	0.0 (0.06)
	-1,+1	0.0 (0.10)	0.0 (0.07)
	BOTH	0.01 (0.10)	0.0 (0.07)

Treatment – planning calculations use CT data for line integrals to transport particles or modify dose distributions based on effective range. Since integration is an averaging process, numerical and spatial resolution diminish in importance. Table 1 summarizes the results of a detailed study to determine practical limits for reduced CT numerical precision and spatial resolution using three different CT slices. The procedure was to calculate line integrals with a 1 mm step size vertically for each slice and tabulate the integrals on a square centimeter grid. This was done for three slices with full resolution (12-bit pixel, about 1 mm x 1 mm x 1 cm) and for various test cases. "4/9" indicates a rounding procedure to reduce the numerical precision to eight bits and allows a CT pixel to be stored in one byte. "-1,+1" indicates three pixel lateral averaging for each integrand. When considered with the integration, this is analogous to a thirty-pixel areal average between vertical grid points. Finally, the last test case used both reduced resolution techniques. The changes from the full-resolution cases are shown with standard deviations in parentheses and assumes a linear relation between CT number and stopping power. In fact, for heavy charged particles in material more dense than water, the values will be even smaller. The average integral change is the average change between a final base case integral and a final test case integral. For the average increase change, the average is over the changes in the increase of all the integrals from one centimeter to the next in depth. Results such as these show that accurate calculations can be retained with at least a factor of eight reduction in the bulk of CT data through four pixel spatial averaging and eight bit numerical resolution.

Resolution reduction of CT image data, as opposed to CT treatment – planning data, is subject to more subjective analysis. Visual comparisons of various images has led to the conclusion that four-pixel averaging and eight-bit precision also retains sufficient resolution and detail in a CT image for accurate evaluation of superimposed dose distributions.

Finally, we note that while these techniques preclude regeneration of a diagnostic quality image, they do allow random access of individual CT data elements. This means that treatment – planning calculations and displays can proceed equally well at any orientation relative to the original CT slice.

MULTIPLE SCATTERING

A major objective of treatment – planning calculations is the accurate prediction of transverse dose distributions as a function of depth and their dependence upon multiple scattering in external appliances and the heterogeneous anatomy of a patient. PIPLAN uses a recursive Gaussian model which is energy, material, and geometry dependent. The transverse distribution at any point is the result of folding together Gaussian distributions from multiple scattering at many points upstream. Although the angular distribution from multiple scattering in upstream regions is used to obtain the radial distribution downstream, in this model the angular and spatial distributions are uncoupled. That is, each scattering region assumes all incident particles are still parallel to the initial trajectory but are spatially distributed about it according to upstream scattering. This feature allows a very rapid recursive expression, but only works well for ideally thin scattering regions. To model thick targets, a modifying function is used which effectively requires that the transverse, spatial standard-deviation from a single thick target equals that obtained from many thin targets of the same total thickness. This function essentially compensates for the uncoupling of the angular and spatial distributions and allows large distances to be traversed in a single cycle, such as air gaps between the range modulator and the patient. The function includes two constants which determine the effective energy-loss of a particle. The net result is a recursive model that is both fast and accurate. The degree of accuracy is illustrated for pions in Figure 3 for an unmodulated beam in water. A typical step size of 0.5 cm was used in this calculation.

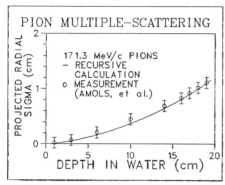

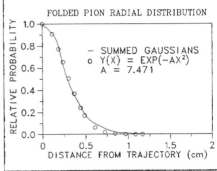

Fig. 3. Comparison of calculation and measurement of projected standard deviation for Gaussian transverse distribution as a function of depth.[1]

Fig. 4. Comparison of Gaussian fit to weighted and summed Gaussian transverse distributions obtained at 5 cm in water for a 3-cm range modulation and 6-cm air-gap.

When beams are range modulated, the transverse distributions at a given point due to different upstream scattering geometries must be added with weights obtained from the range modulation function. Since the sum of Gaussians is not conveniently analytic, the final transverse distribution can be obtained by tracking each ray repeatedly as a function of the range-shifter thickness or by sampling the modulation function for each ray. The first is expensive in time and the second can introduce significant statistical uncertainties in the distal spread peak unless a great number of rays are used. We are currently investigating the feasibility of tabulating for each modulation function a set of parameters at each depth along a trajectory which describe the summed distributions. We find that in most geometries a Gaussian distribution works quite well, as shown in Figure 4. For very large modulation functions, an exponential function gives only a slightly better fit than a Gaussian. If this model is successful, then the precalculated one dimensional dose distributions can be folded through the modulation function and each incident ray will distribute dose radially and in depth as if it had experienced full modulation.

PHASE SPACE SMOOTHING

Another important aspect in predicting transverse dose distributions is accurately representing the phase space of treatment beams, which at LAMPF are non-parallel and contain spatially non-uniform ratios of pions, muons, and electrons. To accurately sample and transport a sufficient number of particles in a reasonable time, two techniques are used.

The first involves measuring a two-dimensional, transverse dose distribution in air and also sampling the true phase space by measuring about 250,000 individual particle trajectories. Then from the particle data, a sub-sample is selected which, by independent calculation, reproduces the dose distribution in air. The particle randomness of the original sample is retained in the sub-sample, but the statistical uncertainty in the transverse dose distribution is reduced to that of the dose measurement. The number of particles in the sub-sample is selected to achieve a desired maximum, statistical uncertainty in PIPLAN calculations. This in turn involves the second smoothing techique.

The relative statistical uncertainty at some point, due to spatially random, overlapping, radial distributions, is inversely proportional to the standard deviation of the distributions and to the square-root of the fluence. Thus for a given uncertainty, there is a direct relationship between multiple scattering and the sub-sample fluence. When the fluence is also given, the uncertainty is determined only by the degree of distribution overlap. Near the patient surface, multiple scattering overlap is small and a minimum radial standard deviation is used to obtain about three percent statistical uncertainty. Normal multiple scattering then yields equal or less uncertainty at depth. Figure 5 compares calculated transverse air scans with the ion chamber measurements for a radial sigma of 0.5 cm, which is the usual minimum. At depth, the multiple scattering sigma exceeds the minimum and the statistical uncertainty is negligible, as shown in Figure 6 for a sigma of 1.2 cm. These results were obtained for a central-axis fluence of only 43 particles per square centimeter. In Figure 7 are shown the transverse scans in a water phantom at mid-peak in a 10-cm spread peak and a central-axis fluence of 50 particles per square centimeter. These curves show essentially no statistical fluctuations and perhaps a small systematic coordinate misalignment.

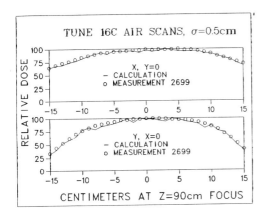

Fig. 5. Comparison of calculation and measurement of air dose on major transverse axes with minimum pencil-beam sigma.

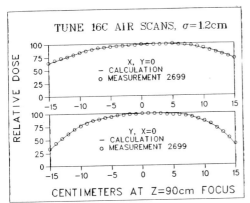

Fig. 6. Comparison of calculation and measurement of air dose on major transverse axes with typical pencil-beam sigma at depth.

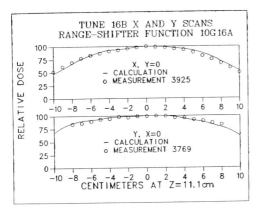

Fig. 7. Comparison of calculation and measurement of water dose on major transverse axes at depth for modulated beam.

CURRENT PROBLEMS

Collimators: Three-dimensional methods of calculation, such as Monte Carlo or three-dimensional ray tracing, must accurately predict dose distributions in complex geometries and materials. This is particularly important in the regions of gross inhomogeneities, such as for a beam collimator. Here PIPLAN exhibits a problem as illustrated in Figure 8. On the left are the depth dose curves for a static rangeshifter. On the right a collimator has also been used and a clear discrepancy between calculation and measurement exists in the entrance region. Preliminary models which attempt to account for this entrance dose with neutrons from pion capture in the cerrobend collimator have not been satisfactory. As shown in Figure 9, when this beam is modulated, the discrepancy accumulates. Monte Carlo calculations are proceeding to aid our understanding of collimator physics.

Dynamic Beam Bolus: Except for strictly parallel beams, bolus design for moving beams and/or patients presents an interesting problem, as schematically illustrated in Figure 10. In the upper left is represented the superposition of a given beam at three different focal points in a target volume, but ignoring the inhomogeneity. Each point in such a composite can be thought of as a point source of beam particles. For bolus, the points of interest are at the patient surface, as represented at the upper right. The bolus at that point must be such that the inhomogeneities are accounted for and that the optimum dose distribution is achieved in the target volume. With unlimited computer resources and time, one could, in principle, perform iterative dose calculations to arrive at the optimum bolus and dose distribution simultaneously. In practice one must settle for something less. Using ray tracing techniques, such as in PIPLAN, one can determine a bolus-thickness distribution for rays passing through the point in question, as indicated in the lower half of Figure 10. Rays which can be made to stop in the target volume give the distribution on the left. Of course some rays may always miss the target volume and collimation or very thick bolus should be used for them, which gives the distribution on the right. The relative number of target-volume stops and misses determine if bolus or collimator is best at a given point. If bolus is used, then the bolus-thickness distribution gives, to first order, the depth-dose distribution under that point due to particles passing through that point. This can be used to select an actual thickness from the distribution depending upon the location of nearby critical structures or various other criteria. Since bolus itself can be very structured and act as a superficial inhomogeneity in highly non-parallel beams, it may be worthwhile to iterate at least once to refine the bolus shape.

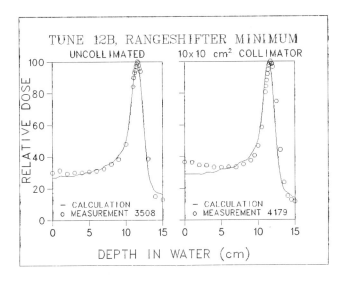

Fig. 8. Comparison of calculation and measurement of
water depth-dose curves without and with collimator.

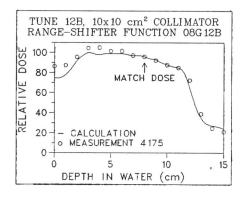

Fig. 9. Comparison of calculation and
measurement of depth-dose curve for collimated and modulated low-energy, medium-
field beam.

In any case, once the bolus is designed, calculations can proceed and the results evaluated.

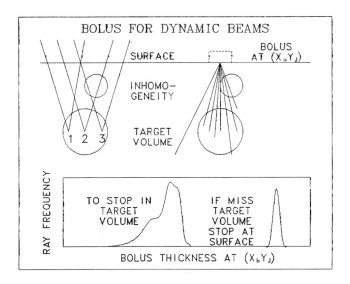

Fig. 10. For overlapping non-parallel beams, bolus-thickness distributions are obtained at each point on the patient surface. The thickness which optimizes the dose distribution is not obvious.

ACKNOWLEDGMENT

The dosimetry data used here was measured with the assistance of University of New Mexico personnel under the direction of A. Smith.

REFERENCE

1. Amols HI et al (1981) Multiple Scattering Distributions for Therapeutic Pion Beams. Phys Med Biol 26(2): 277-289.

PHYSICAL ASPECTS OF THE PION BEAM AT TRIUMF

GABRIEL K.Y. LAM AND LLOYD D. SKARSGARD
Batho Biomedical Facility, TRIUMF, University of British Columbia, 4004 Wesbrook
Mall, Vancouver, B.C. Canada V6T 2A3 and Medical Biophysics Unit, B.C. Cancer
Research Centre.

INTRODUCTION

TRIUMF (TRI-University Meson Facility) is one of the three "meson factories"
that were built in the early seventies to provide meson beams of high intensity
for nuclear physics and chemistry research. The design of TRIUMF is based on a
sector-focussing cyclotron originally proposed by Richardson.[1] The unique
feature of TRIUMF is the acceleration of H$^-$ ions, which enables the simultaneous
extraction of up to four independent beams of different energy and intensity.

As in the other meson factories, the availability of a high intensity π^- beam
has led to studies of the potential usefulness of π^- in cancer radiotherapy,
which was proposed by Fowler and Perkins[2] in 1961. The TRIUMF cyclotron

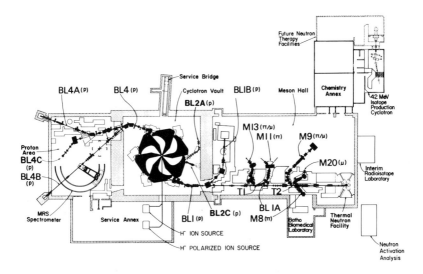

Fig. 1. Layout of TRIUMF. The biomedical beam line is the one designated
M8 in the meson hall.

delivered its first proton beam in June 1975. By November 1979 frequent high intensity proton beams of 100 μA became available, and preliminary patient skin nodule treatment was started. Higher intensity beams are expected to be available in the next year or two as the Π⁻ clinical program develops.

THE BIOMEDICAL CHANNEL

The biomedical channel and the Batho Biomedical Facility are housed in the TRIUMF meson hall, as shown in the site layout in figure 1. We share a common pion production target with two other secondary channels, which limits somewhat optimal design of the pion production target and occasionally presents scheduling conflicts for the use of different target materials.

The biomedical channel is a symmetric beam line based on a design by Harrison and Lobb[3], with two 45° bends. It consists of 5 quadrupoles, 2 dipoles and 2 sextupoles (see figure 2). The channel accepts pions at an angle of 30°C above the forward direction of the proton beam. This angle was chosen because it was the smallest forward angle allowable by the space available around the target. The momentum selection of the channel is Δp/p = 7%, but smaller momentum bites

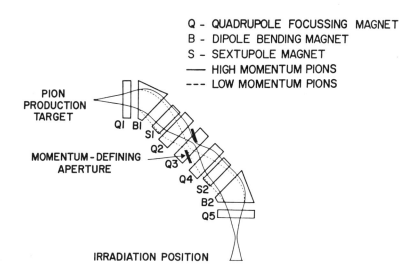

Fig. 2. Schematic of the biomedical beam line, which lies in a plane inclined at 30° to the horizontal above the exit beam.

can be selected using a pair of momentum selection slits at the dispersion plane. A second pair of slits was used to generate sharp lateral cutoff for the irradiation fields.

As the channel was intended as a multi-user facility (physicists, biologists and medical staff), the control system was computerized for simple operation and for protection against misuse. All of the elements (magnets and motors) are controlled through the standard CAMAC[4] interface system by minicomputer. The computer will only execute legitimate commands and instructions, and also conducts continuous routine monitoring of the various parameters. In case of failure or malfunction, the computer will take action to interrupt the irradiation and sends out warning messages and alarms. The computer programming for control[5] uses a macro assembly language and a real time disc-based operating system (Data General RDOS). The control program uses the foreground portion of the computer memory. Since the control program uses only about 10% of the computer time, the background portion can thus be used for handling experiments or data analysis. Normally, the control program in the foreground has priority, but this can be readily reversed for experiments that require special attention. With this foreground and background operation, automatic data taking with various channel settings under computer control is possible. This is especially useful for initial tuning and other beam development.

In order to conserve pions, the total channel length has been minimized to about 7 meters to reduce pion loss due to decay. The beam line is also evacuated to reduce loss due to scattering. This makes tuning difficult because detectors cannot be positioned at various points in the channel. Hence, a systematic tuning method had to be developed using just a pair of multiwire proportional counters and a set of scintillator telescopes positioned at the end of the channel.[6]

The dose distributions of the various beam tunes are measured using an automatic dose mapping system[7] that was developed specifically for the low dose and unstable output during the development stage of the cyclotron. The dose readout is normalized to the number of pions, and hence is immune to beam fluctuations. The dose measurements are made using a 0.5 cc Spokas thimble chamber calibrated in a ^{60}Co beam and using a correction factor of 0.95 for the different W and stopping power of pions.[8]

A system of beam monitors has been developed for the Π^- irradiation, as shown in figure 3. The intensity of the proton beam is monitored at the cyclotron stripper foil, where the H^- ions are converted to protons and extracted. The neutron flux produced near the pion production target is also monitored to give an indication of the intensity of the proton beam for Π^- production. A transmission chamber mounted at the exit end of the pion channel monitors the pion beam intensity as delivered to the treatment room. These 3 monitors seem to provide an adequate system for quick diagnosis of the location of failure, whether it is the cyclotron itself, the primary beam line, or the secondary channel. The transmission chamber is also calibrated to monitor total dose delivered. A second identical transmission chamber, connected to totally independent circuits, is used as a backup system. The lateral drifting of the beam is monitored to a precision of about 1 mm by a quadrant chamber; the readings are continously monitored by the computer, which can recenter the beam by controlling the dipole magnets.

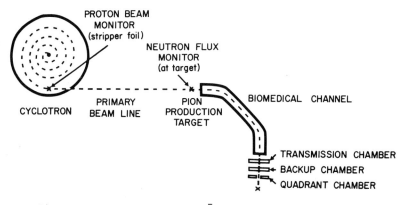

Fig. 3. The TRIUMF biomedical Π^- beam monitoring system.

DEVELOPMENTS FOR HIGHER Π^- FLUX

At present, the TRIUMF Π^- biomedical program is somewhat compromised by the low output of our facility. The pion production has turned out to be only about 60% of what we expected using cross-section data available over 10 years ago. The biomedical channel, moreover, only collects about 70% of its design acceptance, and so we are a factor of about 2 lower in output than expected.[9] Our dose rate at the present cyclotron current of 100 μA proton beam is 3.5 rads per minute per liter volume, so a standard treatment of 125 rads to a liter volume would take almost 40 minutes, which is considered too long for many patients. We are, however, actively trying to increase our pion flux.

Firstly, the TRIUMF cyclotron is capable of delivering more current than the present 100 μA. The present thermal neutron facility beam dump is limiting our operation to about 150 μA.[10] A new beam dump is scheduled to be installed in early 1982, and currents in excess of 200 μA should then be available.

Secondly, it has been shown[11] that the acceptance of the biomedical channel can be increased by a factor of about 2 by adding another quadrupole at the front end of the present channel. For technical reasons, this quadrupole has to be a permanent magnet fabricated from samarium cobalt. Since this magnet will be placed very close to the pion production target, a major concern is the uncertainty of the performance of a permanent magnet in such a high radiation area. Tests for this are being conducted, and if the results are favourable, the installation will proceed. It should be completed early in 1983.

Thirdly, we are also considering a proposal to install a high flux channel similar to the PIOTRON at SIN.[12] This would give us a factor of 15 gain in flux with just 30 to 40 μA from the cyclotron. The cost of such a channel has been estimated at 12 million dollars.[13] This cost is substantial, but such a high flux channel would greatly reduce our demand for high intensity beam from the cyclotron and facilitate beam scheduling and patient accrual.

PATIENT IRRADIATION SYSTEM

With our present flux, however, we are still able to deliver a dose rate of about 18 rads/min to a field size of 4 cm diameter, which is suitable for patient skin nodule irradiation. Eight patients have been treated since November 1979. Most of them received 10 daily fractions ranging from 270 to 330 rads. The skin was irradiated with stopping pions using a plexiglas bolus and a brass ring collimator.

For treatment of deep-seated tumors, we are now developing a more sophisticated system of beam handling. It has been decided to scan using a small, sharply focussed beam to cover different field size requirements. Small spot scanning has the following advantages:

(1) It is easier to produce uniform dose profiles by scanning than by defocussing of magnets.

(2) The inevitable loss of pion flux in collimation will be reduced in spot scanning.

(3) Scanning can cover field sizes and shapes of a larger variety.

(4) Range modulation can be used with spot scanning to produce different range modulation at different locations in the treatment field.

This requires the development of a scanning couch system and a compatible range modulation system.

A sketch of the simple range shifter we have developed for pions is shown in figure 4. The basic component is a 40 cm diameter plexiglas disk onto which additional sector blocks of plexiglas are bolted. The disk is rotated by a stepping motor under computer control to present different thicknesses of

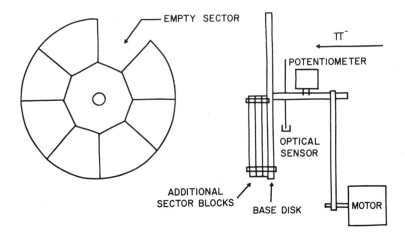

Fig. 4. The TRIUMF biomedical Π^- range shifter. It is based on discrete step range shifting using a rotating plexiglas disc with 8 sectors of different thickness. Left: front view; Right: side view.

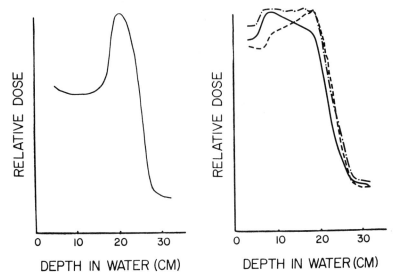

Fig. 5a. Unmodulated depth dose curve.

Fig. 5b. Various depth dose profiles produced by the discrete step range shifter:
uniform flat top (-·-·-)
10% slope up   (-----)
10% slope down (———)

plexiglas to the pion beam.   It will shift the beam in eight steps of 2 cm water equivalence each.   The use of a finite number of range shifting steps to produce extended uniform depth dose profiles was made possible by the development of a mathematical technique to handle linear addition of dose profiles.   Depth dose profiles of various shapes as required for uniform biological effect can also be readily produced, as shown in figure 5.

A scanning couch system has also been developed.   Table 1 gives the specifications for this couch, and the elevation view is shown in figure 6.   The

TABLE 1

SPECIFICATIONS OF SCANNING COUCH SYSTEM

Linear Movement	Total Range
X direction (east-west)	233 cm
Y direction (up-down)	52 cm
Z direction (along beam axis)	92 cm
Rotational Movement	
Main column (in steps of 15°)	180°
Table (continuous)	360°
Table tilt (continuous)	±20°

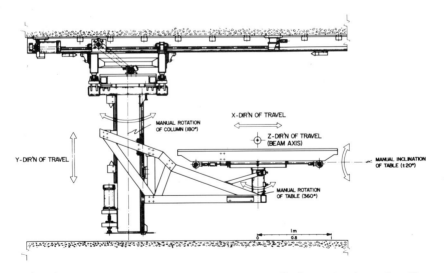

Fig. 6. An elevation view of the TRIUMF biomedical treatment couch.   The various translational and rotational movements are indicated.

system is capable of moving a patient or apparatus weighing up to 1100 lbs. in three dimensions under computer control to a precision of about ½ mm. Together with the range shifter, we will be able to deliver uniform pion beams to any three dimensional volume.

REFERENCES

1. Richardson JR (1963) Design criteria for a 700 MeV cyclotron to accelerate negative hydrogen ions. Nucl Instrum & Meth 24:493-500.
2. Fowler PH, Perkins DH (1961) The possibility of therapeutic applications of beams of negative Π^- - mesons. Nature 189:524-528.
3. Harrison RW, Lobb DE (1973) A negative pion beam transport channel for radiobiology and radiation therapy at TRIUMF. IEEE Trans Nucl Sci NS-20:1029-1031.
4. Costrell L (ed.) (1972) CAMAC: A Modular Instrumentation System for Data Handling. Washington D.C.:U.S. Government Printing Office.
5. Lang H, Harrison RW, Johnson RR, Henkelman RM (1977) CAMAC control of the biomedical Π^- beam line at TRIUMF. Nucl Instrum & Meth 144:589-592.
6. Henkelman RM, Lam GKY, Harrison RW, Poon M, Shortt KR (1978) Tuning of the biomedical negative pion beam line at TRIUMF. Nucl Instrum & Meth 155:317-324.
7. Lam GKY, Henkelman RM, Harrison RW (1978) An automated dose mapping system for the TRIUMF biomedical pion beam. Phys Med Biol 23:768-776.
8. Dicello JF (1975) Dosimetry of pion beams. In Smith VP (ed.), Particle Radiation Therapy. Proc. of an International Workshop, Key Biscayne, Fla. Philadelphia: American College of Radiology.
9. Poon M (1977) Optimization studies of the TRIUMF biomedical pion beam. M.Sc. Thesis, University of British Columbia.
10. Burgerjon JJ (1980) Upgrading of TNF target. TRIUMF Design Note TRI-DN-80-10.
11. Doornbos J (1980) Improvement of M8 intensity with REC quadrupole. TRIUMF Design Note TRI-DN-80-18.
12. Blaser VJP (1976) Erste Erfahrungen mit dem biomedizinischen Pionestrahl des SIN-Einfuhrung und Ausblick. Atomkernenergie 27:146-147.
13. Burgerjon JJ (1981) Cost estimate SIN Piotron. Private communication.

Copyright 1982 by Elsevier Science Publishing Co., Inc.
PION AND HEAVY ION RADIOTHERAPY:
Pre-Clinical and Clinical Studies
L. D. Skarsgard

DETERMINATION OF DOSE DISTRIBUTIONS FOR SCANNED PION BEAMS AT TRIUMF

ROBERT HARRISON
Division of Radiation Physics, Cancer Control Agency of British Columbia,
Vancouver, British Columbia

INTRODUCTION

In the fall of 1981, the computer-controllable 3D scanning couch will be in operation at the TRIUMF biomedical beam line. In the early experiments, we propose to use a small spot (FWHM < 3 cm) beam, scanning the vertical and horizontal directions in a rectangular grid, say, a 7 x 7 array at 1.7 cm spacing to cover a 10 cm square, and to use a dynamic range shifter to cover the required range in depth. It is, of course, possible and desirable to irradiate irregular volumes with such a small spot, but for the present we have confined our interest to rectangular treatment volumes until measurements and experience with simple plans allow us to progress to greater complexity. To calculate the dose distribution of a scanned beam in an inhomogeneous medium, we use the CT-scanner and radiotherapy treatment planning system at the Cancer Control Agency, the largest cancer therapy hospital in B.C. The computer programs we have developed use the electron density information contained in the CT data on a pixel-by-pixel basis to calculate pion dose distributions, but the present paper will discuss calculations performed for a uniform medium, principally because these must be verified by measurements using the scanned beam as soon as the couch is operational. Some results for actual patient scans are presented at this workshop by Dr. Kornelsen.[1]

The Physics Department at the Agency has duplicated the computer and display console used by their CT-scanner (a GE 8800 full-body scanner) then added some extra peripherals such as a printer, a digitizer, and a plotter. CT data may be moved from the scanner to the planning system on magnetic tape or floppy disk, and then GE-supplied software may be used for analysis and measurements of the images.

Pion Beam Model

The beam model that we use to simulate a pion beam is a very simple one: a tabulated depth-dose curve with a cylindrically symmetric Gaussian width transverse to the beam axis.[3,4] The depth-dose curve we use (Figure 1) comes from the central axis depth dose of a large parallel beam that was surveyed with a 1 cc Spokas "tissue-equivalent" thimble chamber. This is the closest

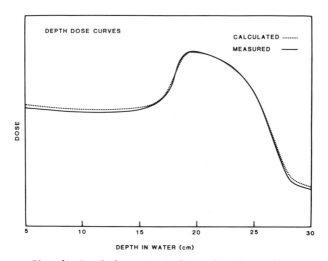

Fig. 1. Depth-dose curve for a broad parallel
pion beam measured with a 1 cc Spokas ionization
chamber, compared to a calculated curve for a
scanned small-spot beam.

situation to the scanned beam available, although measurements with a
parallel-plate chamber that intercepts the whole beam should be done to remove
any effects of beam inhomogeneity. The beam width term in the model arises from
several sources. Firstly, there is the unscattered optic width of the pion
beam,[5] which is as yet not well defined. Preliminary measurements have shown
that this spot size can easily be made too small. That is, at 1.7 cm between
spots, the intensity fluctuation near the surface of the absorber will be too
great if the beam spot is too small. Beam tuning experiments to be carried out
when the couch is ready will decide this component of beam width. Secondly,
there is lateral scatter of the pions in the absorber.[6,7] At each point along
the axis of the spot beam, a summation of the angular scatter from each
overlying volume element is performed. The angular scatter is energy dependent,
so that the lateral scatter from any point depends on both the beam residual
range and the axial distance from the point at which the beam width is being
calculated. Thirdly, there is the beam width contribution of the lateral
scatter in the range shifter. Since the range shifter is of uniform density, an
integral can be evaluated at each depth point in the phantom instead of
performing a sum over volume elements in the range shifter. Figure 2 indicates
the relative importance of these three factors in determining the total beam
width as a function of depth in a typical case.

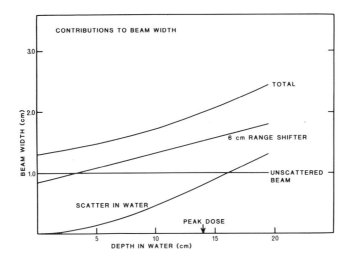

Fig. 2. Contributions to the lateral size of a pencil beam in a typical case.

Results of Calculations

This is a very simple beam model, but it reproduces dose measurements very well, and can easily be tested. A 1 cc Spokas chamber is too large in diameter for good spatial resolution, and the signal from our 0.1 cc chamber is too small for accurate results so we have used x-ray film for beam width measurements, although its insensitivity to LET changes makes it unsuitable for dosimetry. One demonstration the program can provide is to show the effect of an increase in gap width between the range shifter and the absorber, as shown in Figure 3, or the effect of beam shifter thickness for a fixed gap width, in Figure 4. Both of these diagrams include the lateral scatter contributions to beam width but not the unscattered beam width, and curves have been shifted in depth so that the pions stop at the same location on the graphs.

After using this beam model to calculate the dose on a grid due to a scanned beam, the program provides several display aids to examine the distribution. It will plot isodose contours at any dose level as an overlay on the CT image, or will plot depth-dose or transverse dose plots, as in Figure 5. A trackball-controlled cursor also allows the operator to display the calculated dose at any point in the slice.

94

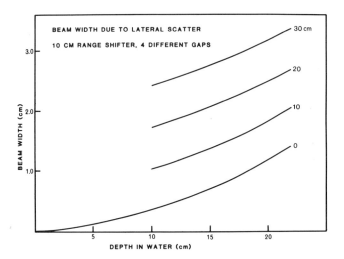

Fig. 3. Changes in pencil beam scattering width
with varying gap width between the range shifter
and the absorber.

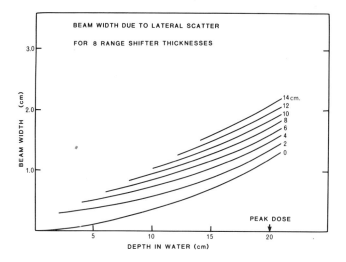

Fig. 4. Changes in pencil beam scattering width
with range shifter thickness.

By calculating the dose distributions for 8 different range shifter thicknesses, we get the series of central-axis depth-dose curves shown in Figure 6. A linear programming algorithm can then select a linear combination of these

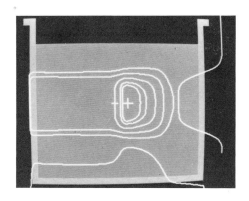

Fig. 5. Video display of isodose curves, depth-dose and cross-sectional dose curves for a scanned beam that has no range modulation.

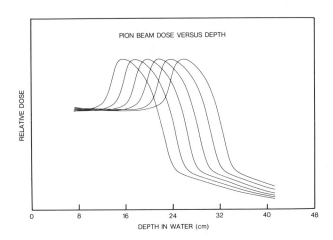

Fig. 6. Calculated central-axis depth-dose curves for a scanned beam at each of the eight range shifter positions.

96

curves that satisfies the prescribed width and shape of the stopping
distribution as required for the specific tumor being treated. A distribution
using the range shifter to provide a uniform dose throughout the pion stopping
region is shown in Figure 7. The isodose and isodensity contours can be plotted

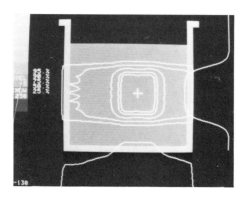

Fig. 7. Video display of dose contours for a
scanned, range-shifted treatment using two
opposed beams.

on a TEKTRONIX pen plotter when the planner is satisfied with the results of his
calculations (Fig. 8), or the video image may be transferred on magnetic tape to
the CT scanner's multi-format camera for photographic hard copy. In actual
treatment, we will normally shape the pion stopping distribution so as to obtain
uniform biological effect throughout the pion stopping region; this will require
reducing the dose at the distal side of the stopping peak.[8,9] In addition, we
will be using parallel-opposed beams wherever possible to correct any residual
differences in biological effectiveness across the peak.

Experimental Verification

The experiments we have been able to perform to date with a scanned beam have
been quite limited, using x-ray film mounted on a 3-D scanner that is normally
used for dose mapping with the thimble ionization chambers. The results of one
experiment are shown in Figure 9. A 7 x 7 array of spots on a 1.7 cm grid was
used to cover a 10 cm square field behind a Cerrobend collimator that was moved
along with the film. The range shifter was not used, and all points along an
edge of the square received 30% extra dose. This is definitely not the most
efficient scheme, because it throws away too many pions in the collimator, but

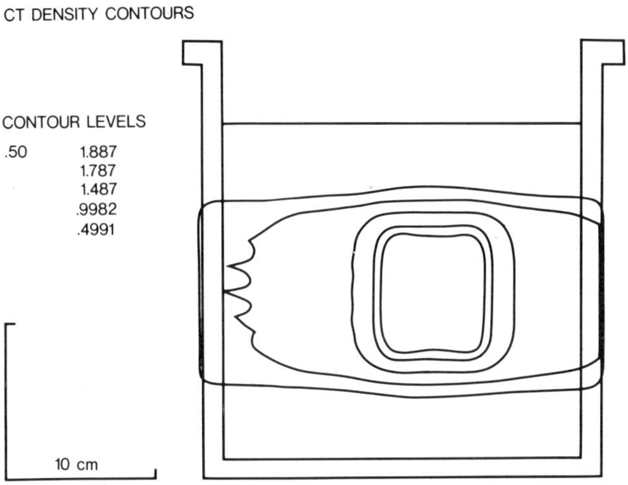

CT DENSITY CONTOURS
CONTOUR LEVELS
.50
1.887
1.787
1.487
.9982
.4991
10 cm

Fig. 8. Pen-plotter output of a treatment plan for parallel-opposed scanned beams.

22 cm
20
18
16
14
12
10
DEPTH
FILM DENSITY
-10
-5
0
5
10
DISTANCE FROM AXIS (cm)

Fig. 9. Measurements of optical density for x-ray films placed perpendicular to a scanned pion beam at several different depths in a water tank.

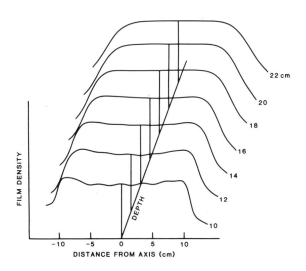

it shows the flatness and uniformity that are achievable using a small spot scanned beam. In this figure, the dose profile at each depth was re-normalized to constant maximum value, so no effect of the pion depth dose is seen.

Future Developments

There are a few unresolved problems with these calculations. For example, the electron contamination of the beam has a smaller lateral scatter than the pion beam so that the calculated beam edges are somewhat too diffuse after the pions have stopped, although the axial dose is still correct. Also, the dose due to star neutrons and other products[10] is spherically rather than cylindrically symmetric for the individual beam spots. The facility for calculating neutron dose exists in the program, but is usually not included because of the difficulty in deciding what fraction of the Spokas-measured dose is due to neutrons and subtracting this from the tabulated depth-dose curve. Since our current goal is to reproduce dosimetry rather than biological effect, we feel this approximation is satisfactory.

Current dose calculations are performed on a single CT slice only, but we plan to extend this to a 3-D calculation shortly. This is mostly a bookkeeping and calculation time problem. At present, a complete dose distribution for a single spot at one range shifter thickness takes 3 seconds, so a full plan in 3 dimensions will still only take about 10 minutes.

REFERENCES

1. Kornelsen RO (1982) Treatment planning considerations on the M8 channel at TRIUMF. In Skarsgard LD (ed.) Pion and Heavy Ion Radiotherapy: Pre-clinical and Clinical Studies. New York: Elsevier/North-Holland (these proceedings).
2. Hamm RN, Wright HA, Turner JE (1975) Effects of Tissue Inhomogeneities on Dose Patterns in Cylinders Irradiated by Negative Pion Beams. Oak Ridge National Laboratory Report ORNL-TM-5088.
3. Lillicrap SC, Wilson P, Boag JW (1975) Dose Distributions in High Energy Electron Beams: Production of Broad Beam Distributions from Narrow Beam Data. Phys Med Biol 20:30 - 38.
4. Li GC, Boyd D, Schwettman HA (1974) Pion Dose Calculations Suitable for Treatment Planning. Phys Med Biol 19:436 - 447.
5. Henkelman RM, Lam GKY, Harrison RW, Poon M, Shortt KR (1978) Tuning of the Biomedical Negative Pion Beam Line at TRIUMF. Nucl Instr Meth 155:317 - 324.
6. Amols HI, Buche G, Kluge W, Matthay H, Moline A, Munchmeyer D (1981) Multiple Scattering Distributions for Therapeutic Pion Beams. Phys Med Biol 26:277 - 289.
7. Watts LJ (1977) A Determination of Multiple Scattering for a Negative Pion Beam. MSc thesis, University of British Columbia.
8. Lam GKY, Henkelman RM, Harrison RW, Skarsgard LD, Palcic B (1979) Uniform Depth Dose Distribution for Biological Irradiation using Negative Pions. Phys Med Biol 24:1243 - 1249.

9. Skarsgard LD, Palcic B, Lam GKY (1982) RBE mapping in pion beams using the gel technique. In Skarsgard LD (ed.) Pion and Heavy Ion Radiotherapy: Pre-clinical and Clinical Studies. New York: Elsevier/North-Holland (these proceedings).
10. Schillaci ME, Roeder DL (1973) Dose Distributions Due to Neutrons and Photons Resulting from Negative Pion Capture in Tissue. Phys Med Biol 6:821 - 829.

TREATMENT PLANNING CONSIDERATIONS ON THE M8 CHANNEL AT TRIUMF

R.O. KORNELSEN
Cancer Control Agency of British Columbia, 2656 Heather Street, Vancouver, B.C.
V5Z 3J3, Canada

The use of CT data is central to treatment planning with charged particle beams in general and negative pions in particular. The relationship between the CT-number of a volume element and its contribution to the path length of a pion may be considered in two parts:

(a) Relationship between CT-number and electron density

(b) Relationship between electron density and pion stopping power.

Experiments were done to relate CT-numbers from our whole-body CT-scanner (General Electric 8800) to electron densities for a selected number of substances in phantoms of 20, 30 and 40 cm diameter. The results of these experiments are shown in fig. 1. The dashed line joining (-1000, 0) and (0,1) would be expected for substances whose atomic number is near that of water. This includes muscle, lung and most other body tissues, excepting fat and bone.

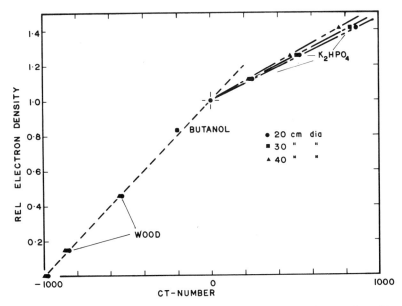

Fig. 1. Electron densities relative to water as a function of CT-number (General Electric 8800).

Since wood has an effective atomic number near that of water (see Table 1), samples of balsa and fir were chosen to simulate lung. Because of photoelectric effect at the CT-scanner energies ($\cong$ 60 keV effective), high-Z materials will result in data points lying to the right of the ideal line and low-Z materials to the left. Butyl alcohol was chosen to simulate body fat (Table 1) and as expected gives a value to the left of the ideal line. Where the

TABLE 1

EFFECTIVE ATOMIC NUMBERS FOR PHOTOELECTRIC ABSORPTION

MATERIAL	Z_{eff}
MUSCLE	7.48
FAT	5.85
WATER	7.43
WOOD ($H_{10} C_6 O_5$)	6.90
BUTANOL ($H_{10} C_4 O$)	6.04

CT-numbers are substantially greater than zero, it is safe to assume that this is due to bone mineral within the volume element. White[1] has suggested $K_2 H PO_4$ solutions of varying concentrations as suitable substitutes for soft and hard bone. As expected, the resultant data points for these solutions lie well to the right of the ideal line. It is of interest that the points are shifted toward the ideal line as the phantom size is increased. This reflects an increase in effective beam energy with filtration and an associated reduction in the photoelectric contribution.

Mass stopping powers for pions of 5, 20 and 80 MeV were evaluated for water, muscle, fat and bone using an expression suggested by Bichsel.[2] The results are shown in figure 2. Proportionality of stopping power to electron density as indicated by the dashed line is expected for muscle. The effect of atomic number is demonstrated by fat and bone.

In the present version of our computer program the conversion of CT-numbers (CTN) to pion stopping powers makes use of the straight line from figure 2, the straight line of unit slope from figure 1 for CTN < 0, and a straight line whose slope depends on phantom size for CTN > 0. This procedure may give rise to an overestimate of pion ranges in fat of up to 5%. However, assuming large regions of fat could be distinguished as such on a CT-scan, it would be easy to take account of this systematic error.

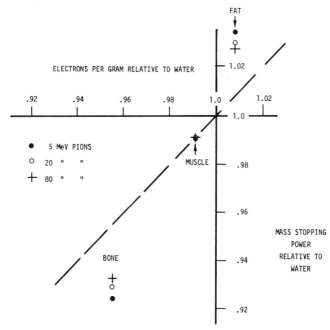

Fig. 2. Pion mass stopping power relative to water versus electron density relative to water.

Figures 3(a) and 3(b) show a scout view and a CT-scan taken at the level of the mid-abdomen in a "lean" patient. Figure 3(c) is a histogram of electron densities derived from the CT-numbers in 3(b). The peak at .4 is due to the flat plywood board under the patient and that near 0 due to pixels containing air just outside the surface. The major constituent is "muscle-like" with small contributions due to fat and bone. Treatment planning in this plane on the assumption of water equivalence would probably not introduce any significant error. Figures 4(a), (b) and (c) show similar data for a section through the pelvis of a "fat" patient. The relatively few pixels with electron density greater than 1 are perhaps surprising. The large peak at .85 suggests that the patient is more nearly fat-equivalent than water-equivalent. In figures 5(a), (b) and (c) taken from a section through the chest the total amount of bone is again small. The peak for lung occurs at about 0.2, a number lower than that usually quoted in the literature. These analyses suggest that bone is less

104

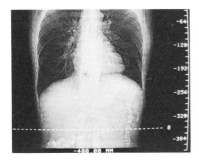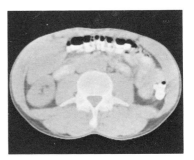

Fig. 3a and 3b. Scout view and CT-scan at the level of the mid-abdomen of a "lean" patient.

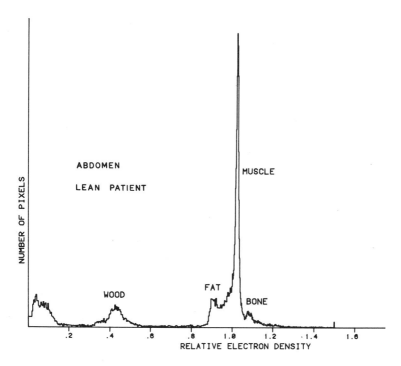

Fig. 3c. Histogram of electron densities derived from CT-scan data.

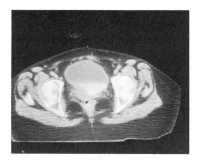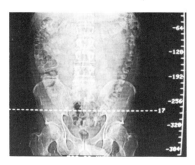

Fig. 4a and 4b. Scout view and CT-scan at the level of the pelvis in a "fat" patient.

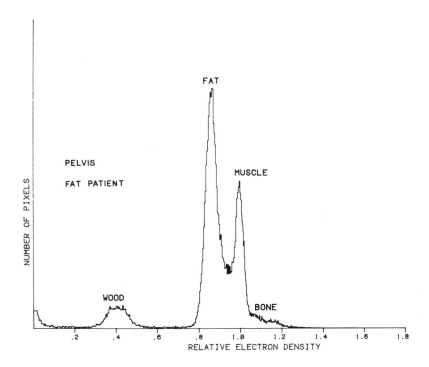

Fig. 4c. Histogram of electron densities.

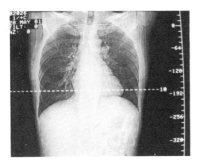 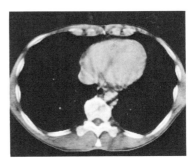

Fig. 5a and 5b. Scout view and CT-scan through the chest.

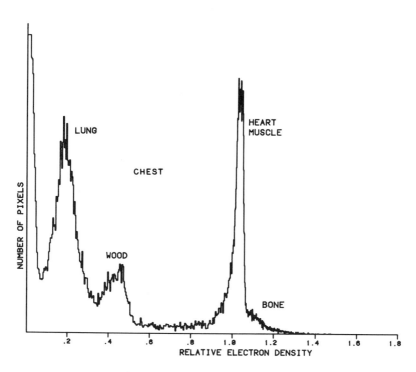

Fig. 5c. Histogram of electron densities.

important than anticipated and fat more important.

The technique for obtaining useful dose-distributions in a water phantom with a scanned spot beam of pions has been described by Bob Harrison in the previous paper.[3] The use of the spot scan technique has a number of advantages in the clinical application, including the following:

(1)   Because the elementary beams are parallel it is possible to maintain a one-to-one correspondence between beam axes and lines on CT-scan slices.

(2)   The lateral flatness at depth can be adjusted by varying the spacing and/or the weighting of the elementary beams.

(3)   The depth dose profile for each spot can be adjusted separately giving flexibility to the shape of the high-dose region.

(4)   The effect of small sharp inhomogeneities is smoothed out by the overlapping beams (see figure 6).

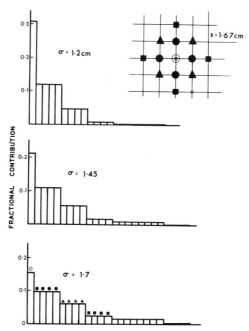

Fig. 6. Fractional dose contributions to a point on an elementary pion beam due to the beam itself and to neighbouring beams. (S is the spacing between beams in the rectangular array, and σ the root-mean-square spread of the pion beam due to multiple scattering, assumed to be Gaussian in shape).

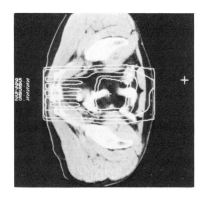

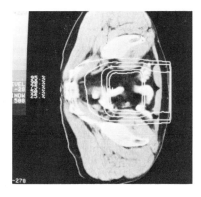

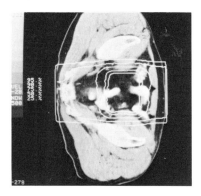

The preparation of a treatment plan for a particular site consists of the following:

(1) A plan of elementary beam positions, weighting factors and range shifting information is produced to give a good distribution in a water phantom.

(2) CT-data are obtained with the patient in the treatment position and with the CT-slices chosen to coincide with the planes containing the elementary beam axes. The effective path length along each beam axis can then be determined using the relationships of figures 1 and 2.

(3) By the use of bolus and/or the range shifter each depth profile is adjusted to cover the appropriate depth interval.

(4) The lateral spread of the elementary beam is assumed to be a single function of effective depth, independent of the distribution of density along the path except for the range shifter and the air gap between it and the patient.

(5) There is no intention, at present, to take account of the variation of charged particle production with tissue composition.

Fig. 7a. Dose distribution to a bladder from 49 elementary posterior beams. Fig. 7b. Distribution due to anterior array. Fig. 7c. Combined distribution.

Figure 7(a) shows the dose distribution to a bladder due to a 10 x 10 cm field made up of 49 elementary beams directed from the posterior. The structure of the beam pattern is noticeable in the entrance region. The distribution due to the anterior field arrangement and the combined distribution due to both posterior and anterior fields are shown in figures 7(b) and (c).

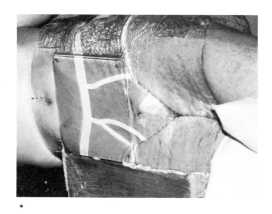

Fig. 8. Patient in vacuum-formed plastic immobilization shell.

The fixed horizontal pion beam puts a severe constraint on patient positioning. Anterior or posterior fields will require that the patient lie on his side. A vacuum-formed plastic shell will be manufactured for each patient and will be used for immobilization during both CT-scanning and treatment (see figure 8). The shell will be physically indexed to the scanning couch, as will other accessories such as bolus and lead-alloy diaphragms.

The total dose to a point in the high-dose region will in general contain a fairly large number of small contributions. This will exaggerate the effect of any uncertainty in the shape of the profile of the elementary beam especially in the low-level "tail" portion. On the other hand, this same feature will serve to "smear out" the perturbations produced by small inhomogeneities in the beam path. It will be necessary to verify the total dose within the scanned beam by direct measurement in a water phantom with a suitable TE chamber.

REFERENCES

1. White DR (1978) Tissue substitutes in experimental radiation physics. Med Phys 5:467.

2. Bichsel H (1968) Radiation Dosimetry, Vol. I, Academic Press, 182.
3. Harrison RW (1982) Determination of dose distributions for scanned pion beams at TRIUMF. In Skarsgard LD (ed.) Pion and Heavy Ion Radiotherapy: Pre-clinical and Clinical Studies. New York: Elsevier/North-Holland (these proceedings).

STANFORD PRECLINICAL MULTIPORT PION RADIOTHERAPY PROGRAM: RELEVANT EXPERIENCE

P. FESSENDEN[1], M. A. BAGSHAW[1], W. HOFFMANN[2], G.C. LI[3], G. LUXTON[4], R. TABER[5],
C. H. C. YUEN[6], H. D. ZEMAN[6]

[1]Dept. of Radiology, Sanford University School of Medicine, Stanford, California 94305, USA

[2]Dept. of Physics, University of Wuppertal, 5600 Wuppertal, 1, West Germany

[3]Dept. of Radiology, University of California, San Francisco, California 94142,'
USA

[4]Dept. of Radiology, University of Southern California, Los Angeles, California 90033, USA

[5]Dept. of Physics, Stanford University, Stanford, California 94305, USA

[6]Varian Associates, 611 Hansen Way, Palo Alto, California 94303, USA

Development of the Stanford Medical Pion Generator (SMPG), constructed to
serve as a prototype multiport pion radiotherapy facility, was sufficiently
complete by 1975[1] to allow preclinical studies in dosimetry[2], microdosimetry[3] ,
and radiobiology[4], to begin. The novel feature, 60 simultaneously converging
pion beams, was made possible by the use of two large 60-segment toroidal
superconducting magnets[5], and the performance of these magnets exceeded their
modest specifications. Since negative pi mesons are produced as secondaries
with nearly equal probabilities over a broad range of angles when energetic
particles are incident on a production target, the large annular toroidal
magnets are well suited to collect efficiently and focus many pion beams simultaneously.

Figure 1 shows the SMPG schematically, indicating the capability of the
system to transport up to 60 beams to the patient tank when pions are produced
by 600 MeV electrons directed on to the target. Each of the beams has geometric convergence from the patient tank window to the SMPG axis. Multiple
scattering of the pions works against this convergence, however, and results
in a peak to plateau ratio of only 2.5:1 for a full momentum-spread (±4.4%)
beam stopping near the center of a 26.5 cm diameter cylindrical water tank.
The multiple scattering in the patient tank entrance window (0.4 mm stainless
steel) coupled with the 50 cm distance from the window to the SMPG axis is a
major contributing factor. This could be reduced significantly by using a
thinner window. A smaller patient tank would also help, but this is impracti-
cal for a clinical system. When all, or many, of the 60 beams are used to
deliver dose to a region near the axis, the dramatic effect of beams entering

112

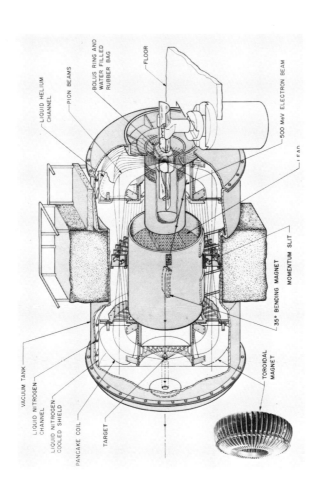

Fig. 1. Schematic of SMPG. (Courtesy of Radiology[1])

from many radial directions is seen in the dose distribution: it is well localized, even with the full momentum spread. For example, Gaussian-type distributions with full width half maxima (FWHM) of 3.3, 3.3 and 5.5 cm in the
X, Y and Z axes, respectively, result for a 5.0 cm long by 1.0 cm diameter
production target and a 22 cm diameter water phantom[2]. The X and Y axes are
perpendicular to the SMPG axis, while Z is parallel to it.

The dose localization advantage gained from the effect of multiple converging beams can cause problems when the pions have less range, since this results
in the peak doses being deposited in regions away from the axis. Under this
condition of a "ring" distribution, there can be severe asymmetries of dose
from one side to the other if the cylindrical water phantom is not aligned
with its axis along that of the SMPG. The requirement to prevent this amounts
to sub-millimeter precision in alignment[2], but is somewhat less severe for
large diameter rings (over 10 cm). This has important implications for actual
patient treatment using the ring scan method, but the stringent requirement
must be strictly met only for alignment of the outside dimension of an overall
cylinderized patient bolus. The alignment of the patient within the bolus is
not as critical, as long as no extensive air gaps between patient and (flexible)
bolus occur. In testing system alignment, the high sensitivity of ring distributions to misalignment (of phantom or superconducting toroids) is a valuable diagnostic tool.

There are compromises in design and utilization of such a system, one of
which is the trade off between pion yield (essentially dose rate) and dose
distribution fall off[2] as a function of momentum acceptance $\Delta p/p$. As the
momentum defining slits are closed down from full ($\pm 4.4\%$) to very narrow
($\pm\frac{1}{2}\%$), the FWHM of a well focused distribution on the axis decreases about
0.8 cm, but the decrease in peak dose rate is nearly a factor of 6. In most
cases this sacrifice in yield would not be worthwhile. However, since the
peaks in ring distributions also sharpen as the momentum slits are closed, it
may be best to use fully open slits except for depositing dose near the edges
of the distribution, where nearly closed slits would be advisable in order to
increase the rate of dose fall-off. This has yet to be explored under a variety of clinically relevant situations, but must be looked at carefully.

There are basically two methods whereby the dose distribution can be enlarged to encompass large (and irregular) volumes: the spot scan and ring
scan methods. (These are discussed and illustrated extensively in another
paper of this conference discussing treatment planning with the PIOTRON multiport pion facility in Villigen, Switzerland[6].) The spot scan spreads the dose

throughout a target volume by raster scanning the patient within a water bolus of rigidly fixed outer dimension. The ring scan method leaves the patient and bolus fixed, but tailors the dose to the target volume by sweeping the pion stopping region radially outward via lowering the current in the superconducting toroid magnets. For an off-center and/or irregular target volume, or for the sake of sparing normal tissues, some of the 60 beams may be closed for all or part of the time. As a simple exercise in the ring scan technique, the SMPG was used to irradiate a hypothetical cylindrical tumor volume in a water phantom[2]. This was done in four discrete steps performing irradiations with rings of diameters equal to 0 (i.e., the focused distribution of pions stopping near the axis), 3.8, 5.5 and 7.5 cm. Since the peak dose rate is reduced for larger diameter rings, the irradiation time (or weighting) is increased for larger rings, being over six times as long for the 7.5 cm diameter ring as for the focus. This procedure produces a uniform (±5%) dose in a cylinder of over 7 cm diameter (radial, or X and Y, direction) by 2 cm high (Z, or SMPG axis, direction). Translating the phantom in the Z direction and repeating the irradiations would increase the Z axis thickness of this cylindrical high dose region.

Of much importance and interest is the question of the radiation quality for different configurations of the pion beams. Because of the rapid geometric convergence associated with multiple beams radially incident from many directions, the contribution to the target volume dose from plateau pions is minimized. (This rapid convergence remains in the SMPG or PIOTRON systems even when, for example, only 10 or 15 beams covering a 60° or 90° arc, are used.) This is a second major advantage, in addition to dose localization, because the low-LET plateau contribution dilutes the beam quality. This feature is particularly apparent for the focused beam configuration, but also contributes to relatively high quality for spread dose distributions[4]. For example, in terms of $\bar{y}_D$, the dose-averaged lineal energy (the microdosimetric analog of LET), the average quality is 58 keV/micron at and near the peak of the focused distribution, and decreases to 49 keV/micron with a variation of ±13% for the simple ring scan spread distribution discussed above.

The advantage with respect to quality for the SMPG type of multi-beam geometry has been corroborated via cellular radiobiology experiments. The studies for the focused configuration give an RBE of about 2.8 (HA-1 Chinese Hamster cells, 85 kV X-ray reference radiation) at 50% survival, and indicate an OER significantly reduced from that using 85 kV. For the spread distribution, the radiobiology measurements made during the limited experimental program indicate RBE's significantly greater than 1.0 (about 2.0, but with a statistical uncertainty of ±30% due to only sparse data being accumulated.) Certainly this is an area in which more experiments are warranted with the PIOTRON multi-beam facility in Villigen, Switzerland.

The work with the SMPG, as well as some cellular radiobiology studies performed by other groups correlated with microdosimetric measurements made by the Stanford group[7] using heavy ion beams at the Lawrence Berkeley Laboratory Biomedical Facility, indicate a generally increasing RBE_{50} with quality $(\bar{y}_D)$. This is shown in Figure 2, presented here to emphasize the importance of

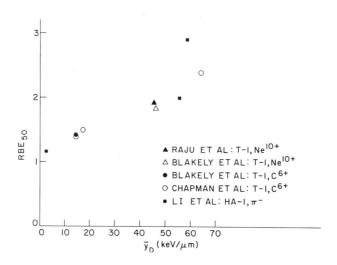

Fig. 2. RBE_{50} for mammalian cell survival vs. $\bar{y}_D$. (Courtesy of Radiation Research[3]. See Reference 10 for sources of data.)

radiation quality considerations. A correlation, or a model, employing only RBE_{50} for mammalian cells and $\bar{y}_D$ is much too simplistic, and of very limited usefulness. What is needed are consistent sets of radiobiology experiments, clinical observations, and microdosimetric measurements all obtained under identical pion (and other) beam configurations, and a thorough analysis including all these data. This must be a long term commitment, since most of the data do not even exist yet, and, at least with respect to clinical data, will not for years to come. However, the effort expended will aid in understanding clinical results, and hopefully eventually assist in the prediction of clinical effectiveness.

The SMPG project was successful in demonstrating the feasibility of the facility to provide simultaneous multi-beam, or multi-port, pion therapy. In addition to the obvious advantage[3] of not requiring more than one patient set up position with the attendant problems of anatomy shift (which would add to those already present from breathing, tumor shrinkage, etc.), the SMPG geometry provides dose localization and radiation quality advantages.

The PIOTRON developed by the Switzerland group, and discussed extensively in six separate contributions to this conference, represents a tremendous advance in bringing sophisticated pion therapy to the clinic. However, as patient treatments progress with this facility, we must continually think ahead and explore means of improving techniques. For example, with both proton[9,10,11] and electron[12,13] produced pion beams, yield is still an important consideration, and ideas to increase yield should be considered. The idea of sweeping the primary beam out of the way when it is no longer useful is probably applicable to both types of pion production, and would allow higher pion yields by dumping the beam away from the patient and toroid regions. Radiation background and superconducting toroid heating would then be less restrictive of higher primary beam currents. It also may result in less internal shielding thereby improving pion yield by virtue of a shorter channel and less loss of pions by in-flight decay. Additionally, extending the technology to achieve even larger acceptance toroidal pion channels, including larger angular and/or momentum acceptance, should be considered and the trade offs in spatial resolution studied. Along with this, research into different pion production target materials, including alloys, may result in higher yields and/or less electron contamination. This work is being done at the facility in Switzerland[14] and should be encouraged.

REFERENCES

1 Pistenma, D.A., Fessenden, P., Boyd, D.P., Luxton, G., Taber, R., Bagshaw, M.A. (1977) Initial Performance of the Stanford Medical Pion Generator.

2 Fessenden, P., Zeman, H.D., Luxton, G., Yuen, C.H.C. (1982) Dosimetry for the Stanford Medical Pion Generator. Int. J. Radiat. Oncol. Biol. Phys. Accepted for publication.

3 Luxton, G., Fessenden, P., Zeman, H.D. (1981) Microdosimetry of Multiport Irradiation with the Stanford Medical Pion Generator. Radiat. Research 85:238-256.

4 Li, G.C., Fessenden, P., Hahn, G.M., Fisher, G., Luxton, G., Bagshaw, M. A. Mammalian Cell Survival Studies Characterizing Multiport Negative Pi-Meson Irradiation with the Stanford Medical Pion Generator. To be published.

5 Boyd, D., Schwettman, H.A., Simpson, J. (1973) A Large Acceptance Pion Channel for Cancer Therapy. Nucl. Instr. Methods 111:315-331.

6 Blattmann, H. (1982) Treatment Planning for Dynamic Therapy at SIN. In Skarsgard LD (ed.) Pion and Heavy Ion Radiotherapy: Pre-clinical and Clinical Studies. New York: Elsevier/North-Holland (these proceedings).

7 Luxton, G., Fessenden, P., Hoffmann, W. (1979) Microdosimetric Measurements of Pretherapeutic Heavy Ion Beams. Radiat. Research 79:256-272.

8 Tsujii, H., Bagshaw, M.A., Smith, A.R., von Essen, C.F., Mettler, F.A., Kligerman, M.M. (1980) Localization of Structures for Pion Radiotherapy by Computerized Tomography and Orthodiagraphic Projection. Int. J. Radiat. Oncol. Biol. Phys. 6:319-325.

9 Goodman, G. (1982) The Pion Therapy Program at TRIUMF. In Skarsgard LD (ed.) Pion and Heavy Ion Radiotherapy: Pre-clinical and Clinical Studies. New York: Elsevier/North-Holland (these proceedings).

10 Knapp, E. (1982) PIGMI: A Hospital-Based Proton Source for Pion Production: In Skarsgard LD (ed.) Pion and Heavy Ion Radiotherapy: Pre-clinical and Clinical Studies. New York: Elsevier/North-Holland (these proceedings).

11 Vécsey, G. (1982) The Piotron. In Skarsgard LD (ed.) Pion and Heavy Ion Radiotherapy: Pre-clinical and Clinical Studies. New York: Elsevier/North-Holland (these proceedings).

12 Loew, G.D., Brown, K.C., Miller, R.H., Walz, D.R., Pistenma, D.A. (1977) Electron Linac Design for Pion Radiotherapy. IEEE Transactions on Nuclear Science 24(3):1006-1008.

13 Tsukada, K., Sato, K., Hayakawa, K., Uetomi, I., Minowa, Y. (1980) Electron Linear Accelerator for the Pion Therapy. U.S.-Japan Cooperative Cancer Research Seminar, Honolulu, Hawaii. Unpulished

14 Crawford, J. (1981) Private Communication.

TREATMENT PLANNING FOR DYNAMIC THERAPY AT SIN

H. BLATTMANN, E. PEDRONI, J. CRAWFORD, M. SALZMANN
Swiss Institute for Nuclear Research, 5234 Villigen, Switzerland

INTRODUCTION

The geometry of the PIOTRON combines the advantages of the physical depth dose distribution, the biological advantages of the stop region with the converging beam geometry present in multiport or rotational external beam radiation therapy. Two modes are available for the 60 beam geometry of the PIOTRON to shape the treatment volume in three dimensions: the ring scan mode and the spot scan mode. Eccentric locations of the tumor inside the body or radiosensitive normal tissue structures may make it preferable to use less than 60 beams, which is possible for both scan modes.

Ring scan mode. For this treatment mode a center of the irradiation is chosen; for the majority of the cases this will be inside the target volume (Fig. 1). Around this center the contour of the patient is made up to a cylinder with material of density one to equalize the material to be traversed by each of the beams to reach the center. The target volume itself is considered to be of homogeneous density, but differences in stopping power on the flight path of the pions are compensated for in the bolus. To compensate

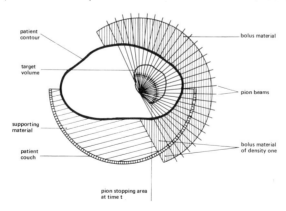

Fig. 1. Ring scan mode, description in the text.

120

for air or fat, material of a stopping power higher than that of water is used; material of lower density is used to compensate for bone. By this method the range for the central axis of each pion beam can be made equal. For the irradiation the patient is aligned in the PIOTRON with the center of the treatment on the axis of the PIOTRON. At the beginning of the irradiation the momentum is chosen so that the pions stop at the center. In the course of the treatment the momentum and therefore the range is reduced, the stopping pions thus forming a ring shaped dose distribution. A scanning function can be found to yield a homogeneous physical or biological dose distribution over the target volume. On the PIOTRON axis the electrons of all the beams used are overlapping, contributing extensively to the total dose. In addition, the overlapping of the pion beams close to the center is also more pronounced than for larger radii, the change of momentum therefore needs to be faster close to the center than further out. Those beams which would deposit their energy outside the treatment volume are stopped by closing the slits. In the third dimension the treatment is done slice by slice by moving

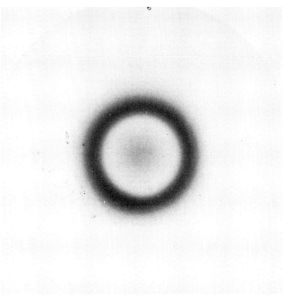

Fig. 2. Radiograph of a ring of 10.5 cm diameter of stopping pions.

the patient on the transporter in the z-direction. As an illustration of the ring scan mode, rings have been radiographed (Fig. 2)
in a cylinder of lucite.[1] In the center of the picture the overlapping of the electron dose of 60 beams produces a spot, the
ring of 10.5 diameter is formed by the stopping region of the
pions. As the target material was beryllium the electron spot is
not very pronounced.

   Spot scan mode. The second method for three-dimensional shaping
is the spot scan mode in water (Fig. 3). For this method a water
cylinder has to be imagined with its axis on the axis of the PIO-
TRON. The momentum is chosen so that all pions stop on the axis and
form a dose spot. Into this cylinder the patient is introduced with
the tumor on the axis of the PIOTRON. To enlarge the irradiation
volume and to adapt the treatment volume to the target volume the
patient is scanned in three dimensions inside the water bolus leav-
ing the outer contour of the bolus fixed. Inhomogeneities are also
compensated for in a solid bolus of density one, attached to the
surface of the patient. Depending on the location of the target
volume this scan mode can also be done with less than 60 beams to
reduce the dose delivered to normal tissue structures in cases of

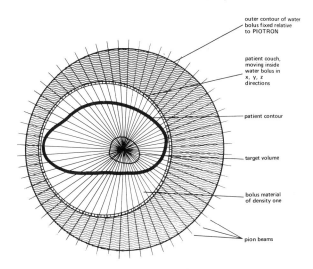

Fig. 3. Spot scan mode, description in the text.

eccentric tumor volumes. Due to the limited freedom for scanning
inside the water bolus for these cases a half moon of polyethylene
is mounted on the water bolus and the water bolus positioned so
that the center of the outer contour of the half moon is on the
axis of the PIOTRON. The water bolus itself is a rubber tube with
a lucite cylinder on the outside and on the inside to accept the
cylindrical patient couch.

Treatment planning procedure. Before the treatment planning[2,3]
for the pion treatment can be done, a series of CT scans of the
region of interest has to be taken at the hospital approximately
40 min. from SIN, with the patient already in the couch used for
irradiation in the PIOTRON. In addition to the scans two scout
views are taken to allow later to confirm positioning before each
treatment. CT scans and scout views are written on magnetic tape
and are transferred to the computer at SIN. On the treatment planning computer the CT numbers are converted into stopping power for
pions. The CT scans are displayed on a colour terminal and the
physician enters the contours of the target volume by means of a
track ball for each CT slice. If the scan mode and the parameters
as number of beams to be used, center of the treatment volume, diameter of the bolus, etc. are chosen, the treatment planning program
calculates the dose distribution assuming homogeneous density. The
compensation necessary in each beam to correct for density inhomogeneities on the flight path are also calculated and can be
printed on a grey tone plotter to scale. When the calculations are
done, the dose distributions are displayed superimposed on the CT
picture in one colour together with the target volume contour in
another colour, the spot positions are also indicated. In the
example illustrated (Fig. 4) a volume has been chosen which in some
slices is separated into two individual volumes. As a help to visualize the three-dimensional target volume the program has an option
to draw an arbitrary projection of the series of target volume
contours and/or isodose contours. Sagital cuts are also available
with the restriction that the resolution in the z-direction is
15 mm corresponding to the spacing of the slices of the CT scans.
Treatment planning can be repeated for other configurations of

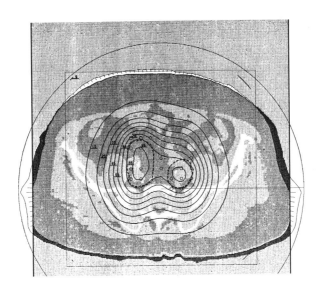

Fig. 4. CT slice with isodose lines and target contours.

beams or for the other scan mode to chose the optimal treatment.
Once the decision on the treatment plan has been taken, a magnetic
tape is produced with the code on it to perform the irradiation by
microprocessors in the PIOTRON. An important part in pion radiotherapy is the exact repositioning of the patient for each treatment in accordance with the position of the patient for the CT
scanning. Having no CT scanner available at SIN a positioner[4] has
been constructed, taking X-ray pictures with a moving source to
achieve the same projection as the scout view taken with the CT
scanner at the hospital. The patient has to be positioned until
both pictures agree well enough.

Dose calculations. The dose calculations are based on measurements of single beams in three dimensions in water. The dose distribution is parameterized by gaussians and dose distributions of
spots composed by overlapping the appropriate number of beams.

Problems for the parameterization of the single beam arise for the tails of the profiles and from the optical properties of the single beam. In the bending plane the stop distribution of the pions is sloped (Fig. 5) which is called the long target effect. There still

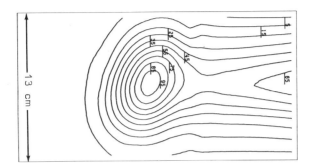

Fig. 5. Dose distribution of a single beam entering from the right the vertical axis is the z-axis, pointing upwards towards the pion production target.

remain unsolved problems in the overlapping of single beams to calculate the dose distribution for spots of various numbers of beams even if the individual variation of the transmission of single channels is taken into account (Fig. 6). The measured dose on the PIO-TRON axis for spots of multiple beams is consistently lower than the calculated dose by about 3 %. If this deviation is taken into account calculations and measurements for beams of 15, 30 and 60 beams agree with measurements to ± 4 % of the peak dose (Fig. 7).

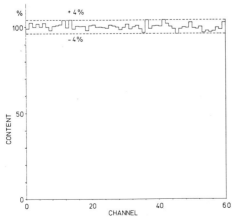

Fig. 6. Variation of transmission of the 60 channels, monitor chamber reading.

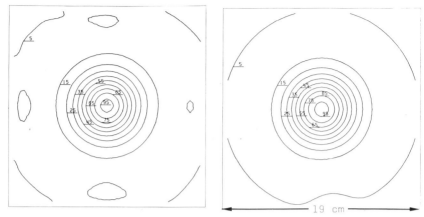

Fig. 7. Comparison between measured (left) and calculated (right) dose distribution for a spot of 59 beams in the 60 cm diameter water cylinder.

Dose calculation for spot scan mode. The dose distribution is stored in a matrix where each element corresponds to the dose on a grid point. The step size of the grid equals the spacing of the spots in the spot scan. The calculation of the dose for a scan is done by changing indices of the matrix elements. For each spot the program calculates the time to remain to yield a homogeneous dose distribution inside the target contour and a minimal dose outside. The irradiation could be done by delivering the calculated dose at these points and closing the slits during the transfer of the patient from spot to spot. This kind of irradiation would be simpler for the calculation but would be time-consuming because of the dead time when the slits are closed, and furthermore, it would be hard on the slits which are not constructed to withstand the number of openings and closings necessary. Therefore, the slits are kept open for the transfer and the dose is calculated for a segment connecting two adjacent spots. If the speed of the transporter is varied in order to deliver the correct dose for each segment of the trajectory a plane of a treatment plan may look as illustrated in Fig. 8. The optimization is done so that the speed never exceeds a prefixed maximum value. On this figure it is also obvious that

126

spots outside the target volume are necessary to achieve a homogeneous dose distribution within the target volume.

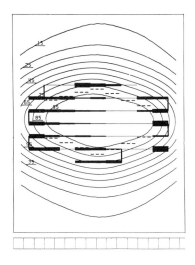

Fig. 8. Example of a plane of a treatment plan with path of the transporter. The width of the track is proportional to the dose delivered on the segment.
Scale divisions below the figure are cm.

Dose calculation for ring scan mode. Due to limited beam time available the necessary measurements as input into the therapy planning program for ring scan mode have not been made yet. Even if the ring scan is done at the beginning with a fixed radius of the bolus, single beams of various momenta have to be parameterized.

Compensation of inhomogeneities. It has been shown by E.Pedroni[2] that compensation of inhomogeneities on the flight path of the pions is more important for ring scan mode, as an error in range results in larger deviations from the planned dose. For spot scan mode there is even the possibility that measurements may show that small inhomogeneities, affecting only part of the beam either need no compensation at all or can be avoided by switching those beams off. An exact compensation cannot be done for the geometry of the PIOTRON. Two sources of error in compensation are the large phase space of the single beam in the z-direction and the resolution achievable in z-direction with the CT scanner in practice. The first problem (Fig. 9) arises from the fact that in each slice of 15 mm thickness the compensation can only be done for this slice, but the pions stopping in this slice are in part traversing ad-

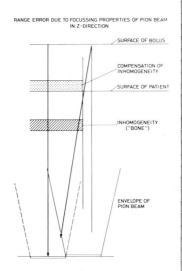

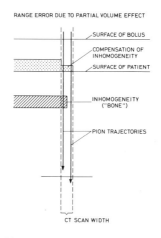

Fig. 9. Errors in range due to focussing of the beam in z-direction.

Fig. 10. Partial volume effect for CT scanning.

jacent slices. The second problem in compensation is the partial volume effect (Fig. 10) in CT scanning. The value measured in a fraction of the 15 mm slice is considered as representative for the whole slice thickness, which is wrong if the inhomogeneity covers only part of the thickness of the slice.

DISCUSSION AND CONCLUSION

It is planned to use both scan modes in clinical applications as both of them have their advantages and their disadvantages. The ring scan mode needs a shorter range resulting in less multiple scattering and less range straggling. As a result the dose-fall-off at the limits of the irradiated volume can be made sharper. There is more high LET contribution in the treatment volume, but it is less uniformly distributed than for the spot scan. Electron contamination is more important, which excludes heavy target materials which would be of interest to increase the dose rate. Of importance at this stage of the project is the larger number of measurements necessary for the input into the therapy planning program

128

and the calibration of the monitor chambers.

For the spot scan mode the maximum range attainable with the PIOTRON is limiting the freedom for scanning in the xy-plane to a circle of 18 cm diameter. In view of the necessity to place spots outside the target volume this is rather modest. Increasing the range would somewhat increase the spot size, making it probably necessary to have a second bolus with smaller outer diameter where a smaller spot size would be of advantage as for head and neck treatments.

The most important problem in connection with the PIOTRON is the limited dose rate. The flux of pions is only low by about 20 % compared to the design goal. The dose rate for a litre volume defined by the 85 % isodose line for the treatment with 60 beams is only about 20 rad/min. This value is further reduced if only 30 beams or less are used, or if shaping is necessary for the ring scan mode. This can only be made up partly by using heavier target materials for the spot scan mode where the electron contamination is less important because of higher momentum and more uniform distribution over the treatment volume.

It can be considered a good step forward, that first dynamic treatments could be performed for homogeneous density and that the measured dose distribution deviates less than 6 % from the calculated dose.

REFERENCES

1 Blattmann H, Salzmann M, Cordt-Riehle I, Crawford J, Hoffmann W, Pedroni E, Shortt K, Tremp J (1980) Integrating Dosimetry Systems for Dose Mapping of Pion Beams. IAEA Proceedings of the International Symposium on Biomedical Dosimetry: Physical Aspects, Instrumentation, Calibration: IAEA-SM-249/35 15 p.
2 Pedroni E (1979) Development of the therapy planning programs for the 60 beam SIN pion applicator. Radiat.Environ Biophys.16: 211-218
3 Pedroni E (1979) BERNO4-Pion Irradiation of a Pancras Tumor. An Example of Therapy Planning for the SIN Pion Applicator. SIN Internal Report TM-65-02: 1 - 94
4 Perret C (1978) Einrichtungen für die Behandlung. SIN Jahresbericht E12-E13

129

THE PION DOSIMETRY PROGRAM AT SIN

M. SALZMANN[1], H. BLATTMANN[1], J. CRAWFORD[1], I. CORDT[2], E. PEDRONI[1], P.G. SEILER[3], K. SCHAEPPI[2]
[1]Swiss Institute for Nuclear Research (SIN), 5234 Villigen, Switzerland
[2]Radiobiological Institute of the University of Zürich, P.O. Box, 8029 Zürich, Switzerland
[3]Laboratory for High-Energy Physics, Swiss Federal Institute of Technology, Zürich (ETHZ), 5234 Villigen, Switzerland

INTRODUCTION

There are several features in pion therapy and especially in therapy with the PIOTRON at SIN, which force us to have a rather complex and sophisticated dosimetric program. The main complications are due to
- the specific dose distribution of a pion beam,
- the variation of the LET mixture within such a beam,
- the fact that we have 60 beams,
- the important problems which occur with the dynamic treatment.

The main components which contribute to the total dose of a pion beam are the dose due to the slowing down of the pions (mainly low LET) and the dose due to protons, neutrons and heavier secondary particles produced at the pion stop position (high LET, *stardose*). In addition the electron and muon contamination contributes to the low LET dose. As is demonstrated in Fig. 1, one therefore expects a spatial variation of the radiation quality within a pion beam. Therefore, our dosimetry system has to fulfill the following requirements:
- The detector systems have to measure the low LET and the high LET dose component separately.
- One needs special equipment to map the dose distributions in three dimensions for a configuration of 1 to 60 convergent beams.
- In order to simulate dynamic treatments for deep-seated tumors in a realistic way, integrating dosimeters and solid phantoms have to be used.
- The monitoring system has to check all 60 beams individually.

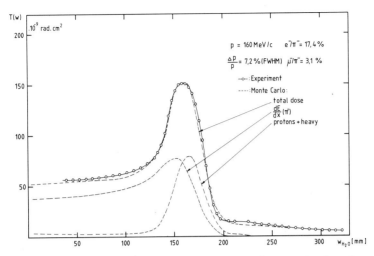

Fig. 1. Dose as a function of depth in water, for a single pion beam (πE3-channel).

MONITORING

Two independent systems, which are based on completely different measuring principles, are used for monitoring.

Pionclock. The pionclock consists of scintillation counter telescopes at four different positions just upstream of the slits. The coincidence rate of the two plastic scintillators in each telescope gives the time base for the irradiations.

Monitor chambers. Near the windows through which the pions enter the treatment tank, 60 parallel plate ionisation chambers monitor the intensity of the 60 beams individually. The ionisation current, which is proportional to the pion rate in each beam, is converted into a digital signal and stored in a PDP 11/45 computer or in a microprocessor. This monitoring system is of very high importance during the treatment because it checks the proper functioning of the slit system by measuring the individual beam intensities right at the position where the beams enter the treatment region.

The 60 monitor chambers give quick and simultaneous information on the beam intensity pattern and therefore can be used to test the symmetry of the PIOTRON (Fig. 2).

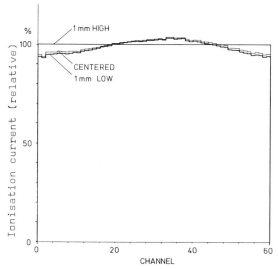

Fig. 2. Histograms of the 60 monitor chamber readings. A vertical shift of the proton beam on the target by ± 1 mm causes a horizontal asymmetry of ± 5 % in the measured ionisation currents. The histogram which showed no asymmetry ("1 mm High") was used to normalize the results of the others individually.

DETECTOR SYSTEMS FOR DOSIMETRY

As has already been mentioned, it is necessary to measure more than just the total physical pion dose. We hope to get a good correlation with the biological effects, if we know two parameters at each point of the dose distribution. These two parameters would ideally be the low LET and the high LET dose. But from the experimental point of view it is much easier to measure the *total physical dose* and *the stardose*. As we will always have to deal with dynamic treatment, we are focusing on integrating dosimeters. In addition the sensitivity of the detectors should be sufficient to accurately measure the dose delivered to a patient in one single fraction, which is approximately 200 rads.

We developed and tested three different systems: (a) film plus activation of aluminium foils, (b) ^{7}LiF-TLD's plus activation of aluminium foils, (c) CaF_2:Tm-TLD's.

Activation of aluminium foils. About 7 % of the pions stopped in aluminium produce a β-active ^{24}Na nucleus.[1] In earlier experiments on a single pion beam we have shown that the aluminium activation

method reproduces the pion stop distribution quite well.[2] We are
of course aware of the problems which may occur due to the neutron
induced activity in the case of much larger irradiation volumes.
For these cases the necessary experiments will be carried out at
the PIOTRON.

In order to get three-dimensional activity distributions we use
a number of large foils (thickness: 0.1 mm) placed between the
slices of a phantom. Within one foil the activity has to be analysed in two dimensions. A new technique has been developed which
allows a quick and simple measurement of two-dimensional activity
distributions.[3] The emitted electrons are detected in two stacks of
multiwire chambers with the foil in between. As the electrons are
emitted isotropically from the foil and only one pair of coordinates is measured at some distance from the foil, one had to find
a method to improve the spatial resolution. This problem can be
solved by applying a large magnetic field perpendicular to the foil
and the wire chamber planes. This leads to a resolution in the
order of 1 mm (Fig. 3).

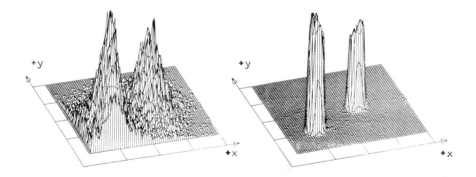

Fig. 3. Two-dimensional analysis of two homogeneously activated
aluminum foils (diameter: 5 cm). The improvement of the spatial resolution by applying a magnetic field of 1.3 T is demonstrated.

This aluminium activation method gives not only the possibility
of calculating a dose which is biologically relevant but we are
able to correct [7]LiF-TLD results and film measurements for the LET
dependence of these detectors.

<u>Film plus aluminium activation</u>. Films have an efficiency which drops rapidly with increasing LET. We therefore tested a combination of a film and a rare earth intensifying screen. In this combination the film in principle records the light from the scintillating material. In order to cover the dose range of several rads to 200 rads we use a very insensitive film in combination with the screen alpha 2 (3M).

Film irradiation has been used successfully since the PIOTRON operation started. It gives quick and qualitative information on beam configurations and asymmetries (Fig. 4). The film results

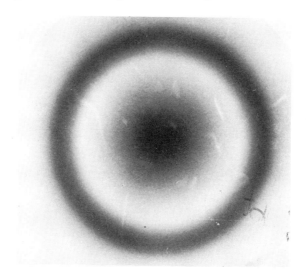

Fig. 4. Irradiation of film. Diameter of lucite phantom: 46.7 cm; momentum: 156 MeV/c (ring distribution); target: 50 mm Mo.

indicate an inefficiency in the region of the stopped pion in the order of 10 %. This inefficiency can be corrected by determining the stop distribution through the activation of aluminium foils in the same experimental setup.

<u>^{7}LiF-TLD's plus aluminium activation</u>. Another pair of detectors which we use is 7LiF powder encapsulated in glass, and in order to

134

correct for the lower efficiency in the high LET region we use the aluminium activation again. This detector pair has been tested for different single beams (Fig. 5).[2] Whether it will work for

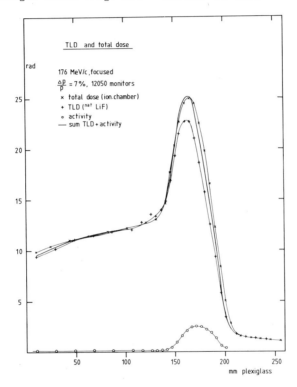

Fig. 5. Correction of [7]LiF-TLD results with the distribution of the aluminium activity for the case of a single pion beam (πE3-channel).

large irradiation volumes as well, can only be checked at the PIO-TRON itself.

CaF_2:TM-TLD's. A special study on CaF_2:Tm material was started on the πE3 single beam and is continuing at the PIOTRON. This material has the unique feature to give information about stardose and total dose simultaneously, because its glow curve has two distinct peaks which vary differently for low LET and high LET dose.[4]

EXPERIMENTAL EQUIPMENT AND PHANTOMS

Water phantom. In order to measure three-dimensional dose distributions we use lucite cylinders of different diameter which can
be mounted on to a water tank and filled with water (Fig.6). The tank
contains a scanner which can be driven in three directions. The
scanner holds an ionisation chamber on a long arm. With this apparatus we control the very time consuming dose mapping in three dimensions automatically with the PDP 11/45 computer for every possible setting of the PIOTRON. Figures 7 and 8 show examples of experimental results. Any asymmetry shows up very clearly in a different maximum value in a ring profile, as is shown in the example
in Fig. 8. In addition to symmetry tests, we use the water phantom
also to study inhomogeneity effects. The optimisation of the machine setting for the first biological experiments and the first
patient treatments was done in that phantom as well.

Realistic phantom. In order to simulate the therapy for realistic cases we built a phantom from solid tissue substitutes.[5] We
limited ourselves to five materials: muscle, fat, hard bone, bone

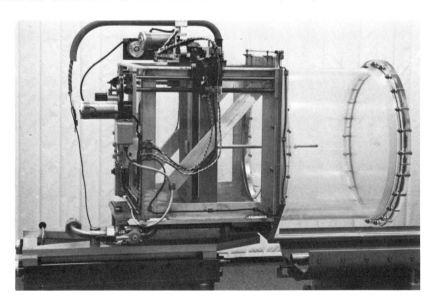

Fig. 6. Water phantom with scanner and ionisation chamber.

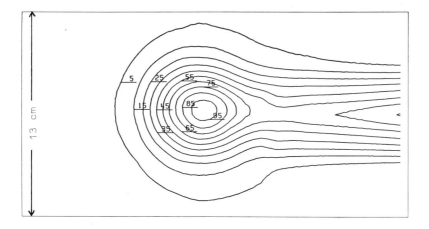

Fig. 7. Isodose plot in a plane along the beam axis of a single
beam of the Piotron (perpendicular to the Piotron axis). The numbers represent the dose percentage of the maximum dose value.

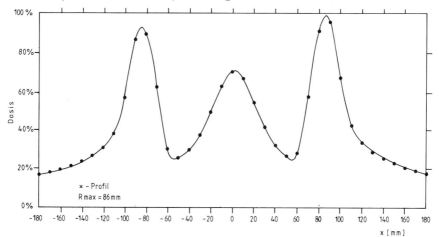

Fig. 8. Profile across a ring distribution along the horizontal direction. Momentum: 156 MeV/c; slits: all 100 % open; target: 30 mm
Be.

marrow and lung. Another material, which is useful for many purposes, is the "rigid water". All materials are based on epoxy
resins. The phantom is built up in slices of a thickness of 1.5 cm
(Fig. 9). The shape of the boundaries between the different tissues is taken from CT-scans of a patient. With this phantom we

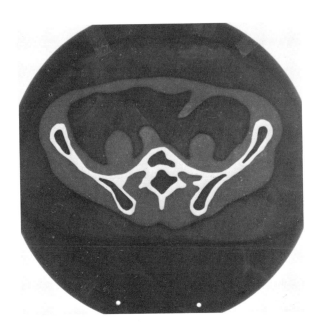

Fig. 9. Slice of the realistic phantom.

simulate dynamic   treatments and measure the resulting dose distributions with one of the detector systems described above.

IN VIVO DOSIMETRY

In the first treatments [7]LiF-TLD's were used routinely for the
in vivo dosimetry. In addition, whenever possible, we had the on-
line reading of an ionisation chamber.

For deep seated tumors we will use a combination of TLD's and
aluminium foils arranged in a tube which can be placed inside the
body, surgically or inside cavities.

In addition to the dosimetric system described above, the beam
optics of the PIOTRON was measured, and a method has been developed
to separate microdosimetric spectra for stopped pions, for pions in
flight, for electrons and muons.[6] In order to get the
necessary biological information at specific points within the dose
distribution we will use mammalian cells embedded in a gel as a
biological dosimeter.[7]

138

REFERENCES

1 Hogstrom KR, Amols HI (1980) Pion *in vivo* dosimetry using aluminium activation. Med Phys 7: 55-60
2 Salzmann M (1979) Measurements at the πE3 single beam correlated
   to dosimetry and therapy planning for the pion applicator at
   SIN. Radiat Environ Biophys 16: 219-223
3 Seiler PG, Wemmers G, Salzmann M, Moline A (1981) Two-dimensional measurement of π⁻ induced beta activity in extended
   foils. Submitted to: Phys Med Biol
4 Hoffmann W, Möller G, Blattmann H, Salzmann M (1981) Pion dosimetry with thermoluminescent materials. Phys Med Biol, in
   press
5 Constantinou C (1978) Tissue substitutes for particulate radiation dosimetry and radiotherapy. Thesis, University of
   London
6 Schuhmacher H, Menzel HG, Blattmann H, Salzmann M (1980) Time-
   of-flight microdosimetry and its application to radiation
   quality studies of negative pions. Proc 7th Symp Microdos 2,
   Oxford/UK, Sept 1980: 1083-1099
7 Skarsgard LD, Palcic B (1974) Pretherapeutic research programs
   at meson facilities. Proc XIIth Int Congr of Radiology 2:
   447-454

COMPUTER MODELING OF HEAVY CHARGED-PARTICLE BEAMS

John T. Lyman
Biology and Medicine Division, Lawrence Berkeley Laboratory, University of
California, Berkeley, California 94720 USA

INTRODUCTION

Computer modeling can be a useful aid when we design experiments for heavy
charged particle beams, particularly if there is a lack of experimental data.
For example, an adequate description of the radiation field is usually not
available. While the size of the field and the range of the primary ions
are known, the quantitative change in beam quality as a function of depth
of penetration is usually not known. Part of this change in beam quality
is due to the difference in energy loss as the ions are slowed down, which
is well understood. Another important factor affecting beam quality is nuclear reactions of the primary ions which cause fragmentation. Secondary
particles produced by these reactions generally continue in the same direction, have a smaller energy loss, and a greater range than the original particle. Qualitatively, the type and energy of these fragments are known.
However, we do not have enough experimental data on beam quality for the beams
of interest.

In designing ridge filters[1] to broaden the Bragg peak for heavy charged-
particle radiotherapy, two types of modeling are used. First, the physical
characteristics of the beam are modeled. These are computer calculations
based on theoretical and empirical considerations that can be used to gain
a better understanding of the physical characteristics of heavy charged particle energy distributions and LET distributions. The second type of modeling
calculates the biological effect of heavy charged particles as a function
of beam quality. When the beam model is combined with a biological response
model, it is possible to predict biological effects that might be observed
when biological systems are irradiated by heavy charged-particle beams. The
biological effect of most interest to the radiotherapists is cell survival.
The results of these types of modeling are used for radiation therapy treatment planning using the heavy charged-particle beams.

METHODS AND MATERIALS

The beam model is based on a computer program (BRAGG) which is used to calculate a Bragg curve of a heavy charged-particle beam[2]. This program is a mathematical model that couples the processes of ionization energy loss and nuclear interactions. The results with the initial program agree very well with experimental data for those cases in which secondary particle production is of minor importance[3]. For the cases in which the secondary particle production is more important, the program has been modified so that the Bragg curves of the secondary particles can be added to the curve of the primary ions[4]. The spectra of the secondary particles used in the calculation is determined empirically by comparing the calculated and the experimental Bragg curves. Additional constraints on the secondary particle spectra are based on measurements of the beam charge as a function of depth of penetration. This is the curve that can be obtained with the use of a Faraday cup[3].

The model that is used to predict the biologically equivalent dose is based on the linear-quadratic cell survival model[5]. We assume that this model will predict the effect of a single fraction of radiation, and that the parameters that affect cell survival are constant for all fractions. The linear and quadratic coefficients both are a function of the beam quality[6].

In order to design a beam modification device (such as a ridge filter) to produce a broad region with a high biologically effective dose, the beam model is combined with the biological effects model in order to predict cell survival as a function of depth of penetration of the beam[7]. The broadened region is produced by superpositioning Bragg curves, each with a different residual range. An iterative method is used to minimize the difference between the desired depth-survival curve and a calculated curve. The resulting dose distribution is a composite curve obtained by the appropriate range shifting of the initial Bragg curve and the proper weighting of the shifted curves.

RESULTS AND DISCUSSION

Bragg curves for carbon, neon and silicon ions have been calculated using the beam model described above. The results are shown in Figure 1, along with the experimental Bragg curves measured at the Bevalac. The curves are normalized so that the initial point is plotted at a value that corresponds to the LET measured in keV/um . The calculations allow the total dose curve

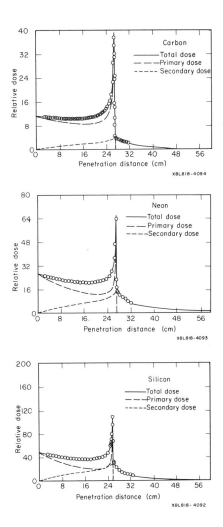

Figure 1. Bragg curves for carbon, neon, and silicon ions showing expected contributions of the primary and secondary ions to the total dose. Total dose calculation is compared to measured dose points.

to be separated into the dose due to the primary ions and the dose due to all the secondary particles. In the region beyond the Bragg peak, the total dose is from the contribution of the secondaries only.

Based on the calculated Bragg curves, depth-dose curves were calculated for a 10-cm spread Bragg peak, which would be isosurvival at the 66% level. These curves are shown in Figure 2. The top panel of the figure shows the predicted depth-survival pattern. All ions give the same survival in the spread Bragg peak; however, outside this region the survival depends upon the particular ion, with the lighter ions showing higher survival. The middle panel shows the dose distributions that are required to produce the depth-survival patterns. Carbon, the lightest of the three ions, has the lowest dose outside the spread Bragg peak; between the proximal and distal peaks carbon shows the greatest slope because of the large relative change in relative biological effectiveness (RBE).

The bottom panel of Figure 2 shows the dose-equivalent distribution. This is the dose distribution a low-LET radiation would have to have to cause the same depth-survival distributions shown in the top panel. The dose distribution is related to the dose-equivalent distribution by the RBE for the appropriate survival level at each point. The dose-equivalent distribution shows that outside the spread Bragg peak region, the lighter ions have the lower effective doses. In the high dose region (or in the spread Bragg peak region) the beams have equally effective doses. The depth-dose curves for each ion show what is already evident from the Bragg curves: as the nuclear charge is increased the fragmentation increases, which is clearly shown by the increase of the secondary dose beyond the Bragg peak. Also, the slope of the physical dose in the spread Bragg peak decreases less rapidly as the nuclear charge is increased. This reflects the fact that the relative change in RBE between the proximal and distal peaks is less for the heavier ions.

These calculations of the dose-equivalent distributions are based on RBE values at survival levels from 100% to 66%. Most values of RBE that are reported for these beams are for a 10% survival level[8]. When the RBE is calculated at the 10% level for the beam quality assumed, the values fall in the middle of the range of the reported values for two different cell systems (Figure 3). At the same dose-weighted LET value, the RBE values for the different beams are not equal because of a velocity dependence of the cell survival parameters[9].

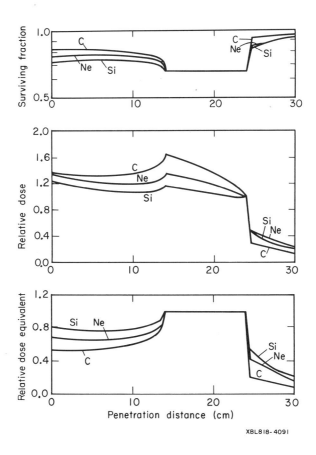

Figure 2. Calculated distributions of cell survival, dose, and dose-equivalent as a function of penetration distance for beams of carbon, neon, and silicon which have been modified to provide a 10-cm region with a high biologically effective dose.

144

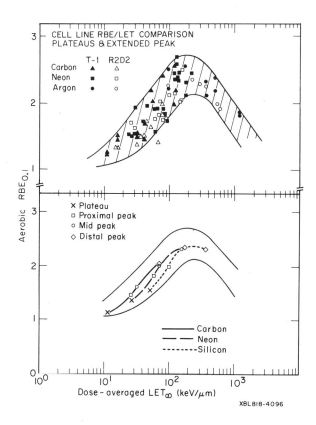

Figure 3. Top panel: Aerobic RBE-10 values vs. dose-averaged LET for two cell lines; data are from plateau and spread Bragg peak measurements[9]. Bottom panel: Calculated RBE-10 values for the carbon, neon, and silicon beams with a 10-cm spread Bragg peak plotted within the limits of the experimental data.

Unless the OER is equal to one, it is not possible to shape a single port depth-dose distribution to be isosurvival for both the aerobic and anoxic cells simultaneously. Therefore, we choose the distribution to optimize the shape of the curve for the aerobic cells. This avoids regions of nonuniform biologically effective dose to the normal cells within the treatment volume for a single port irradiation.

A treatment region that is not isosurvival for the "model" cell can be partially compensated by the use of equally weighted parallel opposed ports[10]. This would be the preferred treatment if the dose to the tumor were the only consideration. However, dose to the surrounding normal tissues outside the treatment volume is also a consideration, as critical structures in the beam path may limit treatment choices. Consider, for example, a treatment volume that is within three cm of a critical tissue that will be irradiated by both the entrance and exit portions of a parallel opposed pair of beam ports (Figure 4). If the tolerance dose for the critical normal tissue is 50% of the desired tumor dose, then the optimal plan might be a pair of parallel-opposed carbon beams equally weighted. If the ion of choice were silicon, it would not be possible to use equally weighted ports without exceeding the tolerance dose to the critical normal structure. A two-to-one weighting factor of the doses would deliver the specified tumor dose and keep the dose to the critical structure below the tolerance dose. This would result in a change in beam quality across the treatment volume which would be undesirable for all but the "model" cells.

CONCLUSIONS

Several conclusions can be drawn from the use of computer modeling in radiotherapy treatment planning with heavy charged-particle beams. The heavier beams will probably have the highest clinical utility when used with (1) short ranges where the fragmentation is minimized or (2) applications where the dose beyond the distal peak is of minimal consequence such as treatments of brain tumors where the treatment volumes frequently include the whole brain.

The use of single port treatments are the most effective means to limit the integral dose. Therefore the single port dose distribution should be optimized to provide a high uniform effective dose distribution throughout the tumor region. This distribution should be based upon the critical normal tissues within the target volume because severe damage to these tissues will prevent the escalation of the dose schedules which will therefore have the consequence of a higher probability of local failure.

146

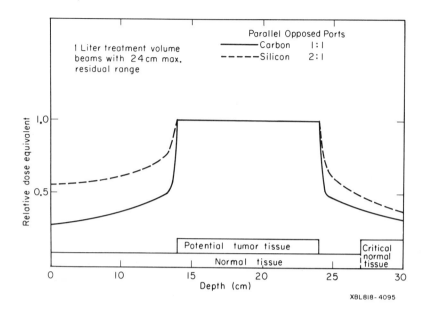

Figure 4. Dose-equivalent distributions for parallel-opposed treatments with carbon and silicon beams. The carbon beam was equally weighted, but the silicon beam was unequally weighted to illustrate the impact on treatment planning of critical structures near the treatment volume.

Multiple port treatments are advised when the critical normal tissue is outside the target volume and the use of a single port treatment would exceed the tolerance dose to the critical normal tissue. Multiple portal plans using parallel opposed ports are advised when the equivalent dose distribution is not uniform within the target volume for both the normal tissues and the tumor tissue. Parallel opposed ports will also provide a more uniform OER across the target volume. This can be important if the anoxic cells limit the probability of local control.

Finally, the use of beams of higher atomic number to achieve a lower OER value must be balanced against the use of lighter beams with their lower probability of fragmentation and better dose distribution.

ACKNOWLEDGEMENTS

These studies were supported by the National Institute of Health (Grant CA19138) and the Office of Health and Environmental Research of the U.S. Department of Energy under Contract W-7405-Eng-48.

REFERENCES

1. Karlsson BG (1964) Methoden sur Berechnung und Erzielung Einger fur die Tie-fentherapie mit Hoch-Energetischen Protonen Gunstiger Dosisverteilungen. Strahlentherapie 124:481-492.
2. Litton J, Lyman J, Tobias C (1968) Penetration of high-energy heavy ions with the inclusion of coulomb, nuclear, and other stochastic processes. Lawrence Berkeley Laboratory Report UCRL-17392 Rev, Berkeley, CA.
3. Raju MR, Lyman JT, Brustad T, Tobias CA (1969) Heavy charged-particle beams. Radiation Dosimetry III:151-199.
4. Chatterjee A, Tobias CA, Lyman JT (1976) Nuclear fragmentation in therapeutic and diagnostic studies with heavy ions. In Shaw BSP, Merker M (eds.), Spallation Nuclear Reactions and Their Applications, pp. 168-191. Dordrecht-Holland: Reidel D.
5. Fertil B, Deschavanne PJ, Lachet B, Malaise EP (1980) In vitro radiosensitivity of six human cell lines. A comparison study with different statistical models. Radiat Res 82:297-309.
6. Chapman JD, Blakely EA, Smith KC, Urtasun RC (1977) Radiobiological characterization of the inactivating events produced in mammalian cells by helium and heavy ions. Int J Radiat Oncol Biol Phys 3:97-102.
7. Lyman JT (1980) Radiological physics considerations for selection of heavy charged-particle beams for biomedical research. In Radiation Oncology, Maria Design Symposium, vol. II:27-41. Medical Accelerator Research Institute in Alberta, Edmonton, Alberta, Canada.
8. Blakely EA (1980) Choice of particle species. In Radiation Oncology, Maria Design Symposium, vol. II:47-93. Medical Accelerator Research Institute in Alberta, Edmonton, Alberta, Canada.
9. Blakely EA, Tobias CA, Yang TCH, Smith KC, Lyman JT (1979) Inactivation of human kidney cells by high-energy monoenergetic heavy-ion beams. Radiat Res 80:122-160.
10. Tobias CA, Lyman JT, Lawrence JH (1971) Some considerations of physical and biological factors in radiotherapy with high-LET radiations including heavy particles, pi mesons, and fast neutrons. In Lawrence JH (ed.) Progress in Atomic Medicine: Recent Advances in Nuclear Medicine vol. 3:167-218.

Published 1982 by Elsevier Science Publishing Co., Inc.
PION AND HEAVY ION RADIOTHERAPY:
Pre-Clinical and Clinical Studies
L. D. Skarsgard

149

TREATMENT PLANNING FOR HEAVY CHARGED PARTICLE RADIOTHERAPY

GEORGE T.Y. CHEN AND SAMUEL PITLUCK
Radiotherapy Section
Division of Biology and Medicine
Lawrence Berkeley Laboratory
Berkeley, California 94720

INTRODUCTION

Over the past three and one half years, the radiotherapy physics group has been involved in the development of pixel by pixel treatment planning for heavy charged particle radiotherapy. The progress, techniques, and further studies required in this endeavor are reviewed in this article. Additional information on the clinical physics of charged particle radiotherapy may also be found elsewhere.[1,2]

PATIENT CT SCANNING

The planning process begins with a CT study of the patient in the treatment position. CT scans are the principle source of information on tumor localization and quantitative data on inhomogeneities. Horizontal charged particle beams are available at both the 184 inch cyclotron and at the Bevalac, and the most common treatment position for lesions of the abdomen and thorax has been the patient seated position. In April 1981, we scanned our first patient in the patient upright mode. The EMI 7070, as shown in Figure 1, is specially modified to permit scanning with the patient immobilized in an upright position. The entire gantry assembly is raised or lowered to permit scanning at various longitudinal positions. The scanner may also be used in the standard patient recumbent position. This is the second of two modified EMI scanners, the first being at the Massachusetts General Hospital.

TARGET CONTOURING

The next step in treatment planning is definition of the target (treatment) volume by the radiotherapist. This is currently achieved through interactively entering target volumes via a joystick while viewing each CT image on a raster graphics display. Other groups[3] have developed procedures where selected slices are contoured and target contours intermediate to these are calculated by interpolation. This is an important feature when dealing with a large number of CT slices. Contour information is essential for two tasks in treatment planning: 1) a set of target contours defines the shape of the treatment aperture and 2)

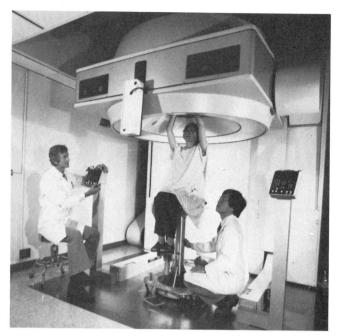

Figure 1. EMI-7070 x-ray CT scanner in patient upright mode.

contour information may be used to design a three-dimensional compensator. In order to design compensators, the water equivalent distance must be known from the distal margin of the target contour to the body entrance surface.

CONVERSION OF CT DATA TO RELATIVE STOPPING POWER

We have used the quantitative information from single energy CT scans to determine the water equivalent path length. The technique is described in detail elsewhere.[4] Briefly, selected reference materials are CT scanned and their relative stopping powers are measured in a charged particle beam. Tissue analogs such as alcohol and water to simulate fat, and solutions of dibasic potassium phosphate and water to simulate various densities of bone are used in the generation of the calibration curve, as shown in Figure 2. The curve is parameterized in two parts: from air (-500 EMI units) to a CT number of 55, a parabola is fit through the data. From CT number 55 to +500, the data are fit to a straight line. Data from the EMI 5005 and EMI 7070 Scanners (scanning at 120 KVP) and the GE 7800 (120 KVP) all appear to lie on the same calibration curve within experimental error.

The accuracy of CT numbers is influenced by a number of factors including size and shape of the object, position within the reconstruction region, and presence of inhomogeneities. Scans of water equivalent elliptical phantoms with internal air holes exhibit local CT number deviations from expected values of 4-5% for air and as much as 7% for water equivalent plastic. Countering these local variations in the practical usage of CT data in treatment planning is the fact that generally one averages over these fluctuations when line integrals from body surface to deep seated tumors are calculated. In a number of clinical situations, we have found that the water equivalent pathlength extracted from a single energy CT scan is within 2% of the measured value.

Phantom studies of the accuracy of single energy CT scans in predicting water equivalent pathlengths have been complemented with a series of studies on the cadaver of a frozen dog. Diodes were implanted in a number of regions in this dog as part of an experiment on radioactive beam localization, performed by Doctors A. Chatterjee, E. Alpen, W. Saunders and myself. Figure 3 shows a diode positioned in the dog's thorax. The path length from a lateral field passes through part of a rib, a collapsed lung, a blood-filled trachea and

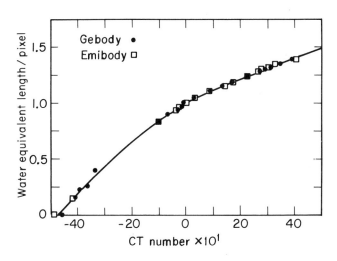

Figure 2. Calibration curve relating CT numbers and water equivalent pathlength

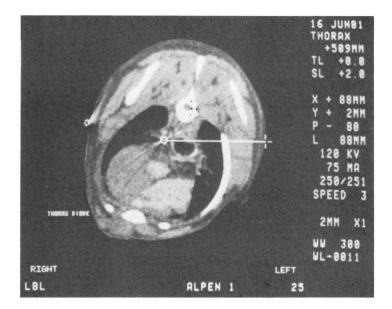

Figure 3. Scan of dog with diode implanted in thorax.

finally into the diode. The geometric distance as measured by the CT Scanner
was 8.8. cm. Using the single energy calibration curve, the CT predicted water
equivalent length was 8.4 cm and the experimentally determined water equivalent
length by a water column scan and diode was found to be 8.5 cm. In a second
measurement, a diode was planted in the dog's brain. The geometric distance
from the entrance surface to the diode was measured to be 6.7 mm, and the CT
estimated water equivalent path length was calculated to be 7.4 cm. The diode
measurement produced a value of 7.5 cm, in excellent agreement with the CT calculated values. These correlations between diode measured residual range in the
dog and CT estimated pathlengths are very recent data, and are still undergoing
detailed analysis. However, they appear to support the use of a single energy
scan technique in relatively simple regions. Dual energy scans may be required
in more complex areas such as in the region of the base of skull.

CT DATA PREPARATION

Although the CT to water equivalent path length problem appears to be well
toward a solution, this does not imply that CT preprocessing of scan data for
treatment planning is by any means totally solved. In Figure 4 both gas and
contrast are present in the gastro-intestinal tract. Literal use of this CT

data would result in errors in compensation design. From the anterior direction, a compensator constructed from exact CT values would compensate for gas and contrast whereas it is likely that neither are present at the time of treatment. For this reason, to insure adequate tumor irradiation, it is necessary to selectively edit these areas from the CT data and replace them with CT values of water. In considering that a possible 20 to 40 CT scans must be examined and edited, it is clear that semi-automatic techniques for this process must be developed. We are investigating the utility of a controlled search algorithm in three dimensions as described elsewhere.[5]

THREE DIMENSIONAL GRAPHICS

Up to this point, we have CT scanned a patient in the treatment position and the radiotherapist has defined the target volume he wishes to treat. At this stage it would be highly desirable to visualize these contours and adjacent normal structures in three dimensions. At LBL, we have been exploring the display of CT derived contours in psuedo-three dimensions on an Evans and

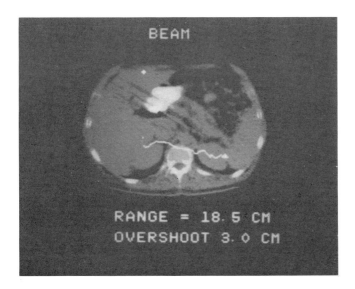

Figure 4. Typical abdominal scan of a patient with pancreatic carcinoma. Gas in bowel results in beam overshoot from anterior field.

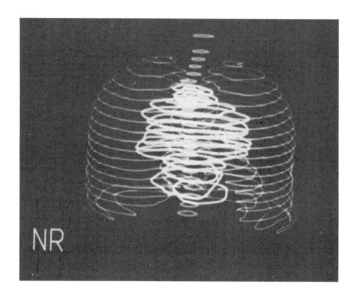

Figure 5. Target contours from sequential CT scans displayed on Evans and Sutherland Graphics unit. Also seen are lungs and spinal cord. The original figure was color coded.

Sutherland Picture System unit. This is a sophisticated vector graphics unit capable of displaying a large number of vectors and rotating them in real time by the manipulation of a dial. Depth cuing is achieved by intensity variation; objects closer to the viewer are brighter. Color may be used to differentiate between different contours. An example of the images possible from the device is shown in Figure 5. This example is intended to display an esophageal target volume, lungs and spinal cord. We see in the definition of the target volume a rather irregular shape, which is due to difficulties in being totally consistent from transverse slice to slice. We plan to develop algorithms which will smooth the entered volumes.

DOSE CALCULATIONS

As Dr. Lyman has described in the previous presentation, the isoeffective central axis depth distribution is the principal planning beam information used for dose distribution calculation. These are shown in Figure 6 for carbon, helium and neon. Both physical dose and isoeffect distributions are currently calculated and samples are shown in Figures 7A and B. In this particular example, a square target volume is indicated and the required compensator to produce this dose distribution is shown adjacent to the external body surface. Variations of approximately 1 cm in the compensator reflect the variation in path length due to some rays traversing a large path length of fat, with a density of 0.92 g/cc. In the abdomen, no substantial inhomogeneities exist (with the exclusion of air) and compensation could be achieved rather readily. However before such fully compensated treatments are implemented a study on variability of abdominal target as a function of the time must first be completed. It must be determined whether target volumes defined on an initial treatment planning scan are indeed valid for the entire course of radiotherapy. We plan to scan a selected number of patients on a daily basis for approximately 5 days and on a weekly schedule of once every 5 weeks in order to determine target volume location and shape variation. Data accumulated from this study will be used to define guidelines in target volume definition which take into account any potential organ shift.

COMPENSATION FABRICATION

Once the treatment plan has been finalized, compensation fabrication must be

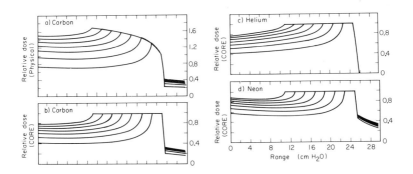

Figure 6. a) family of carbon ridge filtered beams: physical dose; b) carbon isoeffective distribution: c) helium isoeffective distribution; d) neon isoeffective distribution. (CORE: Cobalt 60 rad equivalent)

156

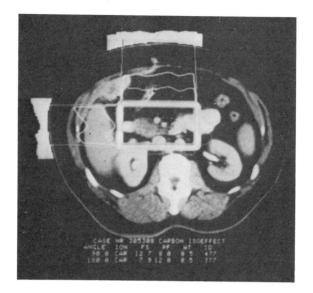

7 a)

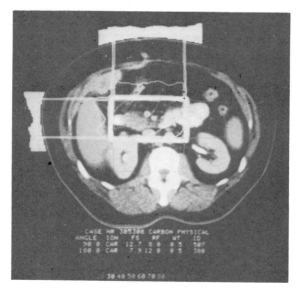

7 b)

Figure 7 a) two field carbon isoeffective dose distribution. The compensator
are shown as light colored regions on the body surface. Tumor is uniformly
dosed to 100%. b) corresponding physical dose distribution. These figures
were reproduced from a graphics display where isodose lines are color coded.

performed. We are developing the capability of milling compensators by computer controlled machines. This technique was first suggested and used by the Massachusetts General Hospital Proton Group. At LBL, computer generated and fabricated compensators are undergoing dosimetric verification. We have used cellulose nitrate, a nuclear track detector, to determine the stopping distribution of heavy ions. The technique of analyzing holes etched in this material was developed principally for heavy ion radiography, a separate project at the Lawrence Berkeley Laboratory. However, this particular technique is extremely well suited for dosimetry in three dimensions for heavy charged particle radiotherapy and we will continue to explore its use in treatment planning verification.

Acknowledgements: This work was supported by NCI Grant 5PCCA19138 and ERDA Contract W-7405-ENG-48.

REFERENCES

1. Thomas R, Perez-Mendez, V, (eds) (1980) Advances in Radiation Protection and Dosimetry in Medicine. New York: Plenum Press.
2. Chen GTY et al. (1981) Heavy charged particle radiotherapy, in Ann Rev. Biophys. Bioeng. 10:499-529
3. Goitein, M (1981) private communication
4. Chen, GTY (1979) Treatment planning for heavy ion radiotherapy. Int. J. Rad. Onc. Bio. Phys. 5:1809-1819
5. Rhodes, ML (1979) An algorithm approach to controlled search in three dimensional image data. ACM Proc. SIGGRAPH 79 Vol. 13 No. 2 pp134-142.

PROBLEMS OF INHOMOGENEITIES IN PARTICLE BEAM THERAPY

LYNN VERHEY AND MICHAEL GOITEIN
Department of Radiation Medicine, Massachusetts General Hospital, Boston,
MA 02114.

INTRODUCTION

The use of pions, protons and heavy ions for radiation therapy is being
investigated at several centers in North America and throughout the world. One
of the prime reasons for the interest in charged particle radiotherapy is the
excellent physical dose confinement potentially achievable with these particles.
The improved physical dose distributions are made possible by the relatively
small amount of multiple scattering and by the rapid fall-off of dose with depth
beyond the end of the Bragg peak. These same physical characteristics make
stringent requirements on the accurate assessment and compensation of inhomogeneities without which quality radiotherapy with these particles cannot be
accomplished. This stands in contrast to the situation for conventional photon
therapy. Figure 1 shows depth dose distributions for a cobalt-60 photon beam
and for an unspecified heavy charged particle ion beam beneath a 3 cm thickness
of bone. In the case of cobalt-60 the dose in the shadow has been reduced by
11% whereas for the heavy charged particle beam the range of the particles in
the shadow of the bone has been decreased by 2 cm making possible a dangerous
underdosing of the target volume. This paper will discuss techniques for assessing the distribution of heterogeneous objects within the patient, of predicting
their effects on dose distribution, and of compensating for their presence in
a way which will minimize their impact on treatment plans.

THEORY

The primary energy loss for charged particles traversing tissues is accomplished by a large number of interactions with atomic electrons, each of which
transfers only a small amount of the incoming particle's energy to the medium.
This electromagnetic energy loss process depends directly on the electron
density of the medium, inversely on the square of the particle's velocity and
logarithmically on the adjusted ionization potential of the medium.[1]

The linear attenuation coefficient for photons is also directly dependent
on the electron density of the material. CT information can therefore be used,
in principle, to plan the depth of penetration of charged particle beams. In
reality, photons of diagnostic energies such as those used in conventional

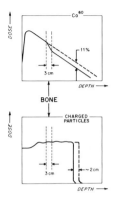

Fig. 1. Depth Dose distributions for Co⁶⁰ (top) and charged particle beam (bottom). Dashed line shows ·dose in homogeneous material, solid line for dose beneath 3 cm slab of bone.

CT machines, suffer energy loss through both photo-electric and compton processes. Therefore the net attenuation is a function not only of the electron density, but also of the distribution of atomic number. However, with the use of tissue analogue materials it has been shown that a simple functional corre-lation between CT number and charged particle stopping power can be found so that scanning patients at a single energy is almost certainly adequate.[2] If necessary, dual energy scanning could be used to disentangle the compton and photo-electric contributions to the attenuation.[3]

The presence of heterogeneous objects shadowing or enclosed within the target volume produces not only a change in range over that which would be obtained from a homogeneous phantom, but also, can produce local perturbations to the dose distribution at boundaries between high and low densities. It has been shown that in the case where the amount of material overlying a heterogeneity is equal to or greater than the water-equivalent thickness of the heterogeneous object, then the maximum amplitude of the dose perturbation beneath an air-tissue interface is 8% for a proton beam.[4] In the case of a bone-tissue inter-face this maximum dose perturbation is even less. For particles heavier than protons the need for overlying material is even more critical. As long as the above-stated rule is obeyed, the effect of interfaces on the dose distributions can usually be ignored.

The effect of inhomogeneities on particle range is, of course, very important. Both proton and heavy ion radiography have been shown to be impressive in their ability to yield high density resolution.[5] This is due to a strong dependence of charged particle fluence on density which should serve as a word of caution in charged particle treatment planning.

TREATMENT PLANNING CONSIDERATIONS

We would now like to discuss some practical treatment planning considerations in the design and use of compensators. It will be assumed that a dual energy technique or a single energy scan has been used to obtain a matrix of pixels of stopping power information for the particle of interest with the patient immobilized in the treatment position. The first and foremost consideration is the difficulty associated with registration of the bolus relative to the patient. As Figure 2a shows, in the absence of multiple scattering, beam divergence and patient motion, it is possible to exactly compensate for an inhomogeneity at a depth with a bolus on the surface.

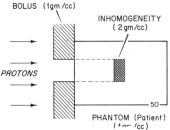

Figure 2a.
Perfect compensation on the surface for an inhomogeneity at depth is shown.

However, when one takes into account the divergence and multiple scattering of the beam particles in the phantom, and more importantly, the potential motion of the phantom relative to the bolus, it becomes obvious that perfect compensation for an inhomogeneity at depth is not possible. Figure 2b, for instance, shows the effect of misregistering the bolus relative to the inhomogeneity, thereby producing an undershoot with a danger of local recurrence on one side and an overshoot which may endanger tissue distal to the target volume on the other side.

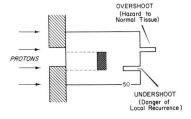

Figure 2b.
Misregistration of the bolus relative to the patient can produce both undershoot and overshoot.

Figure 2c shows an obvious way of planning for potential patient motion by modifying the compensator design to assume a maximum lateral motion of patient relative to the bolus. This has the effect of producing overshoot beyond the target volume in certain areas but also guaranteeing that if the patient motion is truly within the assumed limits that an undershoot is not possible.

One must then consider whether the planned overshoot is acceptable in terms of radiation tolerance.

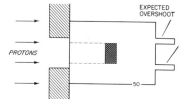

Figure 2c.
To allow for potential patient motion, the bolus must be constructed as if the inhomogeneity were larger. No under-shoot is possible if patient motion is within allowed limits.

Besides patient motion, compensation for heterogeneities is complicated by the existence of beam divergence and multiple scattering. These have the effect of modifying particle trajectories from that which would be predicted on the basis of geometry alone. If one does not take these factors into account when designing the compensator, it again would be possible to underdose certain portions of the target volume.

One further phenomenon which can, in principle, lead to an underdosing in the target volume is insufficient spatial resolution of the CT scan.[6] This fact is demonstrated in Figure 3 where a proton beam is shown incident on five thin slivers of widths between 1 and 4 mm. At the bottom of Figure 3a is the calculated pullback of the proton beam due to the presence of the sliver rela-tive to a homogeneous medium. This calculation is based on CT data from an actual scan of the slivers with a spatial resolution of about 1 mm. In Figure 3b we see the pullback from the CT data after smearing by +/- 2 mm. In 3c, the same data has been smeared by +/- 3 mm. As can be seen, with a CT scan of insufficient spatial resolution, the maximum pullback of the beam due to the slivers is underestimated. This means that if one is not careful the target

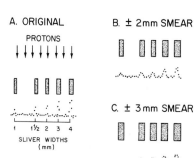

Figure 3.
Proton beam stopping dis-tribution beneath slivers of varying width. (A) Cal-culated from CT scan of +/- 1mm spatial resolution. (B) Calculated after smear-ing CT data to simulate +/- 2mm resolution. (C) Calculated from CT data smeared by +/- 3mm.

volume will be potentially underdosed by a treatment plan which calculates its compensation on the basis of the poor resolution CT scan. Multiple scattering of the beam particles tends to lessen the requirements on spatial resolution. Although 1-2 mm spatial resolution is sufficient for proton therapy and more than adequate for pions, it would be insufficient for heavy ions unless beam divergence is artificially introduced.

The treatment planning program must design the following items for each portal of a patient's treatment: the aperture, which defines the beam shape in two dimensions, the compensating bolus, which defines the beam shape in depth, and the range and modulation of the beam which are determined by the maximum depth and extent of the target volume. In Figure 4 is shown a schematic of a patient contour and a compensating bolus[7] designed without accounting for patient motion or multiple scattering. For the beam trajectory shown, the thinnest element of this section of the bolus would be traversed. However, the fact that 3 or 4 mm of patient motion relative to the bolus is potentially possible means that the particle shown might traverse either of the nearest neighbors to the nominal bolus element. In this case, if the particle would traverse either the neighbor above or below the darkly shaded bolus element, the beam would be pulled back more than intended in that portion of the target volume.

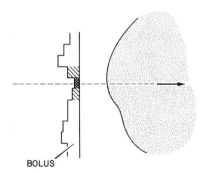

Figure 4.
Schematic of patient
contour and compensating
bolus.

BOLUS

Therefore the bolus design must be modified so that the thicknesses of the nearest neighbors, shown cross-hatched, are set equal to that of the thinnest section of the bolus which is the darkened region in the center. This procedure is followed for all of the bolus elements thereby guaranteeing that if the patient motion is within the expected limits that no portion of the target volume will be underdosed. In Figure 5 is shown a practical application of this principle where a bolus which is designed for a fixed patient contour is smeared by the appropriate amount, producing a possible stopping contour on the right hand section, which is as deep or deeper at each point than the desired stopping contour shown on the left hand section.

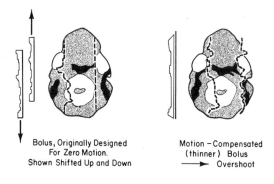

Bolus, Originally Designed
For Zero Motion.
Shown Shifted Up and Down

Motion – Compensated
(thinner) Bolus
——➤ Overshoot

Figure 5.
In left drawing is shown deepest and shallowest limits of high dose region designed without consideration of motion. In right drawing is shown limits of high dose region beneath motion-compensated bolus.

Figure 6 shows how the bolus design is further modified for the effects of multiple scattering. If we look at one small section of patient contour as shown in this figure, we see that the unscattered particle would traverse the blackened central element of this portion of the patient whereas due to multiple scattering, displaced particles may traverse either of the next two nearest neighbors which are shown cross-hatched in the inset to the figure.

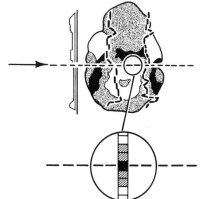

Figure 6.
Blown-up region of CT section shows blackened pixel through which unscattered particle would travel and cross-hatched pixels through which scattered particle could travel. For safety, the lowest density pixel from this set must be chosen.

If the nearest neighbors have an electron density greater than that of the nominal pixel, then that particle may be pulled back and stop short of its intended depth. The bolus design must therefore be modified by assuming that each particle can be displaced on either side of its unscattered trajectory by an amount which is calculable by multiple scattering theory and that the pixel density must be set to be equal to the maximum in that swath of potentially traversed pixels. As shown in Figure 7 this again has the property of guaranteeing no underdosing of the original designated target volume and of producing overshoot beyond that target volume.

MULTIPLE SCATTERING

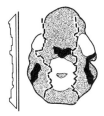 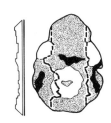

Maximum Density
leads to
Maximum Undershoot

Minimum Density
leads to
Maximum Overshoot

Figure 7.
Left figure shows line of deepest penetration for maximum density assumption. Right figure shows line of deepest penetration for minimum density assumption. Reality should lie between these two.

Finally, in Figure 8 we see the completely smeared bolus design and two separate stopping contours, one which is calculated for the minimum overshoot situation which corresponds to always taking the thickest bolus element and the highest density pixels and the maximum overshoot which corresponds to taking the minimum bolus thickness and the minimum pixel density at each point. The true stopping contour must lie somewhere between these two limits.[7] It is critical when designing a treatment plan and compensator that the uncertainties in the resulting design are calculated and displayed before the treatment plan is accepted. In particular, it is important to know the minimum and maximum possible depths of penetration at each point of the beam and to decide whether both of these limits are acceptable in terms of the tolerance of the patient to radiation.

BOLUS MOVEMENT &
MULTIPLE SCATTERING COMPENSATED FOR

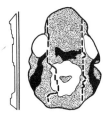 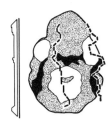

Minimum
Overshoot

Maximum
Overshoot

Figure 8.
Combining effects of multiple scattering and potential patient motion. Left figure shows minimum possible beam penetration, right figure shows maximum possible penetration. Reality should lie between these two.

CONCLUSIONS

The calculations shown have been performed for a proton treatment beam. The principles involved are easily adapted to treatment with pions or heavy ions. However, the differences in the multiple scattering parameters of these particles must be kept in mind. In particular the width of the multiple scattering distribution for pions is approximately 2.5 times as wide as that for protons, whereas for a very heavy ion beam such as neon the width of the scattering distribution is about one fifth that of protons.[8] In the case of pions this may mean that the immobilization constraints are less severe than they are for heavier particles since the multiple scattering will tend to smear out the dose distribution by an amount which is larger than the effects of potential misregistration of the bolus relative to the patient. On the other hand, for heavy ions the opposite is true, namely the fact that multiple scattering is extremely small means that the immobilization of the patient is of primary concern when designing a treatment plan.

For the case of protons our dose distributions are significantly affected by objects as thin as 1-2 mm. This implies that we should strive to immobilize patients to this level to take fullest possible advantage of the dose confinement properties of a proton beam. In Figure 9 is shown a patient immobilized with a thermoplastic mask in the seated position for treatment of a melanoma with our fixed horizontal proton beam. Also visible is the contoured plastic compensator. We have studied intra-treatment motion of patients treated in various positions by comparing pre- and post-treatment radiographs taken along the beam axis.[9]

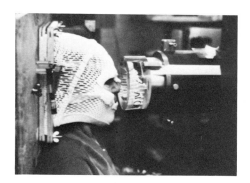

Figure 9.
Patient immobilized in seated position for treatment of melanoma of nasal cavity. Note compensator attached to beam defining aperture.

Figure 10 shows the distribution obtained from a study of five patients treated
in the seated position. The mean movement observed was slightly less than 1
mm although we would normally design our compensator with an assumed maximum
patient motion of +/- 3 mm.

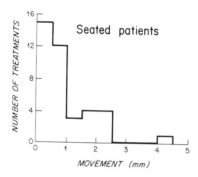

Figure 10.
Distribution of patient motion in plane
perpendicular to beam. Motion determined as difference between pre-treatment and post-treatment radiographic
positions. Mean movement was 0.8 mm
with std. deviation of 0.9 mm and worst
case movement of 4.0 mm for 39 treatments in 5 patients.

SUMMARY

In summary, we would like to emphasize the following points: First, precise
compensation at the surface for a heterogeneity at depth is not possible. Second
the disturbance of the fluence distribution beneath interfaces between air and
tissue or bone and tissue can usually be ignored in practical situations, whereas
the change in range represented by these heterogeneities is clearly very important for particle therapy. Third, the registration of the patient relative to
the bolus is very crucial and one must not only pay great attention to the
immobilization of the patient, but one must be able to evaluate the maximum
potential patient motion relative to the bolus and to modify the compensating
bolus design appropriately. Fourth, the effects of multiple scattering must be
included by either a formal Monte-Carlo calculation through the patient section
of interest or by assuming a range of pixels through which the scattered particle might travel and by accounting for both the minimum and maximum integrated
stopping power for each particle trajectory. Fifth, the acceptance of the treatment plan should be based on an understanding of the range of dose distributions
physically achievable in the actual treatment situation. In particular, this
implies an understanding of the shallowest and deepest possible penetration at
each point of the target volume. Sixth, every effort should be made to verify
the resulting compensating bolus. In reality, this implies treatment planning
of a complicated tissue-like phantom with included heterogeneities based on a
CT scan and followed by an exposure in the particle beam with dose measurements

made at various portions of the phantom. Although some work has been done in this regard, more needs to be done since direct verification of the treatment plan in the patient is normally not possible.

REFERENCES

1. Bichsel H (1972) Passage of Charged Particles Through Matter. American Institute of Physics Handbook, McGraw-Hill, sec. 8, 142.

2. Chen GTY, Singh RP, Castro JR, Lyman JT and Quivey JM (1979) Treatment Planning for Heavy Ion Radiotherapy. Int. J. Rad. Oncol. Biol. Phys. 5:1809-1819.

3. Rutherford RA, Pullan BR and Isherwood I (1976) Measurement of effective atomic number and electron density using an EMI scanner. Neurorad. 11:15-21.

4. Goitein M, Chen GTY, Ting JY, Schneider RJ and Sisterson JM (1978) Measurements and calculations of the influence of thin inhomogeneities on charged particle beams. Med. Phys. 5:265-273.

5. Koehler AM (1972) Medical treatment and diagnosis using 160 MeV protons. In Cyclotron 1972, American Institute of Physics Conference Proceedings No. 9, J.J. Burgerjon & A. Strathdee, eds.

6. Goitein M (1977) The measurement of tissue heterodensity to guide charged particle radiotherapy. Int. J. Radiat. Oncol. Biol. Phys. 3:27-33.

7. Goitein M (1978) Compensation for inhomogeneities in charged particle radiotherapy using computed tomography. Int. J. Rad. Oncol. Biol. Phys. 4:499-508.

8. Goitein M and Sisterson JM (1978) The influence of thick inhomogeneities on charged particle beams. Rad. Res. 74:217-230.

9. Verhey LJ, Goitein M, McNulty P, Munzenrider JE and Suit HD (1982) Precise positioning of patient for radiation therapy. Int. J. Rad. Oncol. Biol. Phys. 8:289-294.

Published 1982 by Elsevier Science Publishing Co., Inc.
PION AND HEAVY ION RADIOTHERAPY:
Pre-Clinical and Clinical Studies
L. D. Skarsgard

SPECIAL TOPICS IN HEAVY ION RESEARCH

C.A. TOBIAS, Wm. CHU, A. CHATTARJEE, E.V. BENTON, J. FABRIKANT, Wm. HOLLEY, J. SCHMIDT, E. BLAKELY AND T.H. HAYES
Department of Biophysics and Lawrence Berkeley Laboratory, University of California, Berkeley

The aim of this paper is to discuss a variety of research areas where heavy ions, because of their physical properties, have useful biomedical applications. Because of limited accelerator time available, some of these fields are still relatively undeveloped. Our aim is to discuss the present status of several of these fields and to point out opportunities for new research. We may classify the special applications of heavy ions into four groups:

(a) diagnostic and structural investigations.

(b) applications of secondary beams.

(c) applications that relate to depth dose distributions.

(d) applications relating to special lesions made by heavy ions in biological material.

A. DIAGNOSTIC AND STRUCTURAL INVESTIGATIONS

Heavy ion radiography.

From the point of view of cancer therapy, attention must be paid to several diagnostic problem areas:

(a) Early diagnostic localization of cancer, before the disease has a chance to disseminate and invade distant normal tissues, is a crucial problem: all too often the first recognition of the existence of tumors occurs only when there is already metastatic involvement.

(b) For precise therapy planning, it is important to know the exact three dimensional boundaries of tumors. If the margin allowed beyond the suspected boundaries of the tumor is not sufficiently large or if there are distant unrecognized extensions of the tumor, then therapy is bound to fail.

(c) When therapy is delivered, it is important to be able to position the patient and the beam in such a manner that the planned dose distribution is actually achieved. If the patient's organs shift between the time of diagnostic studies for therapy planning and actual beam delivery, or if the distribution of gas or air in the body cavities has altered or if the tumor has extended or receded then there is a chance for errors in beam delivery.

(d)   It is desirable to have evidence by independent methods that the beam has been delivered in accordance with the treatment plan and that the right tissues were irradiated.

(e)   Post therapy followup can also benefit from sensitive and accurate measurement of the extent of tumor: it is important to determine at an early time whether or not the desired tumor regression has been achieved and how long tumor growth remains under control.

The range penetration properties of heavy ions make them specially suitable for the support of therapy: two techniques, heavy ion radiography and the use of radioactive beams will allow us in the future to satisfy most of the requirements stated above.

The principles of heavy ion radiography:

The object of heavy ion radiography is to accurately image the distribution of electronic stopping power in the tissues of the body. This aim is achieved by allowing a parallel beam of monoenergetic particles to cross the object to be radiographed, then measuring the spatial pattern of residual range distribution. If a set of residual range distributions are obtained, each with a different angle of incidence of the beam, the obtained data may be mathematically reconstructed to accurately image the three dimensional electron density distribution of the body. The subject has been reviewed in some detail.[1,2,3]

The first heavy ion radiographs were obtained by Benton, Henke and Tobias[4] soon after the initial acceleration of nitrogen beams in the Bevatron. A stack of plastic nuclear particle detectors was mounted behind the subject and the distribution of particle stopping points was imaged on each sheet. Information from the sheets could be integrated to yield the residual range distribution and indirectly the stopping power distribution of tissues. This scheme is shown on figure 1. The first computerized reconstruction of radiographic data from a human subject was performed with helium ions at the 184" cyclotron in 1974 by Crowe and Budinger.[5] They used a stack of multiple wire chambers to obtain the location and residual range of particles. The first high energy neon ion three dimensional tomography of the human head was accomplished at the Bevalac in 1980.

Range energy relationship, straggling and multiple scattering: The passage through water of a parallel beam of monoenergetic carbon ions is shown schematically in figure 2. This figure contains the Bragg ionization curve, the relative flux density of parent carbon particles and the overall flux density of secondary fragments produced by nuclear collisions with nuclei of the absorber. The distribution of stopping points of the particles as function of depth is also shown. This distribution is quite narrow. The accuracy of radiography depends on the narrowness of the distribution; two factors are important: the initial energy spread of the particles emerging from the accelerator and the range straggling due to the statistical nature of energy transfer events.

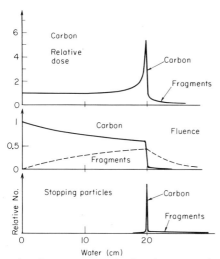

Fig. 1. Top: Bragg ionization curve in water. Middle: Flux density. Bottom: the distribution of stopping particles.

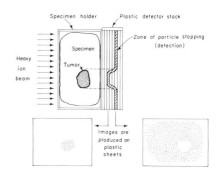

Fig. 2. Schema of heavy ion radiography. The particle beam passes through the object: the stopping points of the particles are recorded in a plastic detector stack. The distribution of etched tracks forms an image in each detector sheet.

The range energy relationships for several heavy ions of radiographic interest have been calculated by Steward.[6] However, if a beam of particles is used, the stopping points show a statistical distribution due to range straggling. For heavy particles the variance of range distributions is between 1 and 0.1% of the range. It is inversely proportional to the square root of the particle mass number, so that neon ions have about 4.5 times smaller straggling than protons.

Another limitation to radiography comes from multiple scattering of the particles. The beam particles scatter off many of the nuclei of the absorber. Consequently they do not move along exactly straight trajectories; instead, the particle stopping points exhibit radial deviations. By the use of phantoms, we have experimentally tested the resolution achievable by various particle beams. In addition, theoretical calculations were also made for resolutions obtainable. In figure 3 the doses necessary for resolving the structure of an object consisting of parallel stripes are given.

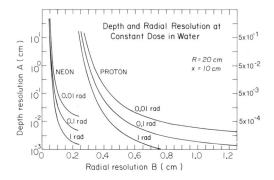

Fig. 3. Depth and radial resolution for beams of 20 cm range for neon and proton particles at various dose levels.

Projection radiography with heavy ions. We have developed a technique for heavy ion mammography.[7] This technique is both quantitative and sensitive to soft tissue density changes. In order to obtain mammograms, the breast was immersed in lukewarm water and gently squeezed between two parallel plastic plates. In this manner the electron density of water could be quantitatively compared to that of mammary tissues. An example of human carbon ion mammograms is given in figure 4. From radiographs and pathological studies[8] we find that the heavy ion number of adipose components of tissues varies between -60 and zero; the normal stroma varies from -10 to +50; carcinomas appear denser and have densities up to +70.

Heavy ion mammograms are characterized by relatively great contrast for small density differences. Figure 5 demonstrates the computer integrated heavy ion radiograms of a subject with a well localized carcinoma. The high contrast obtainable by this method is particularly valuable in women with fibrocystic disease. A dose of about 20 millirad of carbon is adequate for a heavy ion mammogram. This dose is more than 20 times lower than the usual dose necessary for low voltage X ray mammography. When the tumors are small, it is difficult to determine with certainty whether a local density in the radiograph is carcinoma or merely dysplasia. We are developing methods whereby the computer aids in sorting the pixels in the image by density. We can then compare the density spectra of right against left breast, or if two radiographs are taken separated by a time interval, the density spectra can be compared with a view to detect changes that may have occurred as part of the disease process.

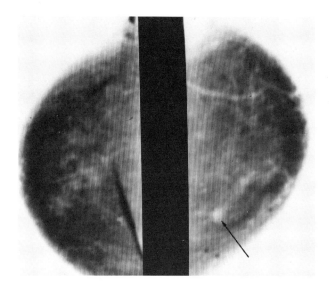

Fig. 4. Radiographic patterns in human breast recorded at 0.1 rad (left) and at 0.019 rad. The images shown are patterns on one of the sheets in the stack.

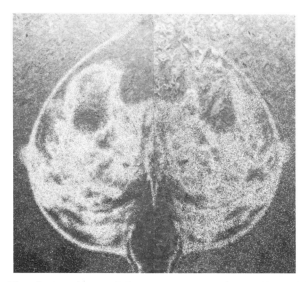

Fig. 5. CRT image of integrated carbon ion radiographs of the left and right breast of a subject. The right breast has a small dense carcinoma (arrow).

Satisfactory techniques have been developed for heavy ion radiography of extremities and of the midsection of the body. In figure 6 are shown neon ion radiographs of a human foot. It can be seen that with heavy ion radiography, the soft tissues, skin, tendons, muscle and adipose tissue can be clearly differentiated. This results from the fact that gradations in bone density are proportional to stopping power changes for heavy ions, whereas with X rays there is a nonlinear relationship.

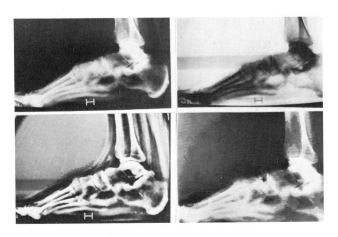

Fig. 6. Four images integrated from the same stack of plastic detectors of a human foot. Since more than 1000 shades of grey are possible, and the human eye can only see 70 shades at one time, each image appears different. At lower left the skin, subcutaneous fat and tendons are clearly visible.

Tomographic reconstructions of heavy ion images. When plastic nuclear detectors are used, it is practical to perform tomography by obtaining a series of pictures at a series of angles. The exposures can be either in thin or in thick slices. If thick slices are avaliable, the mathematical reconstructions can be in three dimensions. Figure 7 is a two dimensional reconstruction of human brain in vitro taken with neon beams at 90 different angles. The noise in these reconstructions at comparable dose levels is usually lower than for X rays: when heavy ions pass through matter, there is no beam hardening problem as is the case when X rays are absorbed by tissue. The statistical reliability of the measurements do not depend on the ratio of quanta between entrance and exit, as in the case of X rays, but rather on the accuracy of range measurements. We are currently engaged in quantitative comparisons of tomography between modalities.

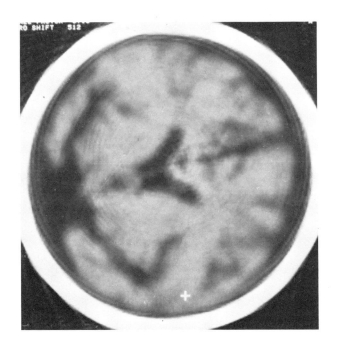

Fig. 7. Tomographic reconstruction of a slice of a human brain specimen. Neon ion radiographs.

Active heavy ion radiography with the MEDUSA. There are many advantages of the passive nuclear detector systems, among which are low background, continuous sensitivity and lack of limitations due to finite detector sizes. Among the disadvantages of passive detector systems are the bulkiness of the detector stacks and the time needed for processing and scanning the stacks. Our laboratory is engaged in a modest program toward the use of active, on line detector systems. Solid state position-sensitive detectors are being developed in our laboratory. Liquid position-sensitive counting systems, such as the argon time projection counters are also of definite interest. We report here on the development of a gaseous multiple wire imaging system.

The MEDUSA (Medical Dose Uniformity Sampler) was initially developed by Alonso et al.[9] to rapidly assess the uniformity of heavy ion fields used in medical research at the Bevalac. It consists of 16 multiple wire chambers deployed in a plane perpendicular to the beam direction. Each chamber has 60 parallel pairs of wires and the directions of the wires in different chambers divide the plane angle of 2Π into 16 parts. The integrated ionization is collected and stored between each pair of wires once for each beam pulse. The 960 measurements thus obtained for each beam pulse are then mathematically reconstructed into a planar image. This instrument can rapidly and with reasonable accuracy image beam distributions.

The Medusa was further developed into an instrument that can image residual range distributions by providing an appropriate range filter and by taking sequential images at different range values. When data of this type were obtained with a subject in the beam positioned to many different angles with respect to the beam direction, it became possible to image three dimensional electron density distributions. At present, the resolution of the device is limited by the wire spacing in Medusa and the size of the objects studied must be smaller than the useful diameters of the wire chambers in Medusa. The first three dimensional reconstructions obtained of a living subject, a dog, are shown as a-p, transverse and coronal slices in figure 8. One can clearly delineate the heart, rib cage, abdominal muscles, sternum, etc. and the visible detail appears to be about half of the wire spacing, or .15 cm.

In summarizing the experience with heavy ion radiography to date, we are impressed by the high electron density resolutions obtainable at very low doses with this technique. With further development of the tomographic techniques, heavy ions should be very useful for early detection of cancer. It is likely that the diagnostician will be aided by computerized preprocessing of the data obtained; many significant density differences show up with the present density scale of 1000 shades of grey. The eventual use of heavy ion radiographic techniques in relation to heavy ion therapy seems desireable: the quantitative stopping powers obtained by this method are the same numbers that must be used in quantitative therapy planning. X-ray tomography can supply some of these numbers when appropriate corrections are made, however near high density gradients it would be preferable to use heavy ion numbers. Active instruments, such as Medusa could be used on line and heavy ion images could be taken with the patient in position for therapy a few minutes before actual therapeutic exposures. The resolution is already good enough to detect unwanted shifts in organs, or volumes filled with gas; if Medusa information was available, appropriate shifts could be made each day in the therapy plan to account for the changes that have occurred in the patient. The information of heavy ion radiography is different from that of other diagnostic modalities and in conjunction with X rays, our diagnostic knowledge would be augmented.

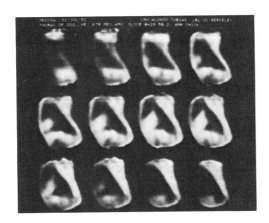

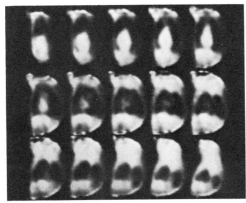

Fig. 8. Three dimensional reconstruction of the thorax of a dog. The Medusa instrument was used with 570 Mev/amu neon beam. 16 slices are shown, each 0.4 cm thick. Anterior-Posterior (top), transverse (middle), and coronal (bottom) sections are shown. Total dose 2.5 rad.

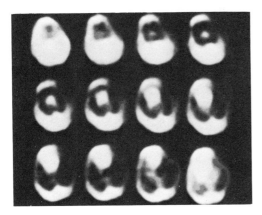

Heavy ion microscopy. There are several obstacles one must overcome in the electron microscopy of biological materials that limit the information obtainable: the wavelength of the electrons limits the absolute resolution, the radiation effects caused by the microscopy beam tend to destroy the structure of the specimen at high resolutions and microscopy must be carried out in vacuum on thin, dehydrated specimens.

The properties of protons and heavier ions are sufficiently different from those of electrons that we believe that heavy ion microscopy might some day become a useful adjunct to electron microscopy. The wavelength of heavy particles is much smaller than that of electrons at comparable velocities, so that the absolute limit to resolution is much lower. Heavy ions travel along nearly straight line trajectories, unlike electrons: because of this, high vacuum and highly dehydrated states are not conditions for effective microscopy. This is an important consideration: dehydration often causes derangement of biological microstructures and one would like to be able to look at fully hydrated cells and subcellular structures at high magnifications. It appears to be desirable to attempt to image biological structures with heavy particles in spite of the drawback that these particles, like electrons, also cause irreversible radiation effects that might alter the structures under observation.

Belanger et al. attempted to use alpha particles for microscopy in 1959.[10] More recently Yang et al.[11] and independently G. Kraft at the GSI accelerator laboratory in Germany developed a simple technique for heavy ion beam microscopy. During the last year Kraft visited Berkeley and we have joined our efforts.[12] We might call the current technique "heavy ion replica microscopy". The procedure, shown in figure 9, is quite simple. A biological specimen is placed on a clean sheet of mica or on a special plastic slab, a "resist". The specimen can be dry, hydrated or even a moist living cell. A beam of highly monoenergetic heavy ions is passed through the specimen and the particles are allowed to come to rest in the plastic. The particle fluence must be high enough so that a sufficient number of particles pass through each picture element to be resolved, and the particle energy should be barely greater than that necessary to cross the thickest part of the object. The resist is then "developed" in a strong hydrolysing agent; each particle produces a conical lesion, the apex of which determines the maximum depth of penetration. If the particle density is high enough, we obtain an etched out replica of the stopping power distribution of the specimen. This is a negative replica: it is shallow where the specimen is thick, and deep where the specimen is thin. A Van de Graaf accelerator or a particle ion source may have sufficient energy to supply

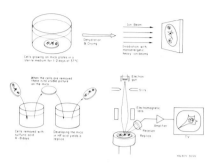

Fig. 9. Procedures for heavy ion
microscopy.

the necessary beam, but usually special efforts must be made to make the beam strictly monoenergetic, and a pure parallel stream of particles.

The replica can be examined by light microscopy or by scanning electron microscopy.[13] With the latter technique care must be taken not to melt and distort the replica. In figure 10 the helium ion replica micrograph of some muntjack chromosomes is shown. Our calculations show that the limiting resolution of this technique depends largely on the straggling and multiple scattering of the heavy particles. We believe that a practical resolution limit might be about 10 x the resolution of the optical microscope. This is an important domain for imaging: electron microscopes have much higher resolution, but often the structural integrity of the specimens is not preserved because of dehydration. The biological phases of the present program are concerned with imaging of chromosomes and of other subcellular particles. We plan to apply the method in a study of chromosome aberrations. It seems feasible to obtain three dimensional information by using tomographic techniques.

Heavy ion replica microscopy might be only the first step in the future field of heavy ion microscopy. It appears quite feasible to develop a heavy ion transmission scanning microscope that would combine high resolution with the ability to measure electron density distribution in tissue. It also seems feasible to use for imaging some of the fluorescent X rays generated in tissues by the beams and to obtain some information on the chemical composition. Finally, it is possible to image the recoil ions sublimed from the surface of the specimen as the particles strike the surface.[14]

180

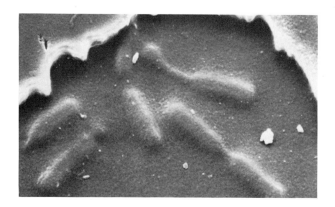

Fig. 10. Muntjack chromosomes with helium beam replica microscopy
using CR-39 plastic. The image seen here is that of an SCM scan.

B. APPLICATIONS OF SECONDARY BEAMS

Collisions of heavy ions with nuclei of resting matter produce a
fragmentation spectrum. Head on collisions often result in a multiplicity of
light and heavy fragments, and if the velocity of the primary projectile is high
enough, these fragments include mesons. The multiplicity of fragments increases
with the velocity of the beam: when this velocity is high, one can often
observe a central "jet" core of fragments travelling nearly parallel with the
beam and other fragments with much wider angular distribution. Many particles
of the jet are assumed to be generated with momenta comparable to that of the
primary projectile. Collisions of this type occur in space flight between
primary heavy cosmic rays and the nuclei of the spacecraft wall, and of the
astronauts; in the interest of safety of spaceflight, it is of interest to
explore the quality of the secondary radiation fields such events create and the
biological effects of the particle jets. Some preliminary studies have been
performed in the USSR by Akoyev.[15]

Radioactive fragments. In glancing collisions, there is usually just one
main fragment: this fragment usually retains a forward momentum very nearly the
same as that of the primary projectile is deposited in the absorber with a
definite range, as shown in an example in figure 11. Of special interest to

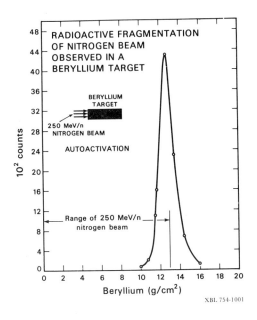

Fig. 11. The distribution of deposited 11-C radioactivity in Beryllium, produced by a 250 Mev/amu 14-N beam.

medicine are radioactive fragments. Carbon beams give rise to 11-C, and one finds 13-N, 15-0, 18-F and 19-Ne among the fragments produced by heavier beams. Tobias et al.[16] described some of the properties of "autoradioactivity". If the charge to mass ratio of the radioactive particles is different from that of the parent projectiles then one can electromagnetically separate a pure radioactive beam. For example Alonzo in our laboratory obtained a focused 19-Ne beam which had about 1% of the primary 20-Ne beam intensity. As is shown in figure 12, the radioactive beams have range energy relationships and Bragg curves similar to the parent beams, except that the energy spread is greater. As a radioactive beam deposits its particles in tissue the velocity of the particles slows down and they pick up electrons prior to coming to a complete stop. In this phase the particles behave as hot atoms, often free radicals or ion radicals, and they undergo chemical reactions with the molecules of biological matter. It might be possible in the future to analyse some of the reactions of radiation chemistry in this manner. After the particles stop in tissue, they become instantly deposited radioactive tracers, suitable for tracing flow or biochemical action. We believe that tracing of blood flow in brain, or measuring the speed of blood flow through heart valves might be eventually feasible. The beam radioactivity should be distinguished from target radioactivity: both are present in tissues exposed to heavy beams; however the target radioactivity produced by radioactive beams is relatively small.

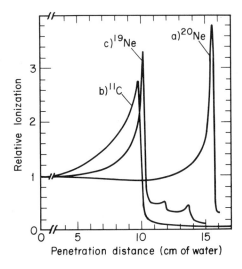

Fig. 12. Typical Bragg curves produced by 11-C and 19-Ne radioactive beams. Small contaminating peaks are shown in the 19-Ne beam. For comparison a stable 20-Ne Bragg curve is also shown.

Chattarjee et al.[17] are exploring the use of radioactive beams for localizing the region where heavy beams are deposited in tissue. If the majority of the deposited beam particles do not translocate, then imaging the distribution of radioactivity can serve to measure the stopping power of tissue and to check the adequacy of beam delivery in therapy. In order to be able to image the distribution of the short lived positron emitting beam particles in tissue, a special coincidence camera was built by J. Llacer (PEBA). The stopping region of a small radioactive beam can be determined within a few seconds with an accuracy better than 0.1 cm depth when the dose delivered by the beam is about 2 rad.

For the future, it appears quite feasible to plan accelerators with sufficient beam intensity to allow the use of radioactive beams for delivering therapeutic doses. The location of radioactivity would be constantly monitored and feedback information from the PEBA camera could be used to adjust the range of the beam while the dose is being delivered. When multiport irradiation is used to reach a small well defined region in the body, as in pituitary irradiation or when administering focal doses to small regions in the brain, the use of radioactive beams might be invaluable.

In the future it might also be possible to use radioactive beams for the synthesis of compounds with carrier free short lived isotopes. As the beam intensity increases, more and more radioisotopes will be available as beams. It is of course also possible to channel stable fragments. For example the use of beams of nuclei with neutron excess have been mentioned as tools of transuranium element research. The availability of such beams depends again on the possibility of having intense primary beams available. Fragment beams with neutron excess might also be useful as sources of fast neutrons with strong forward moments. In one proposal by D. Van Dyke such a beam might be used to scan a heavy metal target in order to obtain a scanned neutron source to be used for neutronography, for activation analysis of the body's elements or for therapy.

C. APPLICATIONS THAT RELATE TO DEPTH DOSE DISTRIBUTIONS

In addition to local therapy of cancer, the Bragg ionization characteristics of heavy ion beams make these uniquely suitable for basic scientific and medical investigations that require high doses in small local regions. There are three distinct types of particle induced lesions:

(a) Focal lesions. These are made deep in tissues by the Bragg peaks of small parallel beams of monoenergetic heavy ions. Sometimes multiple ports are used.

(b) Laminar lesions are usually made by the Bragg peaks of strictly monoenergetic heavy particles. The cross-sections of these lesions can be quite large. The lesions are arranged much like the narrow lamina of the brain: the affected cells are arranged in a sheath, parallel to the outer surface of the skin or to the surface of an artificial bolus.

(c) Knife edge lesions. To produce these, a parallel beam of particles is passed through a thin slit prior to entry into tissue. The lesions simulate the effects of cutting except that there is no bleeding, the effects develop gradually, and the width and severity of the "cut" can be accurately controlled.

Pituitary irradiation. The pituitary gland is located near the geometrical center of the skull in a bony cavity, the sella turcica. After initial studies with rats and primates demonstrated that shaped particle beams directed to the pituitary can safely produce states essentially identical to surgical hypophysectomy[18] pituitary proton and later helium irradiation became the first human therapeutic application of particle beams, beginning in 1955.[19] The first group of patients had metastatic, advancing mammary cancer and a number of significant regressions of metastatic lesions were achieved in this group. We now know that Bevalac carbon beams with their large peak to plateau ratios, and the capability to localize the Bragg peak of radioactive 11-C are probably even better suited for pituitary irradiation than proton or helium beams. In the future, attempts might be made to use radioactive Carbon beams for pituitary Bragg peak therapy of metastatic carcinoma.

Three additional medical studies were carried out at Berkeley on pituitary radiation with helium beams by a group of physicians under the leadership of J.H. Lawrence: treatment of advanced diabetes with vascular disease[21], treatment of acromegaly and of Cushing's disease.[22] The latter two are very successful and are being used routinely: pituitary irradiation for these diseases is being used at Harvard University and in Leningrad, USSR, in addition to Berkeley. The need for controlled statistical studies is indicated in the case of diabetes: the first series indicated that many patients can benefit from this procedure also.

Focal treatments of arteriovenous malformations in brain. Surgical excision or surgical ablation are the methods of treatment for intracranial arteriovenous malformations, vascular fistulae and acoustic neuromas. However when the CNS lesions are inoperable alternative methods are necessary. Conventional radiotherapy has been tried in the past and abandoned. Focal particle irradiation is being tested at the Harvard University proton cyclotron and at Berkeley with helium ions.[23] The particles are aimed at the tree of arterioles supplying the diseased region. The consequence of moderate particle doses and subsequent mild fibrosis is a reduction of blood flow, with a concommitant relief of pressure on the venous side of malformations. The use of Bragg peak treatment usually allows complete protection of essential regions of brain. The study is in its second year.

Focal lesions and homeostatic function. Many of the homeostatic functions of the body are controlled from hypothalamic nuclei. Bilateral ablation of specific sites results in profound alteration of the hypothalamic control of pituitary function and of other properties of the autonomic nervous system. Budinger et al.[24] have recently begun a study of the control of thyrotropic and somatotropic hormones from the hypothalamus. Several years earlier, the effects of focal lesions on the anterior and the posterior hypothalamic nuclei were explored with helium beams. Among the late effects observed were hypothalamic obesity, deficient rate of growth, imbalances in temperature control, capillary fragility, abnormal thyroid function, glycosuria, and behavoural alterations, such as rage. Large doses to the hypothalamus result in complete cessation of appetite and greatly reduced water turnover, hypothermia and eventual death.[18]

Other studies included a search for the regions of brain which control instinctive behaviour in pigeons[25] and a study of the control of water turnover.[26] Local particle irradiation has been shown to result in transient increases in the permeability of the blood brain barrier. This was demonstrated by observing the distribution of intravenously administered fluorescein.[27] Because of all the important functions of the hypothalamus, it is important to protect this region of the brain from high doses in radiotherapy. An important field that remains almost unexplored is the role of the hypothalamus in feedback carcinogenesis of the endocrine glands.

Laminar lesions in brain. The neural elements of the cerebrum and cerebellum are organized in highly differentiated lamina. It has been very difficult to study the anatomical interconnections and functions of each layer, because surgical intervention almost always involves cutting millions of nerve fibres in several adjacent layers. Using low energy monoenergetic heavy ions it has been possible to kill neurons in a very narrow laminar layer in mice and in rats.[28] The neurons with their soma in the lamina with the highest dose perish, but Krueger has demonstrated that injured fibres that cross the exposed layer can often regrow.[29] The long range heavy ions available at the Bevalac make it possible for the first time to produce relatively narrow laminar lesions in the brain of large mammals.

Knife edge lesions. Perhaps the most interesting applications of particle lesions were performed by Gaffey who has attempted to cut the corpus callosum in felis.[30] By directing the heavy ion beam in such a manner as to avoid the hypothalamus and pituitary, he was able to prepare animals without electrical connections between the two lobes of their cerebral hemispheres. In order to be successful, Gaffey had to produce a slit beam of several tenths of cm width. When the lesions are very narrow, the electrical impulses conducted in the fibres of the corpus callosum jump across the injured region. This procedure is entirely bloodless and is not a great hazard for the subject. Gaffey has been working on the foundations of a new therapeutic method for focal epilepsy. He believes that it is possible to electrically isolate the epileptogenic foci from the rest of the brain by using laminar and knife edge lesions and he has performed some intitial experiments to demonstrate the feasibility of this approach.[31]

SPECIAL LESIONS MADE BY HEAVY ION BEAMS IN BIOLOGICAL MATERIAL

In this section we return to the description of heavy ion damage at the cellular and molecular level. At high velocities, the energy density in the track is relatively low, and the particles behave as other low LET radiations. When the energy density in the track is high, higher order free radical reactions become important for the chemical and biological action. These can produce double strand scission in DNA with relatively high efficiency. When the track energy density is high we can also observe changes in the electrical and filtration properties of biological membranes.

Perhaps the most dramatic lesions are observed at very high LET, near the low energy stopping points of the tracks. A single densely ionizing particle is able to produce microscopically observable lesions in cells which have the appearance of channels or tunnels, when observed in the electron microscope.

Sensory and motor effects due to heavy ions. We know that ionizing radiation can cause passive permeability increases in the membranes of living cells. However, it usually takes high doses of X rays to demonstrate the existence of these effects. Madvanath has shown[32] that a single heavy ion, for example low energy accelerated carbon, is able to cause early lysis of cultured human lymphocytes; this effect appears to be related to membrane injury.

A variety of experiments were undertaken with the HILAC accelerator in an effort to demonstrate immediate effects on the nervous system. Individual pulses of 2 millisecond duration of monoenergetic heavy ions (e.g. Helium or Neon of about 6 Mev/amu) were applied to the cornea of conscious rabbits.[33] If the beam intensity was greater than a threshold value, and if the particles penetrated to a depth of about 140 micrometers where the temperature and pain sensing nerve endings reside, then corneal blinking reflexes were observed with a time delay of about 0.2 seconds. The reflex could be observed by electrically recording potentials from a muscle in the eyelid of the subject. The sensitivity of the cornea increased when a drop of the photodynamic dye eosin was placed on the cornea: anesthetic agents abolished the responses. The sensitivity was greatest when the laminar Bragg peak was placed into the receptor region.

It is known that in vivo most afferent nerve impulses originate in receptors or in specialized nerve endings. The cerebrum is usually quite insensitive to light, sound, pain, or extracellular electrical stimulation. Since heavy particle beams penetrate accurately to predetermined locations without the need for surgery, we decided to explore whether or not one could stimulate nerve action at precisely defined locations in brain by directing appropriate external heavy beams to the location. A device was built which could scan small helium beams of about 0.05 cm diameter. A bone flap was removed from the skull of anesthesized rats and trains of stimulating beam pulses were directed to the motor area on one side of the brain. A variety of motions were observed on the opposite side of the animals in response to the beam when the pulses were 2 milliseconds long and were applied at the rate of about 15/second. The responses, some minor and some violent, were elicited more readily when the beam was scanning over the brain during the period of stimulation. These experiments were difficult to conduct at the HILAC, because of the short useful range of the particles. It is planned to carry out similar experiments at the Bevalac.

Visual phosphenes. The American astronauts in the Apollo space flight series, which culminated in the first lunar landing, observed strange light flashes during their space flights. These were bright stars, streaks and clouds that could be seen with the eyes open or closed. Tobias and Budinger[34] demonstrated in high energy neutron and helium beams at the 184" cyclotron, and later with heavy ion beams at the Bevatron[35], that the effects are caused by individual heavy charged particles when these cross the retina. On a small number of volunteer human subjects it was demonstrated that the dark adapted human eye can perceive individual particles, if these have a linear energy transfer greater than about 10 kev/micron. The particles appear as bright bluish stars, straight streaks and occasional branching streaks, perhaps due to particle fragmentation. Earlier, in 1951, Tobias[36] predicted that heavy ions of cosmic rays could cause such phosphenes. The origin of these sensations appears to be in membrane effects caused in several visual receptor cells simultaneously by a single particle as it crosses these cells. Fluorescence of the vitreous fluid does not appear to be the principal cause. X ray phosphenes are different in appearance and in origin: X ray phosphenes appear as a blue or colored background: these apparently require a somewhat sustained radiation field impinging over a substantial part of the retina.

J. McNulty et al.[37] hypothesized that some of the effects observed by astronauts might have also been due to the Cerenkov effect, and this group has carried out several experiments at the Bevalac. We know that particles with velocities below the Cerenkov limit can cause streaks and stars: however, some of the observed phenomena, particularly the appearance of luminous clouds, might nevertheless be due to the Cerenkov effect. Patients who have been treated by helium beams at the 184" cyclotron in the head region, often observe large fluxes of luminous streaks and some of them also reported olfactory sensations caused by the beam. These sensations are instantaneous and are observed only when the beam is on. The odor reported is similar to that of certain detergents. Since we do not fully understand the manner in which either light or ionizing radiations cause sensations and phosphenes, the general area of membrane effects and action potentials is a challenging one for future heavy ion research.

Developmental effects. The effects of individual heavy ions have important consequences to the organism if these strike a location which controls the development and properties of a substantial segment of the organism. Small doses of heavy particles administered to the embryonic forms of organisms can cause macroscopic developmental malformations. In zea mays, individual heavy ions crossing the embryonic plant in a seed, cause multiple necrotic zones, amplified as the plant develops. This effect has been repeatedly observed in plants grown from seeds exposed to very low doses of space radiation (below one rad), in orbital space flights.[38] Very little work has been done in animals; however, an exploratory experiment was performed by Yang[39] using 600 Mev/amu accelerated iron nuclei (Z = 25). After delivering one rad dose on the 13th day of gestation to pregnant mice, about 30% of mouse embryos exhibited severe developmental malformations, whereas none were observed in an equal number of controls. More experiments must be done to obtain more accurate estimates of the magnitude of this effect.

Thermophysical lesions and the hazards of space radiations. It is well known that heavy ions can readily cause lattice dislocations in crystals. Sometimes these dislocations are arranged along the tracks of ionizing particles. In uranium oxide crystals a lesion was observed that is attributed to shock wave effects around the particle track.[40] Nuclear particle detectors are plastic or crystalline materials, where latent damage caused by heavy ions can be developed by etching with hydrolytic agents into macroscopically visible cylindrical holes or conical depressions.[41] It was demonstrated in our laboratory that heavy ions at very high LET can cause similar lesions in certain types of biological materials and that the lesions can grow in size and severity with the passage of time. The retinas of a group of rats flown into orbit were analysed by Philpot et al.[42], who saw lesions in the retina of these animals, which they attributed to the actions of single heavy cosmic rays. At Berkeley, 600 Mev/amu iron particles were used by Malachowski et al.[43] Groups of mice were exposed to low doses of 1 to 10 rad. Several months later the mice were sacrificed and studied by the techniques of scanning and transmission electron microscopy. Both techniques demonstrated lesions of one or more cell diameters, which penetrated through several cell layers. Some of these lesions, termed "tunnel lesions" are shown in figure 13. These lesions are much larger in size than the central hot core of tracks, which initially extend to a radius of about 10 to 20 nanometers away from the center of the track. Biological amplification or factors in the preparation of the specimens might have contributed to the appearance of the lesions observed.

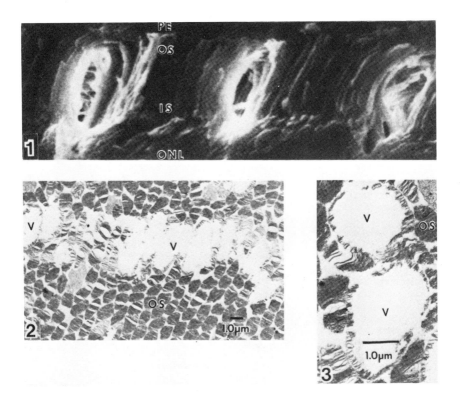

Fig. 13. Top: the appearance of "tunnel lesions" in the scanning electron microscope produced by accelerated iron nuclei in mouse retina. Bottom: the appearance of these lesions in the transmission electron microscope; many visual receptor cells are missing. Malachowski et al.[43]

In an unrelated study, Nelson exposed mouse corneas _in vivo_ to a variety of low and high energy heavy ion beams.[44] The corneas were obtained immediately after exposure, fixed in gluteraldehyde and studied in the scanning electron microscope without any additional etching procedures. Many conical or cylindrical lesions were seen: the diameter of these lesions correlated with the linear energy transfer of the particles and it was demonstrated that each particle can cause a single lesion. No such lesions were seen after various doses of X rays. Typical corneal heavy ion lesions are shown in figure 14. Tobias[45] advanced the hypothesis that such lesions develop under combined action

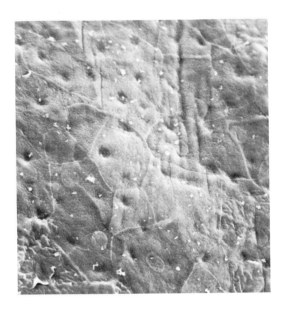

Fig. 14. Lesions at the surface of the mouse cornea
viewed by scanning electron microscopy. The depressions
were caused by single low energy argon nuclei. The
hexagonal outlines of cells and some nuclei are also
seen. From Nelson.[44]

of heat and free radicals; hence the name "thermophysical lesions". We know
that about 85% of the energy transfer from ionizing radiation escapes as heat.
In the core of heavy ion tracks there is so much local energy released that
instantaneously we expect high temperatures and pressures.

The composition of space radiation reflects the elemental composition of the
Universe. Although the dose in a 24 hour day in the solar system away from the
Earth is low, almost half of this is caused by fast heavy ions. The iron group
(atomic number 25) is prominent, but much heavier particles have also been
observed, with atomic numbers up to the 90's. On long space journeys and on the
surface of the moon and the planets, astronauts will be exposed to cumulative
doses of heavy space particles. If individual particles are highly efficient in
causing irreversible lesions in tissues that do not regenerate, then we can
expect a degree of health hazard from cosmic ray primaries. We can also ask how
large the carcinogenic and cataractogenic effects of heavy primaries are. Heavy
ion accelerators are unique facilities for studying space radiation effects.

SUMMARY AND OVERVIEW

We have demonstrated that accelerated heavy ions have potentially important roles in future biomedical research in a variety of fields, ranging from cancer research to brain research and developmental biology. The keys to these applications are in the special physical characteristics of the accelerated particles. The laws governing energy transfer, scattering and depth penetration suggest new applications in microscopy, radiography and nuclear medicine. Particles with high LET cause visual and olfactory sensations. Focal, laminar and knife edge lesions may have future roles in brain radiosurgery. Heavy ions produce special lesions in membranes, DNA and in specialized tissues: these are due to the high local energy density in heavy ion tracks.

REFERENCES

1. Tobias CA, Hayes TL, Maccabee HD, Glaeser RM (1967) Heavy ion radiography and microscopy. In Lawrence Berkeley Laboratory report UCRL 17357:108-120.
2. Tobias Ca, Benton EV, Capp MP (1979) Heavy ion radiography. In Lawrence JH (ed.), Recent Advances in Nuclear Medicine. 5:71-102.
3. Holley WR, Tobias CA, Fabrikant JI, LLacer W, Chu WT, Benton EV (1981) Computerized heavy ion tomography. SPIE Proc Intern Soc Opt Engr 273:283-293.
4. Benton EV, Henke RP, Tobias CA (1973) Heavy particle radiography. Science 182:474-476.
5. Crowe KM, Budinger TF, Calhoon JL, Elisher VP, Huesman RH, Kanstein LL (1975) Axial scanning with 900 Mev alpha particles. IEEE Trans Nucl Sci 63:322-339.
6. Steward P (1967) Calculation of stopping power. Lawrence Berkeley Laboratory Report UCRL-17314.
7. Fabrikant JI, Tobias CA, Capp MP, Holley WR, Woodruff KH, Sickles EA (1980) Lawrence Berkeley Lab Report LBL 11220:347-358.
8. Sommer FG, Capp MP, Tobias CA, Benton EV, Woodruff KH, Henke RP, Holley WR, Genant HK (1978) Int J Invest Radiol 13:163-170.
9. Alonso JR, Tobias CA, Chu WT (1979) Computed tomographic reconstruction of beam profiles with a multi-wire chamber. IEEE Trans Nucl Sci NS-26:3077-3079.
10. Belanger LF and C (1959) J Biophys Biochem Cytol 6:197.
11. Yang TC, Welch G, Tobias CA, Maccabee H, Hayes TL, Crause L, Benton EV, Abrams F (1978) The feasibility of heavy charged particle microscopy. Ann NY Acad Sci 306:322-339.
12. Kraft G, Yang CH, Richards T, Tobias CA (1980) Heavy ion microscopy. Lawrence Berkeley Laboratory Report LBL 11220:375-382.
13. Hayes TL, Tobias CA, Yand CY (1978) Heavy ion microscopy of hydrated cells with SEM imaging of the contact radiograph. Scanning Electron Micros 1:233-239.
14. Macfarlane RD, Torgerson DF (1976) Californium-252 plasma desorption mass spectroscopy. Science 191:990-925.
15. Akoyev IG, Fomenko BS et al.(1971) Determination of biological effectiveness of secondary irradiation with 90 Gev protons. Proc Internatl Cong Protect Against Acult Space Rad, Geneva CERN 233-243.
16. Tobias CA, Chattarjee A, Smith AR (1971) Radioactive fragmentation of N(7+) ion beam observed in a beryllium target. Phys Rev Letters 37A:119-120.

17. Chattarjee A, Alpen EL, LLacer J, Alonso JR, Tobias CA (1980) High energy beams of radioactive nuclei and their biomedical applications. Lawrence Berkeley Laboratory Report LBL 11220:383-388.

18. Tobias CA (1979) Pituitary radiation: Radiation physics and biology. In Linfoot D (ed.), Recent Advances in Diagnosis and Treatment of Pituitary Tumors. New York: Raven Press, 221-243.

19. Tobias CA, Lawrence JH, Born JL, McCombs RK, Roberts JE, Anger HO, Low Beer BVA, Huggins CB (1955) Pituitary radiation with high energy proton beams. Cancer Res. 18:121-134.

20. Lawrence JH, Linfoot JA, Born JL, Tobias CA, Chong CY, Akerlund MD, Manoogian E, Garcia JF, Connell GM (1975). Heavy particle irradiation of the pituitary. In Krayenbuhl H, Masters PE, Sweet WS (ed.), Progress in Neurol. Surg. 6:272-279. Skarger, Basle.

21. Linfoot JA (1979) Heavy ion therapy: alpha particle therapy of pituitary tumors. Linfoot D (ed.), Recent advances in the diagnosis and treatment of pituitary tumors. New York: Raven Press, 245-268.

22. Linfoot JA, Born JL, Garcia JF, Manougian E, Ling RP, Chong CY, Tobias CA, Carlson RA, Lawrence JH (1979). Metabolism and ophthalmological observations following heavy particle supressive therapy in diabetic retinopathy. In Goldberg MJ and Fine SL (ed.), Symposium on the treatment of diabetic retinopathy. Warrenton, Va.: Airlie House, 277-289.

23. Fabrikant JL, Budinger TF, Tobias CA, Born JL (1980) Focal lesions in the central nervous system. Lawrence Berkeley Laboratory Report LBL 11220:399-405.

24. Budinger TF, Linfoot JA, Moyer BR, Lyman JT, Pelletier TL (1977) Brain research with heavy ion beams. Lawrence Berkeley Lab Report LBL 5610:187-197.

25. Fabricius A. (1964) Behavioural effects of radiolesions in the brain of a pigeon. In Haley TJ and Snider RS (ed.), Response of the nervous system to ionizing radiation. Boston: Little, Brown & Co., 708-721.

26. Akerman B, Andersson B, Fabricius E and Svenson I (1960) Observations on the central regulation of body temperature and of food and water intake in the pigeon. Acta Physiol Scand 50:328-336.

27. Van Dyke DC, Janssen P, Tobias CA (1962) Fluorescein as a sensitive semiquantitative indicator of injury following alpha particle irradiation of the brain. In Haley JT and Snider RS (ed.), Response of the nervous system to ionizing radiation. New York: Academic Press, 362-382.

28. Malis LI, Loevinger R, Rose JE (1957) Production of laminar lesions in cerebral cortex by heavy ionizing particles. Science 126:302-303.

29. Kruger L, Clemente C (1964) Anatomical and functional studies of the cerebral cortex by means of laminar destruction with ionizing radiation. In Haley TJ and Snider RS (ed.), Response of the nervous system to ionizing radiation. Boston: Little, Brown & Co.

30. Gaffey CT, Montoya VJ (1973) Split brain cats prepared by radiosurgery. Int J Radiat Biol 24:229-242.

31. Gaffey CT, Montoya JV, Lyman JT, Howard J (1980) Restriction of the spread of epileptogenic discharges in cats by intracranial irradiations. Lawrence Berkeley Laboratory Report LBL 11220:407-414.

32. Madvanath U, Raju MR, Kelly LS (1976) Survival of human lymphocytes after exposure to densely ionizing radiation. In Radiation and the Lymphatic System, 125-139. Ballou IE, Chairman, ERDA Symp. Ser. 37, Washington, DC.

33. Tobias CA (1962) The use of accelerated heavy particles for production of radiolesions and stimulation in the central nervous system. In Haley JT, Snider RS (ed.), Response of the Nervous System to Ionizing Radiations. New York: Academic Press, 19-35.

34. Tobias CA, Budinger TF, Lyman JT (1971) Radiation induced light flashes observed in human subjects in fast neutron, X ray and positive ion beams. Nature, London, 228:260-261.

35. Tobias CA, Budinger TF, Lyman JT (1973) Biological effects due to single accelerated heavy particles and the problems of nervous system exposure in space. Life Sci in Space Res 11:233-245.
36. Tobias CA (1951) Radiation hazards in high altitude aviation. Aviat Med 23:345-372.
37. McNulty PJ (1971) Light flashes produced in the human eye by extremely reactivistic muons. Nature, London 234:111.
38. Slater JV, Tobias CA (1963) Effect of cosmic radiation on seed differentiation and development. Radiat Res 19:219.
39. Yang TC (1979) private communication.
40. Ronchi CJ (1973) The nature of surface fission tracks in UO2. J Appl Phys 44:3575-3585.
41. Fleischer RL, Price PB (1963) Tracks of charged particles in polymers. Science 140:1221-1222.
42. Philpott DE, Corbett RL, Turnbull C, Harrison G, Leaffer D, Black S, Sapp W, Klein G, Savik, LF (1978) Cosmic ray effects on the eyes of rats flown on Cosmos 782, Experiment K-007 Aviat Space Environment Med. 49: Part I, 19-28.
43. Malachowski MJ, Philpott DE, Corbett RL, Tobias CA (1981) Characteristic lesions in mouse retina irradiated with accelerated iron particles. 39th Ann Proc Electron Micros Soc Amer, Atlanta Ga, 590-591.
44. Nelson A (1980) Theoretical and observational analysis of individual ionizing particle effects in biological tissue. Ph.D. Thesis in Biophysics, University of California, Berkeley. LBL Report 11147rev.
45. Tobias CA, Chattarjee A, Malachowski MJ, Blakely EA, Hayes TL In Okada S et al (ed.) Proceedings of the Sixth International Congress of Radiation Research, Tokyo, May 13-19 1979. Tokyo: Japanese Association for Radiation Research: 146-156.

RADIATION BIOLOGY IN VITRO

RBE MAPPING IN PION BEAMS USING THE GEL TECHNIQUE

LLOYD D. SKARSGARD, BRANKO PALCIC AND GABRIEL K.Y. LAM
Medical Biophysics Unit, B.C. Cancer Research Centre and TRIUMF, University of
British Columbia, Vancouver, B.C.

INTRODUCTION

The process of star formation which occurs at the end of negative Π-meson
(pion) tracks results in the release of a variety of short-range, charged
nuclear fragments as well as more penetrating fast neutrons. Both of these
components are high LET and therefore have an associated increased RBE. In the
entrance region, however, pions are lightly ionizing and have a lower RBE. As a
consequence of these properties there are significant geographical variations in
RBE throughout pion dose distributions and these variations are influenced by a
number of parameters:

1. In the pion stopping region the RBE increases with depth to a maximum
   value at the distal edge of the stopping peak, where the fraction of dose
   due to stars is greatest.

2. As the width of the stopping peak is increased the overall or peak centre
   RBE is reduced as a consequence of the greater proportion of passing
   pions and a lower star dose fraction. This is partially offset by the
   increased neutron flux arising from the increased stopping volume.

3. Increasing the field size without altering the width of the stopping peak
   can be expected to increase the RBE, again by increasing the neutron
   flux. For large treatment volumes, it is possible that the neutron dose
   beyond the periphery of the pion stopping volume may give rise to an
   increased RBE in the penumbra region and beyond, although doses will be
   low.

4. The level of e^- and μ^- contamination in the pion beam will also influence
   the RBE throughout the dose distribution, as a result of their low LET
   contributions.

5. Elemental composition of the absorbing tissue may influence the RBE since
   the amount of energy imparted to charged fragments depends upon the
   capturing nucleus. For carbon and oxygen, for example, the dose due to
   charged fragments is quite different.[1]

Some of these effects have already been documented and have been described by
a number of authors.[2-6] They follow directly from the physical properties of
pions described elsewhere in this monograph.[7-9] The situation is complex enough

that it was evident from the outset it would be necessary to do some detailed mapping of the biological effect throughout pion treatment volumes if isoeffective dose distributions were to be obtained. To facilitate such radiobiological measurements with cultured cells, we devised a procedure which has come to be known as the Gel Technique.[10] This paper describes briefly the technique and some recent results obtained on the biomedical pion beam at TRIUMF.

THE GEL TECHNIQUE

The procedure involves irradiating mammalian cells suspended in a stiff gelatin matrix. After irradiation, the gel is sliced and the biological assay carried out. Spatial reconstruction of the biological effect then follows, allowing a detailed and accurate description of the radiobiological properties of the pion beam, as a function of position.

For the studies reported here, Chinese hamster ovary (CHO) cells were used. They were grown in spinner flasks in MEM alpha medium supplemented with 10% fetal calf serum. In preparation for irradiation, the cells were centrifuged and re-suspended in 37°C medium containing 25% gelatin (G8, Fisher Scientific) at a concentration of approximately 4×10^5 cells/ml. At 37°C, this mixture was a viscous fluid which could be poured into ABS (acrylonitrile butadiene styrene) plastic tubes, 30 cm long, 1.2 cm in diameter with a piston at one end. The tubes were then sealed, cooled to 0°C and irradiated in a phantom which also contained 25% gelatin.[5] This ensured that all particle paths traversed equivalent amounts of gelatin, an important consideration since the stopping power of 25% gel/medium is 1.08 x that of water. The entire phantom was placed in an ice water bath during the irradiations. For the experiments described here, the axis of the ABS tube was aligned with the axis of the pion beam. After irradiation, the tube was removed from the phantom, the gel was extruded and sliced, as shown in fig. 1, at intervals of 2 mm or greater along the tube axis. The slices were melted in 37°C medium and appropriate enocula were plated into 5 cm petri dishes for assay of cell survival. After 8 days incubation, colonies were stained and counted.

Gelatin dialysis

Before preparation of the 25% gelatin/medium mixture, it is necessary to extensively dialyse the gelatin to remove toxic products (presumably low molecular weight components such as amino acids, etc.). This is done by preparing a solution of 40% gelatin in hot, double-distilled water, autoclaving it, and then dialysing it for 7 days at 4°C against serum free growth medium.

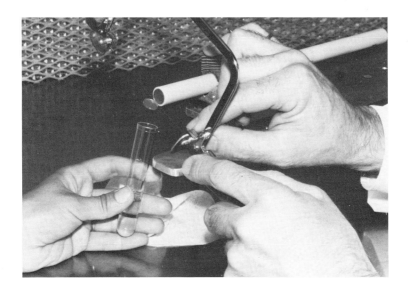

Fig. 1. The gel slicing procedure. The gel/medium is extruded and sliced at intervals of 2 mm or more. Each 2mm slice contains 10^5 cells, which are resuspended by melting the gel/medium in 5 ml of warm medium.

The dialysate is changed daily. The cold dialysis procedure minimized the uptake of water by gelatin and produces a solution that is 27-30% gelatin at the end of dialysis. Additional medium is then added to give a 25% gelatin solution in normal medium (without serum).

TABLE 1

A comparison of the composition of soft tissue and 25% gelatin.

Element	Soft tissue	25% Gelatin/medium
H	10.2	10
C	12.3	12
N	3.5	4.5
O	72.9	73
S,P	0-3	

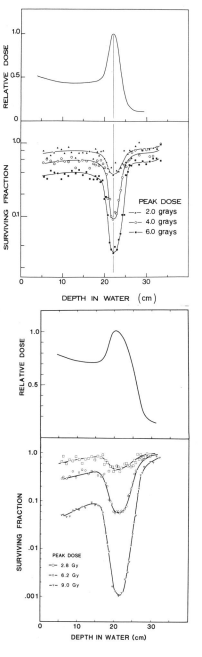

Fig. 2. Pion dose and cell survival vs. depth for a narrow peak, unmodulated pion beam (180 MeV/c). Survival of CHO cells was measured in 25% gelatin/medium at 0°C with a pion dose rate of 0.12 Gy/min. Three survival profiles are shown for peak doses of 2.0, 4.0 and 6.0 Gy.

Fig. 3. Pion dose and cell survival vs. depth for an unmodulated pion beam, momentum slits fully open. CHO cells irradiated in 25% gel/medium at 0°C, pion dose rate 0.16 Gy/min. Peak doses of 2.8, 6.2 and 9.0 Gy.

Although much lower gelatin concentrations would be sufficient to provide a supporting matrix for the cells, solutions containing 25% gelatin are used because their elemental composition matches very closely that of soft tissue, as can be seen in Table 1. Because the yield of pion star products is dependent upon the elemental composition of the absorbing medium, this is an important consideration in the design of an appropriate in vitro test system.[1]

A number of control experiments were carried out which established that the presence of gelatin and the low temperature conditions before and during irradiation did not significantly alter the cellular radiation response.[11]

RESULTS

Figure 2 shows this technique applied to a measurement of cell inactivation along the axis of a beam of relatively monoenergetic pions. The width of the pion stopping peak at 80% of maximum is 2.5 cm (upper frame). The cell survival profiles, shown in the lower frame, easily resolve the abrupt changes in dose which occur at the stopping peak. The three survival profiles shown in this figure represent three gel tubes which received doses of 2.0, 4.0 and 6.0 Gy at the peak of the stopping distribution.

When the momentum slits in the beam line are fully opened to accept pions of all momenta (180 ± 13 MeV/c), the stopping peak is broadened as shown in the upper frame of fig. 3, and the peak-to-plateau dose ratio is decreased. The resulting survival vs. depth profiles for this unmodulated beam are shown in the lower frame of fig. 3 for peak doses of 2.8, 6.2 and 9.0 Gy. In order to maximize our dose rate, this beam tune is used together with the range shifter described by Dr. Lam[7], to provide modulated beams of the desired stopping width and shape.

Figure 4 shows dose and cell survival profiles obtained using the range shifter to modulate the beam tune of fig. 3 to provide a nominal peak width of 10 cm. Although the dose is essentially constant from 9 to 19 cm depth, the cell survival profiles show unequivocally that the RBE increases with depth in the stopping region, even for this extended peak. In all, eight such survival profiles were obtained in this experiment, for a range of peak doses from 1.5 Gy to 9.0 Gy. In order to obtain survival vs. dose responses from such a family of profiles, one can either fit a mathematical model to the data, as we have done[12], or one can construct cross-plots of these data as indicated in fig. 5. This figure shows, in the first frame, the procedure used in obtaining the cross-plots which are given for proximal, centre and distal positions in the stopping peak as well as a position downstream from the peak. The x-ray response measured at the same time on the same cell population is shown for

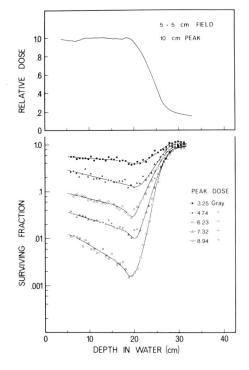

Fig. 4. Pion dose and cell survival vs. depth for a modulated pion beam, generated by range-shifting the beam of fig. 3 so as to produce an extended peak of 10 cm width. Nominal field size 5 cm x 5 cm. Survival of CHO cells measured in 25% gel/medium at 0°C, pion dose rate 0.15 Gy/min.

comparison (270 kVp, half value layer: 1.5 mm Cu). The solid curves in figs. 5(b) to 5(f) represent least-squares fits of the linear quadratic expression

$$\ln S = -\alpha D - \beta D^2$$

to the data shown in each figure. These fitted responses without the data points are grouped together for comparison in fig. 6. It can be seen that the data form a consistent set (the α and β values were fitted individually for each depth) from which RBE values can readily be calculated for any desired survival level.

Effect of Field Size

In order to explore the effect of field size on RBE, a beam tune was developed which gave a depth-dose profile essentially identical to that of fig. 3 (upper frame) but with a nominal field size four times larger, 10 cm x 10 cm. Again a family of survival profiles was generated by irradiating a series of gel tubes to various peak doses. Two of these profiles are shown in fig. 7, compared to results for the smaller field (5 cm x 5 cm). Both sets of data were

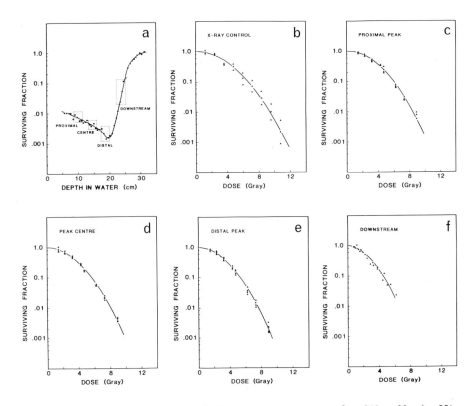

Fig. 5. The construction of Survival vs. Dose responses for CHO cells in 25% gel/medium exposed to x-rays or pions:

(a) Typical pion S vs. depth profile showing data-pooling procedure for cross-plots
(b) 270 kVp x-rays
(c) Proximal peak
(d) Peak centre
(e) Distal peak
(f) Downstream

For pions, data points are those from 8 individual profiles (five of which are shown in Fig. 4) extracted from positions indicated by the frames in (a).

obtained in the same experiment from the same cell population, minimizing systematic errors. The larger field gave consistently lower survival in the peak region for comparable doses, in agreement with the expectation that an increased neutron flux from the larger field would give a higher RBE.

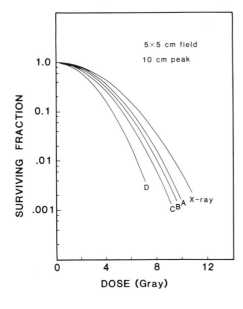

Fig. 6. Summary of the CHO cell survival responses shown in fig. 5 b-f. Only the fitted responses are shown for:
x-rays
Proximal peak pions   A
Peak centre pions   B
Distal peak pions   C
Downstream pions   D

Data are for 10 cm stopping peak, 5 cm x 5 cm field, 0.15 Gy/min.

Again, from families of profiles for each field size, cross-plots were constructed to yield survival vs. dose responses using the procedure illustrated in fig. 5(a). The cross-plots pertaining to the peak centre position for each of the two field sizes are compared in fig. 8; the larger field can be seen to be somewhat more effective. Though the effect is small, essentially the same result has been seen in 4 separate experiments so we are satisfied that the effect is real.

This result led us to question whether larger treatment volumes might lead to higher RBE values outside the treatment volume as well, for example in the beam entrance region, as a result of the greater neutron flux that might be present. To date, however, we have not been able to detect field size dependent changes in RBE in the entrance (plateau) region.

Uniform Biological Effect

The preceding survival vs. depth profiles, obtained from "flat-top" depth dose distributions (uniform dose throughout the peak region), make it clear that if one is to obtain a uniform radiobiological effect to a specified treatment volume with a single pion beam port, the dose profile must be re-shaped,

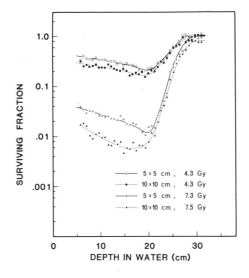

Fig. 7. Dependence of biological effect on pion field size. CHO cell survival vs. depth for pion beams of 5 cm x 5 cm (open symbols) and 10 cm x 10 cm (closed symbols). Pion stopping peak width was 10 cm for both fields (see fig. 4).

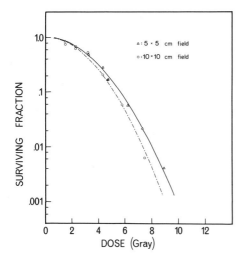

Fig. 8. Survival vs. dose for small field (5 cm x 5 cm) and large field (10 cm x 10 cm) pion beams. Stopping peak width was 10 cm in both cases, uniform dose. This cross-plot was constructed for the peak centre position (see fig. 5d). Data extracted from a single experiment, 15 individual profiles, 4 of which are shown in fig. 7.

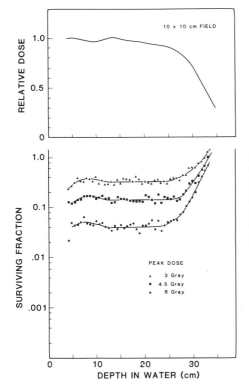

Fig. 9. Pion dose and cell survival vs. depth for a pion beam modulated so as to produce uniform biological effect throughout the stopping region. Nominal field size 10 cm x 10 cm. Survival of CHO cells measured in 25% gel/medium at 0°C, pion dose rate 0.04 Gy/min.

reducing the dose at the distal side of the peak to compensate for the increased RBE. In fig. 9 is shown a "slope-top" dose profile shaped according to the dose response differences of fig. 6. It can be seen that dropping the distal dose by approximately 10% has produced a reasonably uniform biological response throughout the stopping region, at least for the end point used in these experiments: survival of CHO cells following single pion doses. Some verification in vivo is necessary.

RBE SUMMARY

Table 2 presents a summary of RBE values for a few representative dose distributions measured at TRIUMF using the gel technique. Since they are derived from single-dose studies, the RBE values are smaller than will be observed in fractionated dose exposures in vivo.[6,13] A number of general features are evident from these data:

- For all of the stopping distributions, RBE clearly increases with increasing depth in the peak region, as a result of the increasing star dose fraction.
- If the field size is fixed (5 cm x 5 cm) but the peak width is increased from 5 cm to 10 cm, the RBE decreases since passing pions contribute a larger proportion of the dose.
- For a fixed peak width (10 cm) the RBE increases when the field size is increased from 5 cm x 5 cm to 10 cm x 10 cm, presumably due to the increased neutron dose.
- Maximum RBE is observed on the downstream side of the stopping peak where there are very few passing pions and most of the dose is due to stars (the downstream position is taken as the point where the dose is approximately one-half of the peak dose).
- RBE values in the entrance region seem generally to be somewhat greater than 1.0, though values are less accurately known both here and in the downstream position since the doses are lower and the response function is less well defined.

TABLE 2

RBE vs DEPTH for Various Π^- Beams at TRIUMF: Measured in CHO cells at S = 0.1

PION BEAM	RBE				
	Plateau	Proximal	Centre	Distal	Downstream
MODULATED 5 cm Peak 5 x 5 cm Field	1.16	1.22	1.24	1.39	1.48
MODULATED 10 cm Peak 5 x 5 cm Field		1.11	1.18	1.26	1.47
MODULATED 10 cm Peak 10 x 10 cm Field		1.22	1.27	1.32	1.59
UNMODULATED 5 x 5 cm Field	1.10		1.29		1.37

Uncertainties: ± 5% to ± 10% (estimated)

The dependence of RBE on depth in the stopping region and on width of the stopping peak has been observed both at LAMPF[14,15] and at TRIUMF[3-6,12], with comparable results. The field size effect[16] has not yet been confirmed in biological studies elsewhere. One consequence of the field size effect is that it may make the biological effectiveness of different treatment volumes more or less equal, since peak width and field size are parameters which influence the RBE in opposite directions. This would tend to simplify the clinical use of pion beams, since typically the two parameters will increase or decrease in concert when going from one treatment volume to another.

On the other hand, if a mathematical model is to be used to predict the biological effectiveness of new dose distributions, the field size effect described here suggests that the model must incorporate a neutron contribution. The model described by Lam and Henkelman[12] and which we have used in the past would not have predicted the increased effectiveness of the 10 cm x 10 cm field reported here since it characterizes the pion depth dose only in terms of star dose and total dose.

ACKNOWLEDGMENTS

The cooperation of TRIUMF staff in carrying out the pion irradiations is gratefully acknowledged, as is the skillful technical assistance of I. Harrison, D. Douglas, N. McKinney and H. Adomat. The x-ray dosimetry was capably carried out by Dr. R. Kornelsen.

REFERENCES

1. Jackson DF, Lewis CA, O'Leary K, Lam GKY (1982) Molecular effects in pion capture in complex materials. Nature 245:557-560.
2. Raju MR (1980) Heavy Particle Radiotherapy. New York: Academic Press: 356-450.
3. Skarsgard LD, Henkelman RM, Lam GKY, Palcic B, Poon MN (1979) Pre-clinical studies of the negative pi-meson beam at TRIUMF. Rad and Environm Biophys 16:193-204.
4. Skarsgard LD (1979) The biological properties of pions. In Okada S et al (ed.) Proceedings of the Sixth International Congress of Radiation Research, Tokyo, May 13-19 1979. Tokyo: Japanese Association for Radiation Research: 788-801.
5. Skarsgard LD, Henkelman RM, Lam GKY, Palcic B, Eaves CJ, Ito A (1979) Pre-clinical studies of negative pi-mesons at TRIUMF. In Abe M, Sakamoto K, Phillips TL (eds.) Treatment of Radioresistant Cancers. New York: Elsevier/North-Holland: 127-144.
6. Skarsgard LD, Henkelman RM, Eaves CJ (1980) Pions for radiotherapy at TRIUMF. J Can Assoc Radiol 31:3-12.
7. Lam CKY, Skarsgard LD (1982) Physical aspects of the pion beam at TRIUMF. In Skarsgard LD (ed.) Pion and Heavy Ion Radiotherapy: Pre-clinical and Clinical Studies. New York: Elsevier/North-Holland (these proceedings).

8. Dicello JF, Brenner DJ (1982) Radiation quality of beams of negative pions. In Skarsgard LD (ed.) Pion and Heavy Ion Radiotherapy: Pre-clinical and Clinical Studies. New York: Elsevier/North-Holland (these proceedings).

9. Harrison RW (1982) Determination of dose distributions for scanned pion beams at TRIUMF. In Skarsgard LD (ed.) Pion and Heavy Ion Radiotherapy: Pre-clinical and Clinical Studies. New York: Elsevier/North-Holland (these proceedings).

10. Skarsgard LD, Palcic B (1974) Pretherapeutic research programmes at Π^- meson facilities. In Proceedings of the XIII International Congress of Radiology, Madrid, October 15-20 1973, International Congress Series No. 339, Radiology 2:447-454.

11. Henkelman RM, Lam KY, Harrison RW, Shortt KR, Poon M, Lang H, Jaggi BW, Palcic B, Skarsgard LD (1977) Progress during the first year of operation of the Batho Biomedical Facility at TRIUMF. TRIUMF Report TRI-77-2: 1-22.

12. Henkelman RM, Lam GKY (1978) Prediction of biological effect of pion irradiation using the star distribution to determine the high LET dose. In Booz J, Ebriot HG (eds.) Proceedings of the Sixth Symposium on Microdosimetry Brussels, May 22-26 1978 London: Harwood Academic Publishers: 497-506.

13. Douglas BG (1982) Pion beam studies in mice and in pigs. In Skarsgard LD (ed.) Pion and Heavy Ion Radiotherapy: Pre-clinical and clinical STudies. New York: Elsevier/North-Holland (these proceedings).

14. Raju MR, Amols HI, Bain E, Carpenter SG, Cox RA, Robertson JB (1978) Cell survival as a function of depth for modulated negative pion beams. Int J Radiat Oncol Biol Phys 4:341-344.

15. Raju MR, Amols E, Bain E, Carpenter SG, Cox RA, Robertson JB (1979) OER and RBE for negative pion beams of different peak widths. Br J Radiol 52:494-498.

16. Skarsgard LD, Palcic B, Lam GKY (1980) RBE and OER values for the TRIUMF biomedical pion beam. Radiat Res 83:471.

OXYGEN ENHANCEMENT RATIO AND SPLIT DOSE RECOVERY WITH PION BEAMS

BRANKO PALCIC, MLADEN KORBELIK AND LLOYD D. SKARSGARD
B.C. Cancer Research Centre, Medical Biophysics Unit, 601 West 10th Avenue,
Vancouver, B.C. Canada

INTRODUCTION

Stopping negative pions are captured by atomic nuclei which then disintegrate causing "star formation". This results in high LET radiation. Thus, in the pion peak region, one obtains an increased relative biological effectiveness (RBE) as well as a decreased oxygen enhancement ratio (OER). Cellular recovery is also affected; some reports in the literature suggest that there is no cellular recovery in split dose experiments when cells are irradiated with pions in the peak region.[1,2] We have examined these properties (RBE, OER and split dose recovery) with an unmodulated pion beam at TRIUMF and we report in this work a decreased OER as well as a reduced but still significant recovery of cells irradiated with negative pions in the peak region.

MATERIALS AND METHODS

Chinese hamster cells of the CHO line were grown in spinner cultures and were diluted daily. Asynchronous cells were suspended in 10% gelatin in growth medium (gel/med) which is a viscous fluid at 37°C. Aliquots of 0.5 ml of cell suspension (2×10^5 cells/ml) were loaded into 5 ml glass tubes which were then immediately immersed in ice-cold water so that the gel/med suspension hardened. Ice-cold medium, 4.5 ml was then pipetted over the gel/med and the tubes were capped with a silicone stopper.

Hypoxic cells were prepared in a similar way except that more cells were resuspended in 10% gel/med yielding a higher cell concentration (2×10^6 cells/ml). The cells were made hypoxic by flowing purified nitrogen for 2 hours at 37°C over the cell suspension (0.5 ml in 5 ml glass tube). The cells were cooled to 4°C, 4.5 ml of hypoxic cold medium was added to the hardened gel/med and the tubes were sealed with a silicone stopper. This was followed by additional gassing of overlayed medium by bubbling purified N_2 for 1 hour while the samples were kept at 4°C.

A special holder was built from plexi-glass such that glass tubes could be placed at various depths in the pion beam. The tubes were immersed in a 4°C water phantom during irradiation. After irradiation (10 - 25 rads/minute) the tubes were warmed to 37°C and the cells were counted and plated.

For split dose experiments, cells were washed in growth medium after irradiation, placed in plastic tubes and incubated in medium at 37°C in a water bath. The tubes were gently agitated every 5 minutes to keep cells in suspension. At the prescribed times, the incubation was terminated, the cells were centrifuged and re-suspended in 10% gel/med (0.5 ml in 5 ml glass tube). The cells were again cooled to 4°C, overlayed by 4.5 ml cold medium and irradiated with the second dose, as described above.

Following 7 days incubation, the colony forming ability of the cells was determined using standard procedures.

An unmodulated pion beam was used throughout these experiments. Midline momentum for the beam was 180 MeV/c with a spread of ± 7% Δ p/p; x-ray irradiations served as the control (270 KvP, HVL 1.5 mm Cu). The peak width was approximately 7 cm at 80% of the peak dose level. Further details of the beam characteristics at TRIUMF can be obtained elsewhere.[3] Dosimetry for both x-rays and pi-mesons was based on calibrations using Spokas tissue equivalent ionization chambers (0.1 and 0.5 cm^3).

RESULTS

a) RBE for cells irradiated in test tubes

The dose at various depths in the pion beam was measured in a water phantom using an ionizing chamber (figure 1). Test tubes, containing cells in 10%

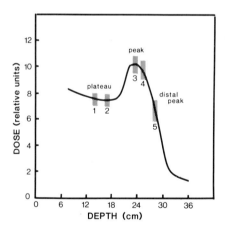

Figure 1: Depth dose profile of an unmodulated beam (midline momentum 180 MeV/c, $FW_{0.8}$ = 7 cm), measured in a water phantom. Cells were placed at the indicated positions on the dose profile such that two samples were in the plateau region, two in the peak region and one in the distal peak region.

gel/med were positioned on the pion beam axis; incoming pions passed through various materials (plexi glass of test tube support rack, glass walls of test tubes, 10% gel/med) before reaching the cells. Corrections were determined for the different stopping powers of these materials compared with water, and the cells then placed at the corrected depths.

The use of glass test tubes instead of gel/med cylinders[4], did not significantly change the survival response of irradiated cells or the measured RBE values for negative pions in this beam tune. An example of the survival response for the peak position when cells were irradiated in glass test tubes is shown in figure 2a and the summary of all experiments using glass tubes is presented in figure 2b. In these experiments, cells received single exposures

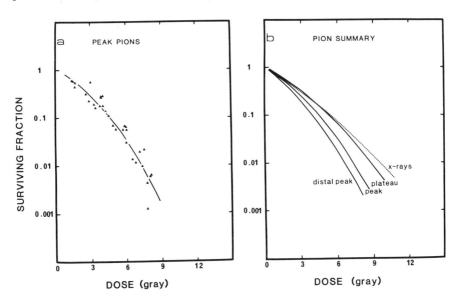

Figure 2: Cells were irradiated at 4°C in 10% gel/med. In figure 2a all experimental points shown were obtained in the pion peak position. The solid curve is the best fit (least squares method) to a linear quadratic function: ln S = aD + bD². In figure 2b a summary of all positions: plateau, peak, and distal peak as well as x-rays is presented. For clarity of presentation, data points are omitted, but the survival curves were obtained from a similar number of experimental points and by the same method as in figure 2a.

to the dose indicated, while cells were kept at 4°C. The dose rate was approximately 20 rads/minute for pion irradiations and 190 rads/minute for x-rays.

For each exposure, two samples were positioned in the plateau region, two in the peak region and one in the distal peak region. From the complete survival curves (figure 2b), the RBE values can be determined at different survival levels. Average values of 1.25 and 1.40 were found for peak pions and distal peak pions, respectively, in the survival region between 0.1 and 0.01. This compares well to the values measured for the same unmodulated pi-meson beam using gel/med cylinders, where values of 1.3 and 1.4 were obtained.[4,5]

b) Oxygen enhancement ratio

The oxygen enhancement ratio was measured in a manner similar to that described above, except that only the peak pion positions were examined. Aerobic and hypoxic samples were irradiated at 4°C with single exposures. Figure 3 shows the results of a typical OER experiment. From the survival curves, the OER values for x-rays and peak pions were calculated at S = 0.1 and

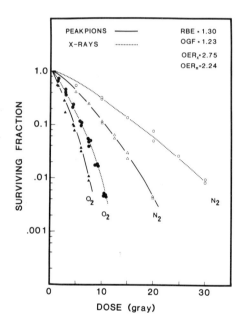

Figure 3: The oxygen enhancement ratio for peak pions and x-rays was measured by irradiation of hypoxic (open symbols) or aerobic cells (closed symbols). Cells were suspended in 10% gel/med during irradiation at 4°.

and S = 0.01 and found to be 2.75 and 2.95 respectively for x-rays and 2.25 and 2.35 for peak pions. One thus finds a decreased oxygen effect with peak pions, to approximately 80% of that obtained with x-rays, yielding an oxygen gain factor (OGF) of 1.24.

Several experiments of this type were performed yielding similar results. The summary of all these experiments as well as the results on the effect of a hypoxic radiosensitizer, misonidazole, in the peak pion region of unmodulated pion beam will be reported elsewhere.

c) Split dose experiments

Split dose recovery was also measured in the peak region and in the plateau region using the same beam tune. Again, cells were placed in 10% gel/med in glass tubes and irradiated at 4°C to the first dose. The cells were then washed free of gelatin, resuspended in growth medium and incubated at 37°C for a prescribed time. At that time the cells were resuspended in 10% gel/med for the second irradiation, also at 4°C. In the first experiment, figure 4, cells were irradiated to two equal doses of the same modality. The exposure dose for each

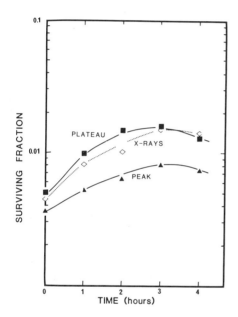

Figure 4: CHO cells were first exposed to a single dose of x-rays, plateau pions or peak pions to decrease surviving fraction to approximately 0.05. Total doses for plateau pions, x-rays and peak pions were 9.4, 10 and 8.1 Gy, respectively). Following the first irradiation, the cells were washed free of gelatin, resuspended in growth medium and incubated at 37°C for the indicated times. The second exposure was then delivered while the cells were again placed at 4°C in gel/med. The second dose was equal to the first dose and was delivered with the same modality.

modality was chosen such that the survival of x-rays, plateau pions and peak pions would be approximately the same if the total dose were delivered in a single exposure. In all cases, including peak pions, split dose recovery is demonstrated. It appears from this and other experiments (not shown here) that the first peak of split dose recovery lies between 3 and 4 hours.

In the second set of experiments, full survival curves were obtained for both single and split dose exposures. For the split dose experiment cells were first irradiated to a dose which decreased the surviving fraction to approximately 0.1 and then, after incubating the cells for 3.5 hours at 37°C under growth

216

conditions, the second dose was delivered to give the full survival curve. The results of a typical experiment are shown in figure 5a and 5b where the survival response of cells to plateau and peak pions is compared. Again, split dose recovery is clearly demonstrated in both cases.

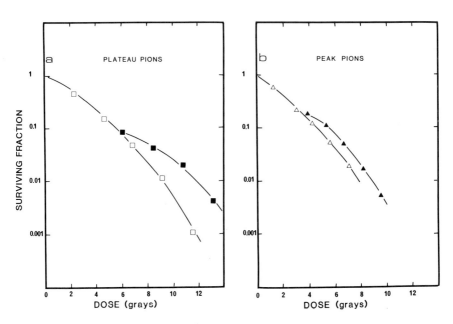

Figure 5: Cells were treated in exactly the same way as described in figure 4. They were incubated in growth medium for 3.5 hours in the split dose experiment (closed symbols). Open symbols represent the survival response for a single exposure experiment. Plateau pions, figure 5a and peak pions, figure 5b.

DISCUSSION

The reduction in OER for peak pions reported here can be compared to other unmodulated negative pion beams. A review of all the data for various endpoints has been recently published.[6] A range of OGF values from 1.2 to 2.0 has been reported[7,8,9,10] for the survival of mammalian cells, although most measured values are in the range 1.2 - 1.5, in reasonable agreement with the value reported here. Factors such as the source of x- or gamma-rays used for comparison and the survival level at which the OER is determined could contribute to differences in OGF values obtained at different laboratories.

Yuhas et al., using a pion beam at Los Alamos, reported that the split dose recovery phenomenon was absent if mammalian cells were irradiated with peak pions.[1,2] They also reported a substantially reduced shoulder in the survival curves obtained in single dose experiments. We have not observed such a complete removal of the shoulder, though pions do seem to reduce it somewhat. Figure 4 and 5, however, clearly demonstrate the presence of split dose recovery, the extent of which is essentially comparable for 10 Gy of x-rays and 9.4 Gy of plateau pions (see fig. 4). For peak pions, recovery is still present though it is significantly reduced.

We found that washing cells free of gelatin, for the period of incubation between fractionated doses was essential in order to demonstrate split dose recovery. If gelatin was present during the incubation period, even recovery from x-rays was completely inhibited. There may well be other conditions associated with handling the cells which could prevent or diminish the magnitude of split dose recovery during this period.

ACKNOWLEDGMENTS

The co-operation of the TRIUMF staff is gratefully acknowledged and in particular the skillful technical assistance of R.W. Harrison, N. McKinney, I. Harrison and H. Adomat. The authors would also like to thank Drs. G.K.Y. Lam and R.M. Henkelman for preparing the pion beam tune and numerous discussions. This work was supported by the B.C. Cancer Foundation and the National Cancer Institute of Canada.

REFERENCES

1. Yuhas JM, Li AL, Kligerman MM (1979) Present status of the proposed use of negative pi mesons in radiotherapy. In Lett JT, Adler H (ed.), Advances in Radiation Biology. New York: Academic Press, 51-83.
2. Kligerman MM, Wilson S, Tanaka Y, Burmester J, Hogstrom KR, Yuhas JM (1981) Response of multicellular tumor spheroids to multiple fractions of negative pi mesons and x rays. Int J Radiat Oncol Biol Phys 7:923-927.
3. Henkelman RM, Lam GKY, Harrison RW, Poon M, Shortt KR (1978) Tuning of the biomedical negative pion beam line at TRIUMF. Nuclear Instruments and Methods 155:317-324.
4. Skarsgard LD, Henkelman RM, Lam GKY, Palcic B, Eaves CJ, Ito A (1979) Pre-clinical studies of negative pi-mesons at TRIUMF. In Abe M, Sakamoto K, Phillips TL (ed.), Treatment of radioresistant cancers. Elsevier/North-Holland Biomedical Press, 127-144.
5. Skarsgard LD, Palcic B (1982) RBE mapping in pion beams using the gel technique. In Skarsgard LD (ed.) Pion and Heavy Ion Radiotherapy: Pre-clinical and Clinical Studies. New York: Elsevier/North-Holland (these proceedings).
6. Skarsgard LD (1979) The biological properties of pions. In Okada S et al (ed.) Proceedings of the Sixth International Congress of Radiation Research, Tokyo, May 13-19 1979. Tokyo: Japanese Association for Radiation Research: 788-801.

7. Raju MR, Richman C (1972) Negative pion radiotherapy: physical and radiobiological aspects. Curr Top Radiat Res Quart 8:159-233.

8. Raju MR, Amols HI, Bain E, Carpenter SG, Cox RA, Robertson JB (1979) OER and RBE for negative pion beams of different peak widths. Br J Radiol 52:494-498.

9. Weibezahn KF, Dertinger H, Schlag H and Lucke-Huhle C (1979) Biological effects of negative pions in monolayers and spheroids of chinese hamster cells. Radiat Environ Biophys 16:273-277.

10. Vainson AA, Shmakova NL, Meshcherikova T, Fadeeva TA, Iarmonenko SP (1977) Radiobiological parameters of pi-mesons. Radiobiologiia 17:874-880.

BIOLOGICAL PROPERTIES OF SINGLE - AND MULTIPORT PION BEAMS: STUDIES ON REPAIR,

RBE AND OER WITH MUTATION INDUCTION (DROSOPHILA), MOUSE FOOT AND MAMMALIAN CELLS

HEDI FRITZ-NIGGLI
Radiobiological Institute of Zurich University
P.O. Box 64, CH-8029 Zurich, Switzerland

Since the end of 1974, when the single biomedical πE3-beam at SIN (Swiss

Institute for Nuclear Research) was available for radiobiological research, a

variety of preclinical studies have been performed. They were restricted by the

dose rates between 3 - 30 cGy/min to very sensitive systems and to experiments

with single doses (see reviews of Fritz-Niggli[1] and Skarsgard[2]). At the end of

1980 the new 60-beam piotron provided multiport pion beams with a dose rate up

to 1 Gy/min and more, and this allowed even fractionation studies.

MOUSE SKIN DAMAGE (EARLY EFFECT)

Since it is assumed that RBE values from experiments on mice skin can be

extrapolated to man, our earlier single dose studies were extended to fractiona-

ted piotron exposures with 5 fractions in 1 week, 6 fractions in 2 weeks, 4,

12 and 20 fractions in 4 weeks, 6 and 30 fractions in 6 weeks[3].

The feet of four mice (NMRI females, 23 - 25 g) were irradiated simultaneous-

ly with peak pions in a 85 % isodose field of 30 mm ϕ. The mice were anesthe-

tised with Pentobarbital and Diazepam. The animals were breathing moist 100 %

oxygen during treatment. Dosimetry by thermoluminescent (TLD) dosimeters. 60

beams were used producing dose rates from 0.7 - 1 Gy/min. The RBE values bet-

ween 1.1 - 1.2 from single piotron doses were the same as obtained with the

single beam[4]. Interesting information could be compiled from the fractionation

experiments with the piotron, as fig. 1 shows. The total dose of 67.5 Gy in

30 fractions yields only a damage score of 1 whereas applied in 12 fractions

in 28 days the skin damage was much higher, score: 2.2. The RBE value against

X-rays (200 kVp) for damage score of 1.5 is 1.5.

The isoeffect curve for a medium skin damage have been calculated according

to the Ellis-formula. The results with peak pions could be fitted with the

curve lying between the curve for X-rays and neutrons (Fig. 2). The exponent for N can be 0.10 and lies between 0.24 for X-rays and 0.04 for neutrons. This value corresponds to the microdosimetric studies of Menzel et al.[5].

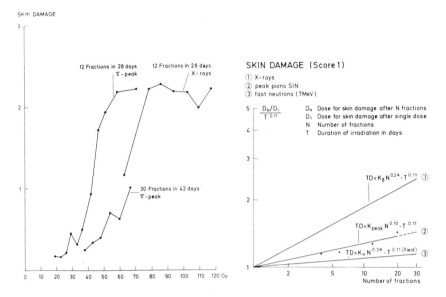

Fig. 1. Skin damage after different fractionation schedule. Scoring after Fowler et al.[6].

Fig. 2. Isoeffect curves according to the Ellis-formula (Fröhlich et al.[3]).

As the experiments were very difficult to perform, unfortunately for X-irradiation only few data exist and RBE-values must be calculated (Tab. 1). The RBE values for single dose are in agreement with data of Raju et al.[7]. The calculated RBE increases with the number of fractions. The observed data agree with the calculations.

	SINGLE BEAM	PIOTRON
single dose (1979)		
peak (0.31 Gy/min)	1.15 - 1.25	peak (1.0 Gy/min) 1.1 - 1.2
(Raju:	1.0 - 1.1)	
plateau (0.2 Gy/min)	0.85	
5 fractions in 7 days		1.5
10 " " 14 "		1.66 (calculation)
20 " " 28 "		1.83 (")
30 " " 42 "		1.93 (")

Tab. 1.
Mouse Skin (RBE)
(Fröhlich et al.[3,4])   Sensitivity depends on O_2 of the breathing air (MF = 1.5 - 2.0)

CELL SURVIVAL (CHINESE HAMSTER OVARY CELLS)

To investigate the biological effectiveness of the piotron over the irradiated focussed field, the gelatine method introduced by Skarsgard and Palcic[8] for the determination of mammalian cell survival was used (Tremp et al.[9]). We thank Prof Skarsgard very much for his help. Suspensions of Chinese hamster ovary (CHO) cells were mixed with a medium containing 25 % gelatine and loaded in a petridish with a diameter of 50 mm. After the irradiation at 20°C (field size for 90 % isodose: ϕ 35 mm in the X- and 26 mm in the Z-axis) pieces of gelatine in the X- and Z-axis (vertical to the Y-axis of the incident beams whereas the Z-axis is along the piotron axis) were cut out, dissolved in warm medium (37°) and appropriate inocula were plated in petridishes. Colonies (> 50 cells) were stained and counted after 8 days. The irradiations with the piotron were made with 15 beams. Thermoluminescent dosimeters, which were put in the X- and Z-axis of the petridish, allowed a simultaneous measurement of doses.

The physical measurements in the different positions correspond very well with the biological data (Fig. 3). The RBE values seem to depend on the cell type and (or) the dose rate (Tab. 2). Some RBE-values have been higher as cited e.g. by Skarsgard[2], possibly due to different experimental conditions. Whereas the data very little within one experiment, they can diverge between different experiments e.g. between 2.0 - 2.8. The aim of further studies will be to find the cause of this variation.

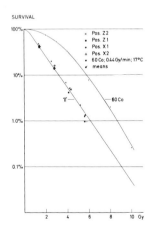

	SINGLE BEAM	PIOTRON (15 beams)
Chinese Hamster: fibroblasts (19/1 subline)		
RBE π(peak) 4.5 - 6.5 cGy/min against 140 kV 4.5 cGy/min	1.3	
π (plateau) against 140 kV	0.8 - 1.0	
CH 0 - (Ovary) - cells		
π peak 0.13 - 0.18 Gy/min, 20° against 200 kV 0.18 - 0.33 Gy/min		
RBE_{50}		1.6
RBE_{10}		1.4
against 60-Cobalt 0.44 Gy/min		
RBE_{50}		2.0 - 2.8
RBE_{10}		1.5 - 1.8
(Skarsgard et al., 1979) π peak 0.12 Gy/min, 0° against 270 kV		
RBE_{50}	1.3	

Fig. 3. Survival of CHO-cells after 60-Cobalt- and peak pion-irradiation (in gelatine for both radiations)

Tab. 2. Cell survival (ability to form macrocolonies)(Tremp et al.[9]) "gelatine" method of Skarsgard and Palcic[8]

GENETICAL AND EMBRYONIC STUDIES (DROSOPHILA MELANOGASTER)

In our opinion several reaction systems in Drosophila (such as genetic and embryonic damage) are eminently suited for testing RBE and OER values, mainly LET differences in treatment volumes. In earlier studies with betatron-rays it could be shown that Drosophila-cells can distinguish between physically not measurable LET differences between photons and electrons. The different stages of Drosophila are small, easy to maintain and to handle. We try to summarize our genetic experiments with the single beam performed in the peak- and plateau-region (Fig. 4). The examination of genetic alteration is also clinically important since the damage to the cell nucleus, in other words genetic damage, is presumed to be the main cause of the subsequent cell death. Fig. 5 represents the analysis according to 2 types of mutations in early germ cells. Interestingly enough, the dose effect curves differ from each other in size and form. They are linear for the complex mechanism of total chromosome loss whereas they are approximately linear-quadratic for the more or less simple mechanism of partial chromosome loss, that means fragmentation. For the induction of chromosome loss the pions dominate over X-rays whereas for the partial loss of a small chromosome region the RBE is less than 1. In Tab. 3 it can be shown that for the induction of recessive lethals the RBE is greater than 1 only for high doses in late spermatids, similar to the data for translocations.

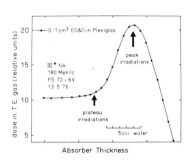

Fig. 4. Position of objects relative to the depth dose curve.

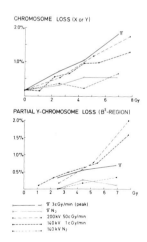

Fig. 5. Induction of chromosome-mutations.

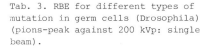

	SPERMATIDS (EARLY) SPERMATOCYTES	LATE SPERMATIDS	SPERMS
RECESSIVE LETHALS			
4.40 - 5.50 Gy	0.4 - 0.9		
10 - 28 Gy		0.6 - 1.3	0.4 - 0.9
TRANSLOCATION			
4.40 - 5.50 Gy	0.4 - 0.7		
10 - 30 Gy		0.5 - 1.2	0.7 - 0.8
CHROMOSOME LOSS (X OR Y)	1.3;OER 3.4		
PARTIAL CHROMOSOME (Y) LOSS (B^S)	0.7		

Tab. 3. RBE for different types of mutation in germ cells (Drosophila) (pions-peak against 200 kVp: single beam).

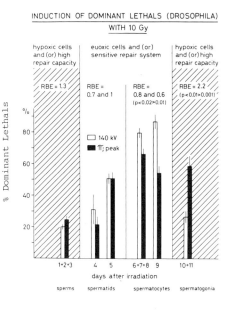

Fig.6. Induction of dominant lethals.

INDUCTION OF DOMINANT LETHALS

The induction of dominant lethals in all stages of germ cells was also tested. Fig. 6 shows some very interesting results. Adult males of Drosophila were irradiated in the peak region of the beam with 10 Gy and mated in successive pairings with virgin females at different days after irradiation. In the first days after irradiation sperms fecundate which had been irradiated as mature and immature sperms; on the following days sperms fecundate which had been irradiated as spermatids and spermatocytes. The induction of mutations with irradiation of sperms and spermatogonia is significantly lower than with irradiation of spermatids and spermatocytes. It is obvious that the RBE changes for different cell stages. So it is < 1 for the sensitive stage of spermatids and spermatocytes: otherwise, in sperms and spermatogonia, it is > 1. It is possible that the high sensitivity of spermatids and spermatocytes is a consequence of higher oxygen tension. Indeed the OER for 140 - 200 kVp irradiation is very high, reaching a factor of 8. Star pions, which are less dependent on oxygen, are not as effective as low-LET radiation in these cell stages. On the other hand they have a higher RBE (> 1) in radioresistent, presumably hypoxic cells such as sperms and spermatogonia. According to our working hypothesis,

224

which we will present soon, the cells could also differ in repair capacity.

Extensive studies on the intrinsic sensitive stages of early spermatids showed interesting results. In Fig. 7a the dose-effect curves for X-rays in air and nitrogen are presented. In a nonparametric determination of modifying factors according to Kellerer and Brenot[10] we found the following estimations of OER in dependence on dose (Fig. 7b). The OER value lies inside the non hatched region. This field is limited by the given data of probabilities of error in %. The OER is surely higher than 2 and could reach a value of nearly 5. The OER values for peak pions are smaller (Fig. 8a, 8b). The RBE in air is less than 1 (Fig. 9a, 9b) and N_2 over 1 (Fig. 10a, 10b). In table 4 the data are summarized.

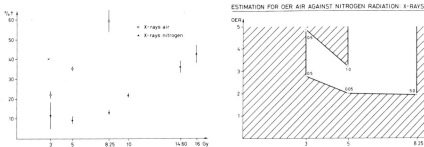

Fig. 7. Induction of dominant lethals by X-rays in air and N_2.
a) dose effect curve.   b) OER

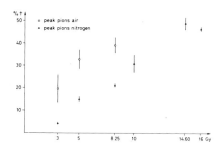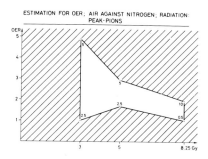

Fig. 8. Induction of dominant lethals with peak pions in air and N_2 (πE3).
a) dose effect curve.   b) OER

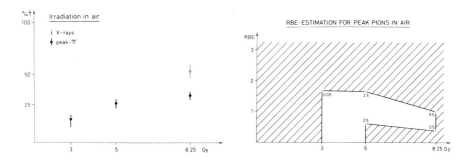

Fig. 9. Induction of dominant lethals with X-rays and peak pions in air (πE3).
a) dose effect curve.   b) RBE

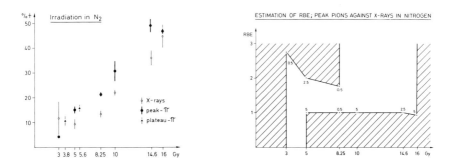

Fig. 10. Induction of dominant lethals with X-rays and peak pions in N$_2$ (πE3).
a) dose effect curve.   b) RBE

	PIONS (PEAK)		PIONS (PLATEAU)	
	RBE	OER	RBE	OER
SPERMATOGONIA	2.2			
SPERMATIDS (EARLY) (ADULTS) 10 Gy)	0.6 - 0.8 IN AIR			
(PUPAE) 3 - 16 Gy)	∼ 1 IN AIR	1.8 - 3.0	< 1	∼1.3-1.9
	1.3 - 2.1 IN N$_2$			

Tab. 4. Induction of dominant lethals in germ cells (RBE and OER); (single π –
beam; 4 - 5 cGy/min).

226

POSSIBLE SELECTIVE DAMAGE OF REPAIR SYSTEM BY HIGH LET-RADIATION; CONCLUSIONS

These experiments and others showed following facts. The RBE of peak pions depends on the system used. In intrinsicly resistant and (or) repair resistant and (or) anoxic systems the RBE values for peak pions are over 1. In intrinsicly sensitive and (or) repair sensitive and (or) euoxic systems the RBE values can be 1 or less.

These facts lead us to the working hypothesis that high LET-radiation can act not only through primary events but can damage the repair system itself, even of cells with high repair capacity (Fig. 11). When the repair system is sensitive, low LET can also damage it and the RBE could be 1.

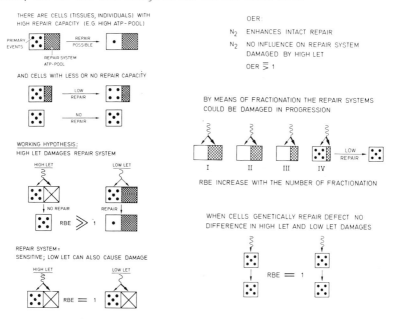

Fig. 11. The influence of LET and O_2-tension on repair.

As experiments with repair deficient cells (genetically repair deficient mei-9-embryos of Drosophila) showed, nitrogen can enhance intact repair. When the repair system is damaged by high LET, nitrogen can not modify and the OER would be low. Further, the increase of RBE by increasing fractionation of high LET radiation can be explained in terms of a chronic damage to the repair system. When cells are genetically repair deficient, no difference in high and low LET damage would be seen as the newest experiments with induction of dominant lethals showed. The repair deficient cells can not register LET-differences.

As said before, RBE values depend also on the oxygen tension of the cells which can influence the production of reactive molecules like peroxides.

In conclusion the problems of RBE can be well described by a two system theory (Fritz-Niggli[11]) which gives more importance to the conditions and characteristics of the reaction systems than to physical modality. One system (high LET RBE = 1 or < 1) is characterized by intrinsic radiosensitivity. Its repair system can be vulnerable, so that low LET and high LET can damage it leading to a RBE of 1. (Table 5).

	RBE	EXAMPLES
SYSTEM I		
intrinsic radiosensitive		
repair system vulnerable,	= 1	normal cells
high and low LET can damage it		(skin, small intestine)
and (or) high O_2-tension	$\gtrsim 1$	spermatids
more reactive molecules produced by		
low LET than by high LET		
SYSTEM II		
intrinsic radioresistent	$\gg 1$	
repair system resistent,		tumor cells?
only high LET damages it		spermatogonia
and (or) low O_2-tension	$\ggg 1$	
only high LET can produce peroxides		

Tab. 5. Explanation of the different RBE values (< 1 till >>) for peak pions.

A high oxygen tension in this system can also lead to a gain for low LET in producing e.g. peroxides and therefore to a RBE even less than 1. The other intrinsic radioresistant system is characterized by a resistant repair system, damagable only by high LET and (or) low oxygen tension.

Since the healthy cells belong mostly to the euoxic and modifiable system (high oxygen tension and (or) vulnerability of repair system as well as intrinsic radiosensitivity) with low RBE of peak pions, and the tumor cells to the other hypoxic and rigid systems with high RBE, this phenomenon could be of great value for clinical application.

ACKNOWLEDGEMENTS

The author is grateful to C. Büchi, E. Fröhlich, P. Schweizer, J. Tremp and J. Zehnder for co-working, P. Binz, E. Frei and T. Suda for skillful technical assistance and H. Blattmann, I. Cordt and K. Schäppi for dosimetry. We thank the Swiss Cancer League and the Swiss National Foundation for Scientific Research for supporting this project (grant No. 3.436.-0.78).

228

REFERENCES

1. Fritz-Niggli H (1979) The suitability of negative pions for radiotherapy: 4 years preclinical research with the biomedical πE3-beam at SIN. Rad and Environm Biophys 16: 185-192.
2. Skarsgard LD (1979) The biological properties of pions. In Proceedings of the Sixth International Congress of Radiation Research, Tokyo, May.
3. Fröhlich EM, Binz P, Blattmann H, Fritz-Niggli H, von Essen CF, Josuran F, Schärer U, Zehnder J (1980) Fraktionierte Hautbestrahlungen bei der Albinomaus mit Peak-Pionen. SIN Jahresbericht 1980:74.
4. Fröhlich EM, Blattmann H, Pfister L, Cordt I, Zehnder J, Fritz-Niggli H (1979) Preclinical Radiobiology with pions: RBE-values for mouse skin damage as a function of single dose of pions. Rad and Environm Biophys 16:289-294.
5. Menzel HG, Schuhmacher H, Blattmann H (1978) Experimental microdosimetry at high-LET radiation therapy beams. In Proc. of the Sixth Symp on Microdosimetry Brussels. Booz J, Ebert HG (eds), EUR 6064:563-578.
6. Fowler JF, Kragt K, Ellis RE, Lindop PJ, Berry RJ (1965) The effects of divided doses of 15 MeV electrons on the skin response of mice. Int J Radiat Biol 9:241-252.
7. Raju MR, Carpenter S, Tokita N, DiCello JF, Jackson D, Fröhlich EM, von Essen C (1981) Effects of fractionated doses of pions on normal tissues: part 1. Mouse skin. Int J Radiation Oncology Biol Phys 6:1663-1666.
8. Skarsgard LD, Palcic B (1974) Pretherapeutic research programmes at negative pion facilities. In International Congress Series No. 339. Radiology 2:447-454.
9. Tremp J, Blattmann H, Fritz-Niggli H (1979) Cell Survival over the depth profile after irradiation with a negative pion beam. Rad and Environm Biophys 16:267-272.
10. Kellerer AM, Brenot J (1973) Nonparametric determination of modifying factors in radiation action. Radiat Res 56:28-39.
11. Fritz-Niggli H (1968) Die Bedeutung des Repairsystems für die relative biologische Wirksamkeit von Strahlen verschiedener Qualität; eine Zwei-System-Theorie. Strahlentherapie 135/2:202-212.

Published]982 by Elsevier Science Publishing Co., Inc.
PION AND HEAVY ION RADIOTHERAPY:
Pre-Clinical and Clinical Studies
L. D. Skarsgard

BIOLOGY OF BEVALAC BEAMS: CELLULAR STUDIES

ELEANOR A. BLAKELY
Biology and Medicine Division, Lawrence Berkeley Laboratory,
University of California, Berkeley, California 94720 USA

INTRODUCTION

At the Lawrence Berkeley Laboratory, particle beams with both unmodified and extended Bragg peaks are being characterized radiobiologically in track segment experiments for the purpose of selecting parameters that will be useful to clinical radiotherapy trials. This paper summarizes RBE (relative biological effectiveness) and OER (oxygen enhancement ratio) values measured with human cells in vitro irradiated with high-energy charged particle beams of carbon, neon, silicon, or argon. Preliminary cellular experiments designed to discriminate the biological response to primary beam fragmentation are also described. An analysis is presented of the medical implications of high LET radiation modalities based on their physical and biological characteristics.

METHODS

Cell techniques

The cell culture and oxygen depletion techniques used in the monolayer experiments have been described in detail[1]. Briefly, two days prior to irradiation, about 7.0×10^4 exponentially growing human T-1 cells were plated on to 35-mm diameter glass petri dishes. Twenty minutes prior to irradiation, the dishes were taken from the incubator, the medium was removed by aspiration, 0.3 ml of fresh medium was added, and each dish was individually placed into specially designed aluminum and glass chambers.

The gas environment within the chamber can be changed from aerobic to hypoxic using nitrogen gas. Each sample was flushed with gas at 160 to 240 cm^3/min for 20-30 minutes. A gas mixture of 95% air + 5% CO_2 was used for the aerobic samples, and 95% nitrogen + 5% CO_2 for the hypoxic samples. Just before irradiation, the chambers were sealed with a slight positive pressure of 25 to 38 cm of water.

After the irradiation, the cells were trypsinized, resuspended, counted, plated, and incubated at 37°C for 10 to 12 days. The colony-forming ability of the cells was scored by staining the cultures with 1.0% methylene blue, and the clones that contained at least 100 cells were scored as survivors. Colony counts on four or more plastic petri dishes were averaged for each data point. Eight or more dishes were used for control and high-dose samples.

Dosimetry

The dosimetry for the heavy charged-particle irradiation was performed using the transmission parallel-plate ionization chambers described by Lyman and Howard[2]. The alignment of equipment on the optical bench, and the methods used to ensure uniform dose distribution across the radial diameter of the beam have been described for the cell monolayer technique[1]. The characterization of the beams with respect to mean LET and to dose contribution from primary particles and fragments has been published[1,3,4].

The Bragg curves for both the monoenergetic and extended Bragg peaks are plotted for each ion in Figures 1 and 2. In addition, recent silicon ion Bragg curves are plotted in Figures 5 and 6. Simulation of parallel-opposed fields was accomplished by cross-firing beams using a method described in the left panel of Figure 4 for the 570 MeV/u argon beam. The range positions indicate the location of track-segment survival studies: the Bragg plateau is designated "0," the preproximal peak is "P," the proximal peak is "Q," the midpeak is "R," and the distal Bragg peak is "S." For the cross-fired exposures, an additional set of survival curves was measured with approximately half the dose from stopping "S" position particles and the rest from stopping "Q" position particles. The cross-fired experiment was called "T" and simulated the "cross-fired" proximal and distal peaks. For cell monolayer experiments, the range segment studied was quite narrow (on the order of μm).

X irradiation was done with a Philips RT 200/250 X-ray unit operated at 225 kVp and 15 mA with a total filtration of 0.35 mm Cu and a half-value layer of 1.08 mm Cu. The dose rate was usually 380 rad/min, measured with a calibrated Victoreen condenser 250 R-meter at a target distance of 24 cm. The exact gas delivery method and geometry used for the heavy-ion exposures were duplicated for the X-ray experiments. X-ray OER values of 2.9 ± 0.3 were obtained at the 10% survival with these methods.

Calculation of RBE and OER values

RBE and OER parameters were calculated from dose ratios at the same level of effect, for example the 10% survival level. Survival data were computer-fitted by least-squares regression analysis to the linear quadratic[5] and repair-misrepair[6] models of cellular inactivation. In most cases replicate experiments were pooled for each beam range studied. RBE and OER values were calculated from the appropriate ratios using the best fits. RBE values for extended Bragg peak beams were referenced to 225-kVp X rays.

The RBE parameter was highly dependent on the cell survival level selected for the comparison. Both the aerobic and hypoxic RBE values in the Bragg peak increased rapidly at low dose. Cell survival measurements were much more accurate at high dose, for example the 10% survival level, compared to lower doses. However, clinically significant doses lie near the 50% survival level. RBE values at both levels will be discussed, but the inherent statistical limitations should be considered when values of RBE-50 are cited.

RESULTS

Figures 1 and 2 summarize carbon, neon, silicon, and argon beam OER and aerobic and hypoxic RBE measurements made with the human T-1 cell line at 10% survival. In these plots, the top panels are the measured Bragg ionization curves for beams with monoenergetic and extended peaks. Both the aerobic and hypoxic RBE values (middle panels), and the OER values (lower panels) are plotted as a function of range.

Figure 1 presents data for the monoenergetic and 10-cm extended peak of a carbon beam with an initial energy of 400 MeV/u, and also a 308 MeV/u carbon beam with a 4-cm peak. The monoenergetic data demonstrate that the OER remains high and the RBE low over the greatest part of the beam's range. However, within the last two centimeters of range, the values quickly change, with the hypoxic RBE at 10% survival reaching a maximum of 3.9 ± 1.0 and the OER dropping to a low of 1.6 ± 0.3 at the closest range studied upstream of the Bragg peak.

When the Bragg peak of the 400 MeV/u carbon beam is spread to 10 cm with a spiral ridge filter, particles are stopped over the last 10 cm upstream of the peak and this causes a reduction of the oxygen effect and an increase of the RBE over a broader region of the range. The physical dose is deliberately sloped to give less dose in the distal peak, where the particles are most effective. An evaluation of the success of two filter designs for isoeffect-

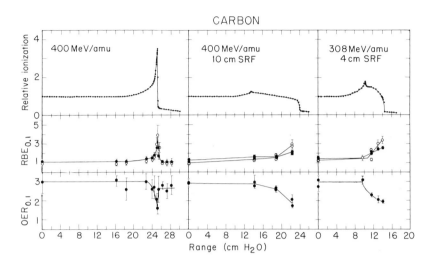

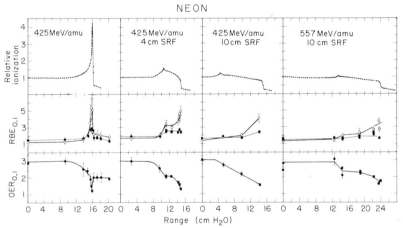

Figure 1. Composite figure of physical Bragg ionization curves and aerobic (solid symbols) and hypoxic (open symbols) RBE-10 and OER-10 measurements as a function of range for monoenergetic and 4-cm and 10-cm extended Bragg peaks of neon and carbon beams produced at the Bevalac. Biological data are based on human T-1 cell survival in vitro. Error bars are 95% confidence limits for monoenergetic beams and 50% confidence limits for extended Bragg peaks.

iveness at the 50% survival level for this cell line is presented in the Discussion. The RBE and OER data from the 10% survival level are presented here for illustrative purposes.

The results from the 308 MeV/u carbon beam with a 4-cm peak show that the RBE is somewhat higher and the OER lower over this shorter extended peak than was measured for the 400 MeV/u beam with the longer peak. This trend is common to most of the beams. The lower the initial beam energy, the higher the RBE, and the lower the OER over the full width of the extended peak. In most cases, however, the RBE is lower and OER higher in the proximal peak than in the distal peak of each beam.

Neon data are summarized in a similar way in the lower portion of Figure 1. The 425 MeV/u monoenergetic neon data are similar to the carbon data, except that the RBE and OER values change earlier upstream of the neon peak and attain a maximum hypoxic RBE of 5.3 ± 1.3 and a minimum OER of 1.2 ± 0.2. The data for the 425 MeV/u neon beam with the 4-cm filter show that the OER is less than 2.0 and that the hypoxic RBE is greater than 3.0 over most of the peak region. At a 10% survival level, these effects are less pronounced for the 425 MeV/u and 557 MeV/u beams with the 10-cm peak. The RBE values are somewhat flattened, but the OER values are still suppressed.

Figure 2 illustrates the monoenergetic and 4-cm extended peak RBE and OER data as a function of range for argon beams with an initial energy of 570 MeV/u. The monoenergetic argon data are unique in that the hypoxic and aerobic RBE values are maximized in a broad peak of several centimeters that lies upstream of the physical Bragg peak. The hypoxic RBE value at 10% survival drops significantly from 4.4 ± 0.6 at 1.2 cm upstream of the Bragg peak, to 3.0 ± 0.6 at the closest peak position. The aerobic RBE value drops from 2.6 ± 0.2 to 1.5 ± 0.2 over the same range. The 4-cm extended-peak argon data show a rather flat aerobic RBE response, but the hypoxic peak RBE values are high and lead to a low OER (about 1.4) across the entire filter.

The argon aerobic RBE is maximized, not at the distal peak, but rather in the preproximal peak region; the hypoxic RBE values peak in the middle of the filter. The RBE drops off beyond this region in the very high LET distal peak because of an overkill effect. The maximally effective LET spectrum for argon appears to be located in the preproximal peak region. RBE characteristics as a function of range are the major consideration in the design of ridge filters. About half of the ionization in the monoenergetic argon peak is due to fragments of primary argon ions. The unique LET spectra and primary beam fragmentation properties of argon are therefore quite different from the carbon and neon beams of similar range that have been studied.

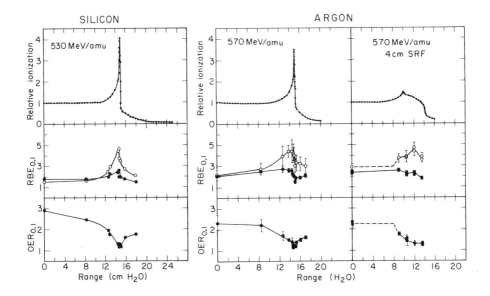

Figure 2. Composite figure of physical Bragg ionization curves and aerobic (solid symbols) and hypoxic (open symbols) RBE-10 and OER-10 measurements as a function of range for monoenergetic and 4-cm and 10-cm extended Bragg peaks of silicon and argon beams produced at the Bevalac. Biological data are based on human T-1 cell survival in vitro. Error bars are 95% confidence limits for monoenergetic beams and 50% confidence limits for extended Bragg peaks.

The monoenergetic 530 MeV/u silicon ion data are also presented in Figure 2. Aerobic and hypoxic RBE values at 10% survival are less than 2.0 over the first 12 cm of range. At depths greater than 12 cm, the RBE-10 values quickly increase, and reach a maximum within the last two centimeters of the Bragg peak. The maximum hypoxic RBE-10 is 4.8 ± 1.2; the maximum aerobic RBE-10 is 2.5 ± 0.3. The OER value at 10% survival in the entrance plateau of the silicon beam is 3.0 ± 0.4. The OER values decrease slowly with depth, and then beyond 12 cm of range quickly drop to a low of 1.2 ± 0.2 in the Bragg peak.

The RBE and OER values from carbon, neon and argon monoenergetic beams[1] are plotted in Figure 3 as a function of beam range. Silicon data from two preliminary experiments are also included. Silicon appears to have potential for therapeutic use because it combines advantageous physical properties of both argon and neon. Like argon, it has low OER values, but because silicon generally produces less fragmentation and has less overkill effect than the argon beams, it has an effective depth-dose distribution that is more like neon.

The cell survival data obtained with the cross-fired technique using carbon, neon, silicon, and argon beams of about 14-cm range are drawn in Figure 4. Where the Bragg peaks from the two opposing beams overlap, the peak-to-plateau dose ratio is magnified without increasing the plateau entrance dose. The overlapping peaks also served to average the number of stopping particles across the entire peak, thus making both the dose distribution and the LET distribution in the peak region more uniform.

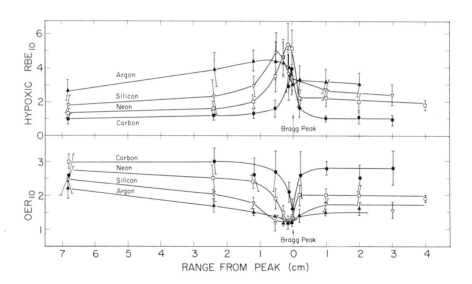

Figure 3. Range dependence of hypoxic RBE and OER at 10% human cell survival in vitro for 570 MeV/u argon, 530 MeV/u silicon, 425 MeV/u neon, and 400 MeV/u carbon beams.

236

SIMULATED CROSS-FIRED BEAMS

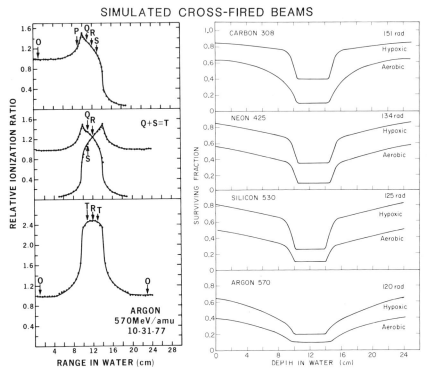

Figure **4.** Isoeffectiveness of extended Bragg peaks. Left: Physical Bragg ionization curves for single-port and simulated cross-fired dual parallel-opposed port 570 MeV/u argon beams for cell monolayer exposures in vitro. Right: Human T-1 cell depth survival curves following simulated cross-fire of carbon, neon, silicon and argon beams for hypoxic and aerated cells with a 4-cm extended Bragg peak. The oxygen effect in the "tumor" is smallest for silicon and argon.

Figure 5 summarizes results from recent silicon-ion beam experiments. RBE and OER values measured at specific ranges of the 670 MeV/u silicon beam with the 10-cm extended Bragg peak are depicted in the lower panel of Figure 5. Notice that the OER is still high at 2.6 ± 0.2 in the entrance plateau and it diminishes to 2.0 ± 0.4 in the proximal peak, 1.8 ± 0.2 in the midpeak, and 1.4 ± 0.2 in the distal peak. The cross-fired parallel-opposed position yielded an OER of 1.6 ± 0.2 which means an averaged OER between 1.6 and 1.8 could be achieved across the extended peak in parallel-opposed fields of this beam. Aerobic RBE values for each of the range positions studied were quite similar to the

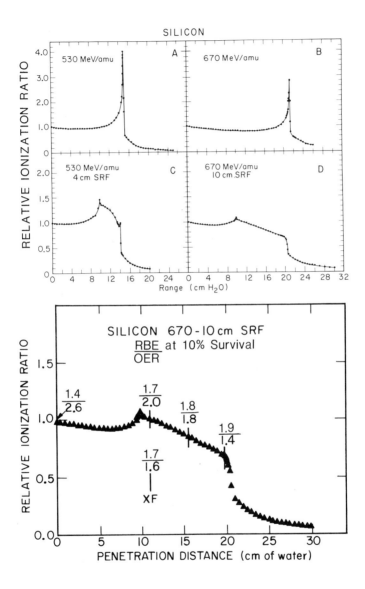

Figure 5. Silicon Bragg curves and 10% RBE and OER values for the 670 MeV/u beam with a 10-cm extended Bragg peak.

neon RBE values ranging from 1.4 ± 0.2 in the plateau at 10% survival and 1.7 ± 1.2 to 1.9 ± 0.2 across the extended peak. Survival curves measured in the simulated dual parallel-opposed position of the 530 MeV/u silicon beam with a 4-cm extended peak (where the beam peaks overlap) yielded an RBE-10 of 2.0 ± 0.2 and an OER-10 of 1.4 ± 0.2. The OER-10 for the cross-fired silicon peak is more similar to the argon cross-fired OER of 1.3 than to the neon cross-fired OER of 1.8.

Additional silicon-ion beam experiments have been designed to evaluate primary beam fragmentation effects on cell killing in vitro under aerobic and hypoxic conditions. Silicon-ion beams of four different initial energies ranging from 320 to 670 MeV/u were accelerated at the Bevalac. Monolayer track-segment cellular survival was measured at residual range positions indicated for each of the silicon beams shown in Figure 6. In conjunction with these biological experiments, J. Llacer conducted physical experiments using silicon-germanium detectors to identify the particle composition and LET at specific residual ranges where biological measurements were made[7]. E. V. Benton irradiated plastic nuclear-track particle detectors under the same specific beam conditions to evaluate particle track diameters for independent LET determinations[7].

We are particularly interested in what effect an increased fragmentation component has on cell killing. Exposing cells at the same residual range of silicon beams of a low and a high initial energy makes this comparison possible. Two beams with different initial energies can be chosen which have the same primary component, but different levels of fragmentation. In addition, cell killing measurements in the plateau of the Bragg curve permit a study of high-LET primary beam without contaminating fragmentation effects.

DISCUSSION

Range filters are designed to extend the effective Bragg peak region by accumulating stopping particles over the broad dimensions required in radiotherapy in order to provide a region of isoeffective cell killing. Several parameters must be considered, including the beam characteristics of energy deposition and fragmentation, the model for cell inactivation that is used to predict the low dose response in the mixed LET radiation fields, the specific radiosensitivities of the cell lines selected for the modeling and their RBE-LET dependence, and the dose level desired for the isoeffect.

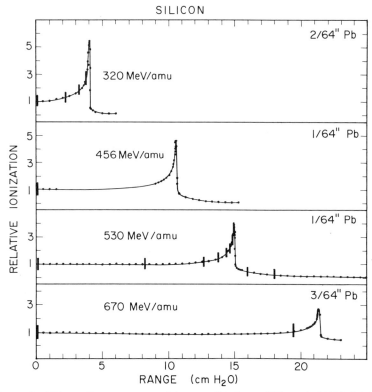

Figure 6. Silicon Bragg curves of beams with four different initial energies:
320, 456, 530 and 670 MeV/u. Residual range positions are designated where
track segment cell monolayer measurements of RBE and OER were made.

Most of the range filters presently in use at the Bevalac are ridge filters
that John Lyman designed based on physical beam parameters and available biological data. As cellular data accumulated with the initial filter designs,
the information was used to design better filters. A representative biological
dose-response profile was developed, and several filters of a newer spiral
design were tooled to extend Bragg peaks to a width of 4 or 10 cm. In some
cases, the same filter can be used for isoeffective killing because the physical and biological properties of two beams are similar enough; this appears

to be true, for example, for carbon and neon particles. In other cases, however, different particles require different filters to achieve similar iso-effective killing across the extended peak. For example, the fragmentation properties of argon are different enough from the other ions to require a flat instead of a sloped dose across the filter.

In order to demonstrate the isoeffectiveness of the available filters using a single cell line (T-1), we used the repair-misrepair (RMR) model for cellular inactivation to computer fit heavy-ion survival data by least-squares regression, and to calculate aerobic RBE values at the 50% survival level. The RMR model was selected because it yields a fit to cell survival data that is representative of fits made with other available models, but has other characteristics useful for analytical interpretation[6].

The RBE-50 values for the various ranges studied were multiplied by the measured physical dose at each range studied. The resultant normalized biologically effective dose (BED) is plotted over each of five Bragg curves of physical dose in Figure 7. The same 4-cm and 10-cm ridge filters were used for each beam studied. The data for the carbon and neon beams with 4-cm peaks show fairly good success in attaining uniformity of aerobic cell killing across the peak. However, the corresponding OER values plotted below each Bragg curve, and the corresponding hypoxic BED values (not shown), demonstrated that it is not possible to design filters to simultaneously achieve isoeffectiveness for both aerobic and hypoxic cells. The OER values across the carbon beam 4-cm extended peak region are around 2.0 and the neon midpeak OER values are similar, although the OER decreases to about 1.6 in the distal neon peak. The 308 Mev/u carbon and 425 MeV/u neon beams with 4-cm extended peak are, in general, very much alike in terms of the measured parameters at this range for this cell line.

The BED and physical dose plots for the longer-ranged 400 MeV/u carbon beam with the 10-cm spiral ridge filter are depicted in the upper right hand panel of Figure 7. There is quite a bit of scatter in the replicate estimates of RBE-50 in the proximal and midpeak regions, and less scatter in the distal position. However, the filter design of physical dose appears to slightly overcompensate for effective dose in the distal peak. More physical dose in the distal end of the peak is needed for isoeffectiveness across the full range of the peak. The OER for this long-range carbon beam is rather high, averaging about 2.5 to 2.6 over the 10-cm width.

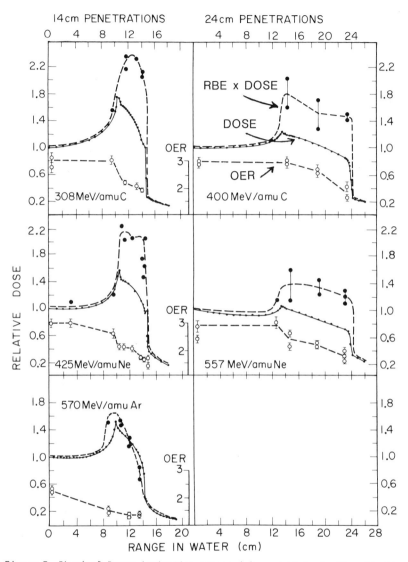

Figure 7. Physical Bragg ionization curves (•), and biologically effective dose (●) and OER (○) at 50% survival as a function of range for heavy-ion beams with 4-cm extended Bragg peaks at 14-cm range penetration, and with 10-cm extended Bragg peaks at 24-cm range penetration.

The BED and physical doses for the 557 MeV/u neon beam with the 10-cm spiral ridge filter are plotted in the center right hand panel of Figure 7. Data from two replicate monolayer experiments show scatter in the neon proximal and midpeak too; however, the isoeffect is somewhat flatter across the 10-cm of the extended peak. The OER values across the peak of this beam average about 2.1 to 2.3, and range from 2.3 ± 0.2 in the proximal peak to 1.6 ± 0.1 in the distal peak.

The final panel in the lower left of Figure 7 presents the 570 MeV/u argon OER values, physical dose, and BED values as a function of range. This beam is different from the others; for the 4-cm filter design, the BED is quite similar to the physical dose, except it is slightly less effective in the distal end of the peak. However, the normalized peak-to-plateau dose ratio is still quite advantageous (about 1.5) in the narrower region straddling the physical proximal peak. This beam is also unique because of its extremely low OER, which averages about 1.4 across the entire width of the peak, including the preproximal and distal regions. The 4-cm filter design appears to be adequate for the carbon and neon beams, but it is not optimal for the argon beam. The BED distribution can be optimized for the argon beam by using a spiral ridge filter design with a much less sloped physical dose. The 10-cm filter design appears to slightly overcompensate for biological killing in the distal peak of the 400 MeV/u carbon and 557 MeV/u neon beam.

The coordinated evaluation of physical characteristics of particle beams by both active and passive detector techniques has been quite useful to the interpretation of beam composition effects on biological measurements. The most extensive study with this collaborative approach has concentrated on silicon ions because the fragmentation effects are significant (although less than for argon ions), and peak LET values are quite close to the critical 100 keV/μm level.

Preliminary biological data in Figure 8 show that silicon OER measurements are similar for all beams at an LET near 100 keV/μm if the primary beam component is the same, no matter what the silicon fragmentation component is. Preliminary physical measurements show that the highest percentage of silicon fragments is composed of aluminum and magnesium. There are also smaller fragments (e.g., Z less than 6) with much lower LET, but their contribution to cell killing is much less. The LET values of the large fragments are high, and therefore do not greatly dilute the primary beam LET. For example, the LET of the silicon fragments in the 530 MeV/u beam is approximately 80% of

the LET of the primary silicon ions near the Bragg peak. A similar comparison
for the 425 MeV/u neon beam shows that the LET of the neon fragments is approximately 40% of the LET of the primary neon ions.

Future experiments will examine fragmentation effects with neon beams of
various initial energies. The percentage of primary beam fragmentation is
significantly reduced for neon compared to silicon ions of similar range, and
the admixture of low-LET fragments with primary neon ions of high LET may demonstrate more dramatically a fragmentation effect of mixed LET beams. This
may be especially true for the LET range encompassed by the stopping neon ions.
Results pooled from physical and biological experiments indicate that silicon
ions may be optimal for simultaneously obtaining a high RBE and a low OER.
The physical basis underlying the biological effects of silicon ions appears
to be that the LET distribution of the fragments is high enough to elicit
optimal cell killing of aerobic and hypoxic cells. Studies are planned to
maximize the high LET component of the silicon beam, and these studies will
guide the development of particle beam delivery dynamics that are under consideration for clinical purposes.

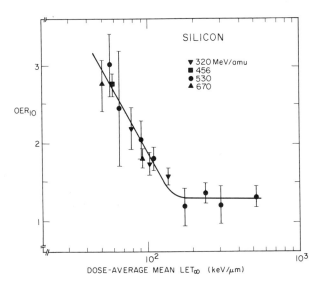

Figure 8. OER values at 10% survival as a function of dose-average mean LET
for silicon ion beams of four different initial energies.

CONCLUSIONS

In general, the results of single-port and dual-opposed port exposures of human T-1 cell monolayers in vitro may be summarized as follows:

1. All charged particle beams studied have superior physical depth-dose advantage over conventional treatment modalities at the same tissue penetration depth.

2. For both beam penetration depths studied (14 and 24 cm tissue range), the midpeak-to-plateau physical dose ratio decreases slightly with increasing atomic number of the particle.

3. Midpeak-to-plateau ratios of biological effectiveness (relative to 225 kVp X rays) for all particle beams studied are greater than one, with a maximum advantage observed for the 14-cm range neon and carbon beams.

4. Midpeak-to-plateau oxygen gain factors are greater than one for all four beams, with the greatest advantage observed for the argon and silicon beams.

5. Dual opposed-port exposures of particle beams demonstrate that more uniformly low OER values, and reduced survival, can be achieved simultaneously over the cross-fired extended Bragg peak region compared to single-port exposures.

6. The cross-fired exposures eliminate some of the imperfections in the spiral ridge filter design, and permit a reduced entrance and exit dose for an equivalent tumor dose from a single-port exposure.

The evaluation of the therapeutic advantages of heavy ions led to a comparison of these beams with other available therapy modalities. The two most important treatment needs are to deliver high killing dose to a localized tumor target while sparing normal tissue lying in the treatment volume, and to reduce the radioresistance of hypoxic cells. Figure 9 is a vector representation that has been constructed for conventional low-LET sources and high-LET radiation modalities (protons, neutrons, negative pions, helium, carbon, neon, silicon, and argon ion beams.).

The vector plots were made to describe the treatment of two targets, a 10 cm x 10 cm field at 10 to 14 cm tissue depth (upper panel), and a 10-cm x 10-cm field at 14 to 24 cm tissue depth (lower panel). The most therapeutically advantageous position on the vector plot is located at the lower right quadrant. For the smaller, more shallow target volume (seen in the upper panel of Figure 9), it appears that 308 MeV/u carbon, 425 MeV/u neon, and 65 MeV negative pion beams are superior in their BED ratio, with the neon beam having

245

VECTOR REPRESENTATION OF THERAPY MODALITIES

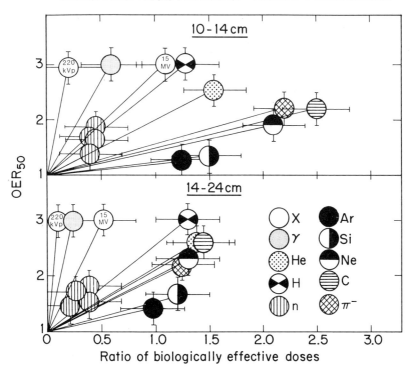

Figure 9. Vector representation of therapy modalities for treatment of: a
small, shallow field (upper panel) and a large, deep field (lower panel).
In vitro cell data from several papers were used to construct this plot.
The ratio of biologically effective doses is equal to the ratio of the RBE-50
x physical dose in the peak divided by the ratio of the RBE-50 x physical dose
in the plateau[8-59].

a slightly lower effective dose ratio but a superior OER advantage. Argon (570 MeV/u), silicon (530 MeV/u), and several neutron energies (5-25 MeV) have the best OER advantage, and argon and silicon beams are better than neutrons with respect to effective dose ratio.

Helium ions and protons show an enhanced BED ratio, but are most similar to the low-LET radiations with respect to OER, which gives them an intermediate place in the vector plot. For a larger, deeper tumor (low half of Figure 9), the relative placement of each of the therapy modalities changes, except for the location of the 187 MeV/u proton and 228 MeV/u helium data which do not change much with increased range. At the deeper range, the 400 MeV/u carbon and 228 MeV/u helium beams are quite similar to each other, as are the 557 MeV/u neon beam and 85 MeV pion beam. The neutron beams and low-LET modalities have deteriorated considerably in their effective dose ratio; however, the neutron OER remains very low. Argon (estimated for a 700 Mev/u beam) and 670 Mev/u silicon data are as low or lower on the OER scale than the neutron beams, with the additional advantage of being more than a factor of two better in effective dose localization.

In summary, track-segment human-cell experiments have been carried out in vitro with carbon, neon, silicon, and argon beams at 14 and 24 cm depth penetration. The results of these experiments substantiate the conceptual basis for the physical and radiobiological advantages of accelerated heavy-ion beams in cancer therapy. If one only considers the BED ratio, accelerated carbon beams appear to be the best modality for situations corresponding to therapy needs. However, the depth-dose distributions of all other heavy particle beams tested, as well as pions, are markedly better than the effective depth-dose ratios that can be achieved with neutrons, X, or gamma rays. A significant depression of the OER at the various depths required for therapy has been achieved with silicon and argon beams, while these beams still retained advantageous BED ratios. The depression of the oxygen effect with silicon or argon ion beams is as great or greater than can be achieved with neutrons or pions, or with heavy ions of lower atomic number. Cell experiments are underway to explore the biological consequences of primary beam fragmentation, and these studies will guide the development of particle beam delivery dynamics for clinical purposes.

ACKNOWLEDGEMENT

The author is grateful to Drs. C.A. Tobias, F.Q.H. Ngo, T.C.H. Yang, and N.W. Albright for their valuable consultations in the preparation of this

manuscript. Excellent technical assistance was provided by P. Chang, L. Lommel,
I. Madfes, L. Craise, O. Oleszko, and K. Smith. The outstanding cooperation
of members of the LBL Biomedical and Accelerator Division staff, including
the Bevalac operations crew is also gratefully acknowledged. The author also
thanks R. Stevens for drafting figures, L. Hawkins for typing, and M. Pirruccello
for editorial assistance. This work was supported by Public Health Service
Grant CA-15184 awarded by the National Cancer Institute, DHEW, and the U. S.
Department of Energy under contract No. W-7405-Eng-48.

REFERENCES

1. Blakely, EA, Tobias CA, Yang TCH, Smith KC, Lyman JT (1979) Inactivation
   of human kidney cells by high-energy monoenergetic heavy-ion beams. Radiat
   Res 80:122-160.
2. Lyman JT, Howard J (1977) Dosimetry and instrumentation for helium and
   heavy ions. Int J Radiat Oncol Biol Phys 3:81-85.
3. Blakely EA, Ngo FQH, Chang PY, Lommel L, Tobias CA (1980b) Silicon: Radiobiological cellular survival and the oxygen effect. Lawrence Berkeley
   Laboratory Report LBL-11220:119-124.
4. Blakely EA, Ngo FQH, Curtis SB, Tobias CA (In press) Radiation biology
   of heavy ions: Cellular studies. In Lett, JT (ed.), Advances in Radiation
   Biology. New York: Academic Press.
5. Chadwick KH, Leenhouts HP (1973) A molecular theory of cell survival. Phys
   Med Biol 18:78-87.
6. Tobias CA, Blakely EA, Ngo FQH, Yang TCH (1980) The repair-misrepair model
   of cell survival. In Meyn RE, Withers HR (eds.), Radiation Biology and
   Cancer Research. New York: Raven Press.
7. Alonso JR, Benton EV, Chu W, Llacer J, Richier J, Tobias CA (1980) Instrumentation for measuring heavy-ion fields. Lawrence Berkeley Laboratory
   Report LBL-11220:21-34.
8. Barendsen GW, Koot CJ, Van Kersen GR, Bewley DK, Field SB, Parnell CJ
   (1966) The effect of oxygen on impairment of the proliferative capacity
   of human cells in culture by ionizing radiations of different LET. Int
   J Radiat Biol 10:317-327.
9. Barendsen GW (1968) Response of cultured cells, tumors and normal tissues
   to radiations of different linear energy transfer. Curr Top Radiat Res
   4:295-356.
10. Berry RJ (1971) Hypoxic protection against fast neutrons of different ener-
    gies. A review. Eur J Cancer 7:145-152.
11. Berry RJ, Andrews JR (1964) The response of mammalian tumor cells in vivo
    to radiations of differing ionization densities (LET). Ann NY Acad Sci
    114:48-59.
12. Bewley DK, Cullen B, Field SB, Hornsey S, Page BC, Berry RJ. (1976) A
    comparison for use in radiotherapy of neutron beams generated with 16 and
    42 MeV deuterons on beryllium. Br J Radiol 49:360-366.
13. Blakely EA, Tobias CA, Ngo FQH, Yang TCH, Smith KC, Chang PY, Yezzi MJ
    (1978) Comparison of helium and heavy ion beams for therapy based on cel-
    lular radiobiological data. Int J Radiat Oncol Biol Phys 4:Suppl 2: 93-
    94 (Abstract).

14. Blakely EA, Tobias CA, Ngo FQH, Curtis SB (1980a) Physical and cellular radiobiological properties of heavy ions in relation to cancer therapy applications. Lawrence Berkeley Laboratory Report LBL-11220:73-86.
15. Broerse JJ, Barendsen GW, van Kersen GR (1968) Survival of cultured human cells after irradiation with fast neutrons of different energies in hypoxic and oxygenated conditions. Int J Radiat Biol 13:559-572.
16. Chapman JD, Blakely EA, Smith KC, Urtasun RC (1977) Radiobiological characterization of the inactivating events produced in mammalian cells by helium and heavy ions. Int J Radiat Oncol Biol Phys 3:97-102.
17. Chapman JD, Blakely EA, Smith KC, Urtasun RC, Lyman JT, Tobias CA (1978) Radiation biophysical studies with mammalian cells and a modulated carbon-ion beam. Radiat Res 74: 101-111.
18. Curtis SB, Schilling WA, Tenforde TS, Crabtree KA, Tenforde SD, Howard J, Lyman JT (In press) Survival of oxygenated and hypoxic tumor cells in the extended-peak regions of heavy charged-particle beams. Radiat. Res.
19. Dertinger H, Lücke-Hühle C, Schlag H, Weibezahn KF (1976) Negative pion irradiation of mammalian cells. I Survival characteristics of monolayers and spheroids of Chinese hamster lung cells. Int J Radiat Biol 29:271-277.
20. Fu KK, Phillips TL (1976) The relative biological effectiveness and oxygen enhancement ratio of neon ions for the EMT6 tumor system. Radiology 120: 439-441.
21. Gerner EW, Leith JT (1977) Interaction of hyperthermia with radiations of different linear energy transfer. Int J Radiat Biol 31:283-288.
22. Gerner E, Leith J, Boone M (1976) Mammalian cell survival response following irradiation with 4 MeV X rays or accelerated helium ions combined with hyperthermia. Radiology 119: 715-720.
23. Goldstein LS, Phillips TL, Fu KK, Ross GY, Kane LJ (1981) Biological effects of accelerated heavy ions. 1. Single doses in normal tissues, tumors, and cells in vitro. Radiat Res 86:529-541.
24. Gragg, RL, Humphrey RM, Meyn RE (1976) The response of Chinese hamster ovary cells to fast neutron radiotherapy beams. I. Relative biological effectiveness and oxygen enhancement ratio. Radiat Res 65:71-82.
25. Hall EJ (1974) RBE and OER values as a function of neutron energy. Eur J Cancer 10:297-299.
26. Hall EJ, Astor M (1979) The oxygen enhancement ratio for negative pi mesons. Int J Radiat Oncol Biol Phys 5:66-60.
27. Hall EJ, Bird RP, Rossi H, Coffey R, Varga J, Lam YM (1977) Biophysical studies with high energy argon ions. II. Determinations of the relative biological effectiveness, the oxygen enhancement ratio and the cell cycle response. Radiat Res 70:469-479.
28. Hall EJ, Kellerer AM, Rossi HH, Lam, YM (1978) The relative biological effectiveness of 160 MeV protons. II. Biological data and their interpretation in terms of microdosimetry. Int J Radiat Oncol Biol Phys 4:1009-1013.
29. Heyder IR, Pohlit W (1979) Radiobiological data for clinical dosimetry in pion tumor therapy. Radiat Environ Biophys 16:251-260.
30. Leith JT, Arcellara V, Lyman JT, Wheeler KT (1975) Response of a rat brain tumor to irradiation with accelerated neon ions. Int J Radiat Biol 28:91-97.
31. Leith JT, Smith P, Ross-Riveros P, Wheeler KT (1977) Cellular response of a rat brain tumor to a therapeutic neon ion beam. Int J Radiat Biol 32:401-407.
32. Li GM, Hahn GA, Fisher P, Fessenden P, Bagshaw M (1979) Interaction of negative pi-mesons with x-irradiation. Presented at the 6th International Congress of Radiation Research, May 13-19, Tokyo Japan (Abstract).

33. Lücke-Hühle C, Blakely EA, Chang PY, Tobias CA (1979) Drastic G_2 arrest in mammalian cells after irradiation with heavy ion beams. Radiat Res 79:97-112.
34. Mill AJ, Lewis JD, Hall WS (1976) Response of HeLa cells to irradiation with negative pi-mesons. Br J Radiol 49:166-171.
35. Ngo FQH, Han A, Utsumi H, Elkind MM (1977) Comparative radiobiology of fast neutrons: Relevance to radiotherapy and basic studies. Int J Radiat Oncol Biol Phys 3:187-193.
36. Ngo FQH, Blakely EA, Tobias CA (1981) Sequential exposures of mammalian cells to low- and high-LET radiations. I. Lethal effects following x-ray and neon-ion irradiation. Radiat Res 87:59-78.
37. Phillips TL, Fu KK (1976) Biological effects of 15 MeV neutrons. Int J Radiat Oncol Biol Phys 1:1139-1147.
38. Phillips TL, Fu KK, Curtis SB (1977) Tumor biology of helium and heavy ions. Int J Radiat Oncol Biol Phys 3:109-113.
39. Raju MR (1980a) Heavy particle radiotherapy. New York: Academic Press.
40. Raju MR (1980b) Radiobiologic properties of pions and heavy ions. A comparison. J de L'Assoc Canad des Radiol 31:26-29.
41. Raju MR, Gnanapurani M, Madhvanath U, Howard J, Lyman JT (1971) Relative biological effectiveness and oxygen enhancement ratio at various depths of a 910 MeV helium ion beam. Acta Radiol 10:353-357.
42. Raju MR, Gnanapurani M, Martins BI, Howard J, Lyman JT (1972a) Measurement of OER and RBE of a 910 MeV helium beam using cultured cells (T-1). Radiology 102:425-428.
43. Raju MR, Gnanapurani M, Richman C, Martins BI, Barendsen GW (1972b) RBE and OER of negative pi-mesons for damage to cultured T-1 cells of human kidney origin. Br J Radiol 45:178-181.
44. Raju MR, Dicello JF, Trujillo TT, Kligerman M (1975) Biological effects of the Los Alamos meson beam on cells in culture. Radiology 116:191-193.
45. Raju MR, Amols HI, Bain E, Carpenter SG, Cox RA, Robertson JB (1978) A heavy particle comparative study. Part III. OER and RBE. Br J Radiol 51:712-729.
46. Raju MR, Amols HI, Bain E, Carpenter SG, Cox RA, Robertson JB (1979) OER and RBE for negative pion beams of different peak widths. Br J Radiol 52:494-498.
47. Rini FJ, Hall EJ, Marino SA (1979) The oxygen enhancement ratio as a function of neutron energy with mammalian cells in culture. Radiat Res 78:25-37.
48. Robertson JB, Williams JR, Schmidt RA, Little JB, Flynn DF, Suit HD (1975) Radiobiological studies of a high-energy modulated proton beam utilizing cultured mammalian cells. Cancer 35:1664-1667.
49. Roots R, Yang TC, Craise L, Blakely EA, Tobias CA (1980) Rate of rejoining of DNA breaks induced by accelerated carbon and neon ions in the spread Bragg peak. Int J Radiat Biol 38:203-210.
50. Schilling, WA, Curtis SB, Tenforde TS, Crabtree KE, Lyman JT, Howard J (1977) Comparison of the radiation response of rat tumor cells exposed at various positions in the extended Bragg peak of heavy-ion beams. Radiat Res 70: 642-643 (Abstract).
51. Skarsgard LD (1979a) The biological properties of pions. In Okada S, Imamura M, Terashima, T, Yamaguchi H (eds.), Proceedings, Sixth International Congress of Radiation Research. Tokyo, Japan: Japanese Association for Radiation Research.
52. Skarsgard LD, Henkelman RM, Lam GKY, Palcic B, Eaves CJ, Ito I (1979b) Pre-clinical studies of negative pi-mesons at Triumf. In Abe M, Sakamoto K, Phillips TL (eds.), Treatment of Radioresistant Cancers. Amsterdam: Elsevier/North Holland Biomedical Press.

53. Tobias CA, Alpen EL, Blakely EA, Castro JR, Chatterjee A, Chen GTY, Curtis SB, Howard J, Lyman JT, Ngo FQH (1979) Radiobiological basis for heavy-ion therapy. In Abe M, Sakamoto K, Phillips TL (eds.), Treatment of Radioresistant Cancers. Amsterdam: Elsevier/North-Holland Biomedical Press.
54. Todd, PW (1967) Heavy ion irradiation of cultured human cells. Rad Res Suppl 7:196-207.
55. Todd P, Martins BI, Lyman JT, Kin JH, Schroy CB (1974) Spatial distributions of human cell survival and oxygen effect in a therapeutic helium ion beam. Cancer 34:1-5.
56. Todd, P, Shonk CR, West G, Kligerman MM, Dicello J (1975) Spatial distribution of effects of negative pions on cultured human cells. Radiology 116:179-180.
57. Tremp J, Blattmann H, Fritz-Niggli H (1979) Cell survival over the depth profile after irradiation with a negative pion beam. Radiat Environ Biophys 16:267-272.
58. Ueno Y, Grigoriev YG (1969) The RBE of protons with energy greater than 126 MeV. Br J Radiol 42:475.
59. Weibezahn KF, Dertinger H, Schlag H, Lücke-Hühle C (1979) Biological effects of negative pions in monolayers and spheroids of Chinese hamster cells. Radiat Environ Biophys 16:273-277.

Copyright 1982 by Elsevier Science Publishing Co., Inc.
PION AND HEAVY ION RADIOTHERAPY:
Pre-Clinical and Clinical Studies
L. D. Skarsgard

EFFECTS ON MAMMALIAN CELLS OF FRACTIONATED HEAVY-ION DOSES

FRANK Q.H. NGO[*], Ph.D.
Division of Biology and Medicine, Lawrence Berkeley Laboratory, University of
California, Berkeley, California 94720, USA.

INTRODUCTION

In this paper we discuss the effects on cultured mammalian cells of fractionated doses of high-LET heavy charged particles at several hundred MeV/amu.
First, the effects of protracted doses of unmodified heavy-ion beams of several
different mean LET's are described. Various techniques were employed including
colony-forming assay, the use of asynchronous and synchronized cell populations,
incubation of irradiated cells at various temperatures, and analysis of postirradiation cell progression kinetics by flow-microfluorometry. Collectively,
these methods facilitate our interpretations of fractionated-dose survival
responses in terms of redistribution of cell-stage density, perturbation of
cell progression, repair of sublethal damage, and potentiation in cell killing
– a phenomenon that was observed with split-dose irradiation of particles of
LET greater than 80 keV/μm.

In the second part, results are presented to show the extent to which the
effects of split doses influence the RBE at the plateau and mid-peak of a
filtered 670 MeV/amu neon-ion beam with a 10 cm spread-out Bragg peak currently used for radiotherapy. The concept of dose-fractionation gain factor will
be discussed.

MATERIALS AND METHODS

Radiations

All heavy ions employed in the present study were produced at the Bevalac
heavy-ion facility of the Lawrence Berkeley Laboratory. The Bragg ionization
curves of the unmodified 400 MeV/amu carbon, 425 MeV/amu neon, and 570 MeV/amu
argon ion beams, used for the fundamental studies are depicted in Figure 1.
The dose rates for these beams ranged from 3 to 8 Gy/min.[**] A 670 MeV/amu
neon-ion beam whose Bragg peak was extended to 10 cm width by a ridge filter

---

[*] Present address: Radiobiology Laboratory, Department of Molecular and Cellular
Biology, Research Division, The Cleveland Clinic Foundation, Cleveland, Ohio
44106, USA.

[**] Abbreviation: Gy for gray; 1 Gy = 100 rad.

252

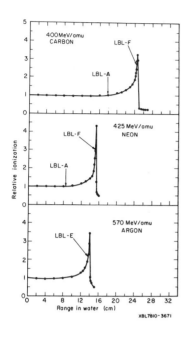

Fig. 1. The Bragg ionization curves of three charged particle beams ^{12}C, [20]Ne, and [40]A produced at the Berkeley Bevalac. The arrows indicate the positions along the Bragg curve where cell monolayers are irradiated.

mechanism with a field size 20 x 20 cm, currently used for cancer therapy, was employed to evaluate the net effects of split dose irradiation on RBE at the plateau and mid-peak regions. Because of the large field, the dose rate of this beam was reduced to 0.35 to 0.5 Gy/min. Figure 2 shows the Bragg ionization curve of this particle beam. The heavy-ion dosimetry has been described elsewhere[1,2].

Low LET radiations used included x-rays and γ-rays. A 250 kV x-ray unit was operated at 225 kVp, 15 mA, with a 0.35 mm Cu filter and a half-value leayer of 1.00-cm Cu. The dose rate of x-rays, measured with a Victoreen, was usually 2.7 Gy/min. The γ rays were from a ^{60}Co unit with dose rate of 7.62 Gy/min, as measured by Fricke dosimetry.

Cell culture and irradiation procedure

Chinese hamster lung fibroblast V79 cells were used in this investigation. The preparation for exponential-growth cultures, medium and antibiotics used, and the irradiation procedure were as described previously[2]. The cells exhibited a mean cell-cycle time of about 11 hours which can be subdivided into 0.5 hr for mitotic stage, 1.5 hr for G_1, 7.5 hr for S, and 1.2 hr for G_2, as estimated by tritium pulse-labeled experiments. For experiments where synchronous populations were used, mitotic cells from a large number of T-flasks were shaken off by a mechanical shaker, collected and plated, and they were allowed to resume growth in a CO_2 incubator at 37°C. For most experiments, cells were trypsinized postirradiation and single cells were plated into T-flasks containing fresh growth medium for the colony-forming assay. A colony composed of 50 cells or more at day 6 after irradiation was considered as a survivor.

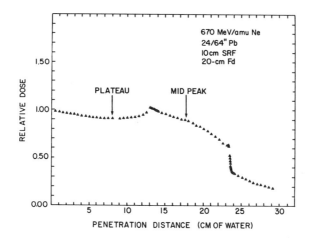

Fig. 2. The Bragg ionization profile of 670 MeV/amu ^{20}Ne ions with its Bragg peak spread out to 10 cm by a spiral-ridge filter system. The arrows indicate the positions where monolayers of cells were irradiated.

Flow-microfluorometry (FMF)

This procedure determines the distribution of cells at various stages of the cell cycle by direct measurement of the DNA content of each individual cell. The measurements were made by using a fluorometer with an argon-ion laser at the Laboratory of Chemical Biodynamics of the Lawrence Berkeley Laboratory.

The preparation of cells for FMF measurements was as described by Lücke-Hühle[3]. The percentage of cells in each stage G_1, S and G_2 + M was calculated using a computer program made available to us by Dr. J. Bartholomew.

RESULTS

Basic studies of dose-fractionation effects

For basic studies of the dose-fractionation effects we conducted experiments using heavy-ion beams with no ridge filter. The LET spectrum of each of these beams is less complex thus allowing a more meaningful study of the effects as a function of LET_∞.

Single- and split-dose experiments were performed with a carbon, neon, and argon ions at selected positions at water equivalent depth. The positions designated LBL-A and LBL-F of the carbon and neon particles, shown in Figure 1, were chosen to represent the Bragg plateau region and the peak region of each particle beam. For the argon particles, only one position, LBL-E, near the Bragg peak was used. The mean LET_∞ values, according to the calculations of Tobias[1], were 16 keV/μm and 85 keV/μm at LBL-A, and LBL-F respectively, for the carbon beam, and 38 keV/μm and 234 keV/μm at LBL-A and LBL-F respectively, for the neon beam, and 245 keV/μm at LBL-E for the argon beam.

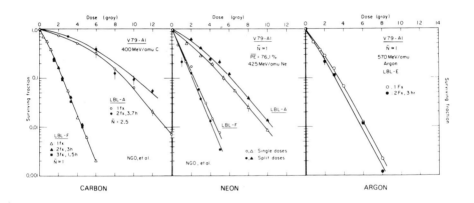

Fig. 3. Survival data for asynchronous V79 cells irradiated with single doses (open symbols) and equal-size fractionated doses of ^{12}C, ^{20}Ne, and ^{40}A at the Bragg curve positions as defined in Figure 1.

Figure 3 shows the survival data of asynchronous V79 cells irradiated with single acute graded or split doses of each of these charged particle beams at the positions indicated. For the carbon particles, while repair of sublethal damage was seen with split-dose irradiation at the plateau position, no difference in survival was detected at the peak position between radiation schemes with single doses, two split doses, or three split doses at a total dose up to 4.2 Gy. For the neon particles, split-dose repair was also seen at the plateau position. However, at the neon peak position, split-dose irradiation separated by 3 hours showed a small, yet significant enhancement of cell killing compared with the results due to single-dose irradiation. A similar enhancement seemed to be indicated by split-dose exposures at the argon peak. Note that for the V79 cell line used in this investigation, the peak RBE is found at LET_∞ = 150 keV/μm, approximately. Thus, the LET's at the neon peak and argon peak po-

sitions are in the over-kill region of biological effectiveness with respect to
cell inactivation.

Figure 4 shows another experiment on split-dose effects with the carbon beam,
purposely choosing a higher total dose for the exposure at the peak position.
Cells were subsequently allowed to grow in fresh medium postirradiation without trypsinization in order to avoid possible artefacts due to the enzyme effect. Although the peak and plateau ion doses selected do not kill to the
same survival level, the data, as shown, confirm the split-dose repair in the
plateau and demonstrate a two-dose potentiation for the Bragg peak exposures.

Since the enhancement of potentiation effect following split-dose irradiation is of great interest in fundamental radiation biology, we pursued this
subject further with the neon beam.

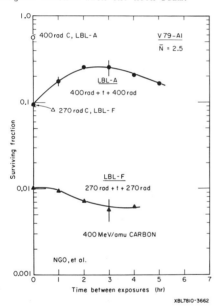

Fig. 4. A comparison of split-dose
effects on the survival of asynchronous populations of V79 cells
exposed to a plateau region (LBL-A)
and a peak region (LBL-F) of an
unmodified ^{12}C beam. At zero time,
the surviving fraction corresponds
to cells which have received the
sum of the split doses with no delay.
N denotes the averaged cell multiplicity.

In our experiments with synchronized populations of V79 cells, we have shown
that there is a small variation with cell-cycle stage in the survival response
to the high-LET neon-peak particles, in a manner qualitatively similar to that
seen with x-rays[4]. Furthermore, it has been reported that high-LET particles
block proliferating cells in G_2 and M stages more effectively than do low-LET
radiations[3,5]. G_2 and M stages are the more radiosensitive stages in the V79
cell cycle[4]. Therefore it was of interest to ask to what extent the killing

potentiation seen with the split-dose experiments using high-LET radiations was due to a radiation-induced cell synchronization effect. In order to answer this question the following experiments were performed.

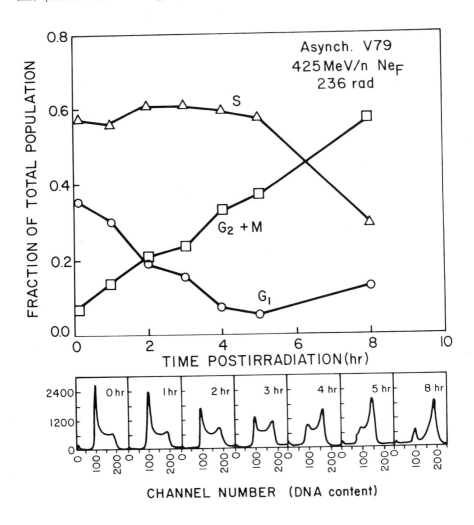

Fig.5. Flow-microfluorometric analysis of cell progression kinetics following a single exposure of ^{20}Ne at a Bragg peak region (LBL-F). Bottom: Histograms showing the relative cell number vs DNA content at various times postirradiation. Top: An analysis of the change in fraction of the total cells in G_1, S, and G_2 + M stages as a function of time postirradiation.

In the first experiment we measured the cell progression kinetics following a dose of neon-peak particles using flow-microfluorometry. The bottom panel of Figure 5 shows the postirradiation changes in DNA histograms of asynchronous populations of V79 cells irradiated with 2.36 Gy of the neon ions. The top panel of Figure 5 summarizes such changes by showing the redistribution of each subpopulation G_1, S, and G_2 + M, with time. It can be seen that within the first 8 hrs postirradiation the G_2 + M population increased steadily, while at the same time the G_1 population decreased steadily for 5 hrs postirradiation. These data suggest that there is a time-dependent enrichment in the net amount of the radiosensitive G_2 + M cells after a single neon dose. In appearance these results support the explanation that cell synchronization caused by a first conditioning dose may play a role in the observed split-dose potentiation. However, it should be noted that the FMF procedures used here apply to all cells scored, and consequently the results do not prove per se that synchronization effects are the same for surviving and non-surviving cell populations.

To compensate for this deficiency inherent in the FMF measurements, a second experiment was conducted. In this experiment, we utilized the property of V79 cells that they would not progress further at hypothermic temperatures. Figure 6 shows the survival data when cells were irradiated with two doses of Bragg peak neon ions separated by various incubation times at 37°C, 22°C, or 4°C. The plating efficiencies (PE) indicated that there was no cytotoxic effect on the unirradiated cells due to the low temperature treatments. The data clearly show that the potentiation effect required a few hours to develop during the 37°C incubation interval. It reached a maximum in about 4 to 6 hours and diminished at a fractionation interval of about 9 hours. At 22°C or 4°C, a smaller degree of potentiation is detectable. The elimination of cell progression effects has not entirely eliminated the potentiation effect. These results are consistent with the interpretation that two-dose potentiation is attributable to at least two distinct cellular phenomena. One of these is radiation-induced cell synchronization as discussed above. The other is radiation-induced sensitization. The existence of the latter phenomena was further tested by using partially synchronized cell populations.

In these experiments, synchronized cell populations obtained by the mitotic selection method were irradiated with a single neon dose as they traversed through the cell cycle. This so-called survival age response was then compared to that which resulted from split-dose irradiation. In the latter situation, cells were exposed to half of the dose at a particular cell stage and then to the second half at various times later, during which the cells were incubated at 37°C.

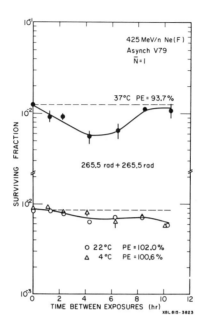

Fig. 6. The temperature-dependency of the two-dose potentiation in cell killing after Bragg peak (LBL-F) ^{20}Ne irradiation. The dashed lines indicate the surviving fraction expected when cells receive a single dose equal to the sum of the two doses. PE denotes plating efficiency.

Figure 7 shows that data from two independent experiments. In each experiment cells of the same age in their cycle were separated into four groups. Two groups were irradiated with single and split dose of neon particles at the peak region (LBL-F); the other two groups of cells were irradiated with single and split doses at the plateau region (LBL-A) of the same beam. Results from the neon plateau exposures were used here to assure the quality of the synchrony and to measure the repair capacity after the exposure to a lower LET radiation source. On the left-hand panel, the data show: (1) Single-dose age response curve was much flatter for the peak neon irradiation than it was for the plateau neons. This difference is expected on the basis of the difference in LETs at these two depth positions. (2) With the peak neons, the split-dose response curve for cells which received their first dose at late G_1 or early S stage was below the single-dose age response curve (closed circles). This

means that irradiated cells which should have moved into a more resistant phase
of the cell cylce actually became more sensitive to the second dose. This indicates that there is true sensitization due to the high-LET split-dose exposures
when the starting population is irradiated at this early stage of the cycle.
This interpretation holds so long as cells at this particular stage are not
being appreciably blocked by the first dose from further progression at 37°C.

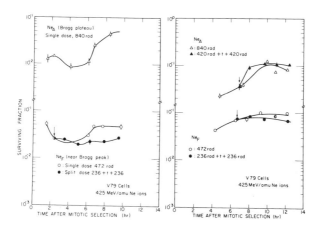

Fig. 7. Further demonstration of split-dose potentiation using partially synchronized cell population and Bragg peak (LBL-F) ^{20}Ne ions.

The data shown on the right-hand panel of Figure 7 pertain to the effects
of split doses for cells irradiated at a later stage, about seven hours
after mitosis. For either plateau neon or peak neon, the differences between
single and split dose treatments were small, if significant. The directions of
the differences, however, appear to be consistent with the results observed with
asynchronous cells (Figure 3). The potentiation marginally detected with peak
neon irradiation (lower curves) is certainly smaller than that shown on the
left-hand panel. This may reflect a cell-cycle stage dependence of the effect,
or may be due to a greater repair of sublethal damage for this cell population.
The latter is expected if cells at late S have a greater capacity for repair
than cells at G_1 or early S do, as was found after x-irradiation by Sinclair[6]

260

and by Whitmore et al[7].

The effect of split dose exposures on the RBE of a clinical heavy ion-beam

In the second part of this work, we were interested in knowing the extent to which the split-dose repair and potentiation observed with a pristine beam are modified in the extended beams currently used in cancer treatments. A 670 MeV/amu neon-ion beam, with a 10-cm spread-out Bragg peak, 20 x 20 cm field as enlarged by a 24/64" Pb filter was employed. This beam configuration was designed for deep-seated malignant diseases with relatively large volume. The depth-dose profile of this beam is illustrated in Figure 2. Exponentially-growing cells in monolayers attached to 25-cm^2 plastic T-flasks were irradiated at the plateau and mid-peak positions as shown. The calculated dose-average LET values at these depth positions are 27 keV/μm and 69 keV/μm*, respectively. Results were compared to data obtained from identical treatment schemes with ^{60}Co γ-rays.

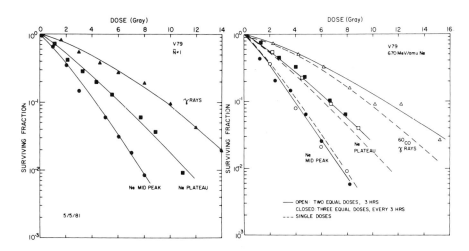

Fig. 8. Survival data of asynchronous V79 cells irradiated with single (left) and fractionated doses (right) of ^{60}Co γ-rays, or ridge-filtered 670 MeV/amu ^{20}Ne ion particles at the plateau and the mid peak positions as indicated in Figure 2. All the curves were fitted to the data by eye. For comparisons, the single-dose survival curves from the left-hand panel are shown as dashed curves on the right-hand panel.

---

*J.T. Lyman, Lawrence Berkeley Laboratory, private communication.

Figure 8 shows the survival data from a self-contained experiment. The data shown on the left-hand panel were obtained for single graded doses, and those on the right-hand panel were obtained for 2 and 3 fractionated doses. For γ-irradiations, only single and two doses were given. Between two consecutive exposures, the fractionation time was 3 hrs at 37°C. All the dose-survival curves were fitted to the respective data points by eye. For comparison, the single-dose survival curves from the left are given on the right by the dashed curves. It is apparent that for γ and plateau-neon irradiation the short-interval fractionation schemes result in higher survival compared to the corresponding single-dose responses. This indicates there is a net repair of sublethal damage between the fractionated exposures for each of these radiations. For the plateau neon, no further increase in survival was detected when the number of fractions was increased from 2 to 3. The apparent lack of further repair for 3 fractions was probably due to a partial cell synchronization effect.

In contrast to the situation with γ rays and the plateau neon ions, there appears to be little or no difference in the survival responses among the single, 2 and 3 fractionated irradiation with the mid-peak neon ions. It seems that the potentiation observed with the unmodified Bragg peaks of carbon, neon, and argon was only marginally seen in the extended Bragg peak of this high-energy neon beam.

The RBE values at three survival levels (50%, 10%, and 5%) for single and 2-dose exposures of the plateau and mid-peak neon ions are summarized in Table 1. Note that on dose fractionation the RBE values were increased appreciably for the mid-peak neon. It is apparent that the increase in RBE is due to the different effects of dose fractionation between the mid-peak ions and γ rays, and is strongly influenced by the effect associated with γ rays. On the other hand, for the plateau neon, there is little change in RBE with dose-fractionation. This is due to approximately the same amount survival increase per unit absorbed dose on dose fractionation between the plateau neon and γ rays. The significance of these results is perhaps better represented by the peak-to-plateau RBE ratio, for which the γ-ray effect is cancelled out. Here one sees a modest gain (on average, RBE ratio increases from 1.45 to 1.67) due to a reversal of the fractionation effect between plateau and mid-peak.

In practice, it is often useful to plot RBE against dose per fraction. This type of analysis is shown in Figure 9. The RBE curves here illustrate the general features characterized in Table 1.

262

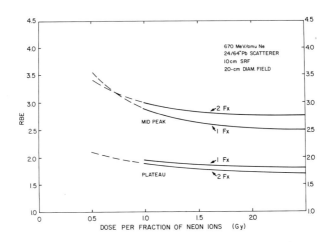

Fig. 9. The RBE of 670 MeV/amu ^{20}Ne ions with respect to ^{60}Co γ-rays as a function of dose per fraction of the heavy ions for single- and two-dose exposures. The curves were derived from the survival curves shown in Fig. 8.

TABLE 1

RBE CHARACTERIZATION OF AN EXTENDED 670 MeV/amu NEON-ION BEAM

	S/S_o	RBE^*_{pt}	RBE^*_{pk}	RBE_{pk}/RBE_{pt}
SINGLE	50%	1.84±0.03	2.72±0.10	1.48 (0.06)
DOSE	10%	1.57±0.04	2.24±0.07	1.43 (0.06)
	5%	1.50±0.01	2.17±0.06	1.42 (0.04)
3 HR	50%	1.87	3.22	1.72
SPLIT	10%	1.65	2.73	1.65
DOSE	5%	1.63	2.68	1.64

* w.r.t. ^{60}Co

Note: The RBE values for V79 cells irradiated with single graded doses or split doses of a 670 MeV/amu neon beam. These values were calculated from the survival curves shown in Fig. 8. The RBEs for the single dose treatment were the average from two independent experiments, accompanied by the standard deviations between the two experiments. Subscripts pt and pk refer to the plateau and mid-peak positions indicated in Fig. 2. The ratio RBE_{pk}/RBE_{pt} indicates the relative biological effectiveness of the mid-peak neons with respect to the plateau neons.

DISCUSSION AND CONCLUSIONS

Repair and potentiation

We have demonstrated that when hamster V79 cells were irradiated with heavy
ions of a few hundred MeV/amu, repair of sublethal damage occurred during the
interval which separated the two radiation doses. Repair was observed in the
cases where the two consecutive doses were from low-LET (γ-rays) (Fig. 8) or
from intermediate-LET (16 to 38 keV/μm) (Fig. 3). But, repair was not demonstrable with two doses of high-LET radiations (Figs. 3 and 8). On the contrary,
a potentiation was found in the latter situations, particularly with unmodified
Bragg peaks. Experimental results from three techniques including flow-microfluorometry, arresting irradiated cell progression between exposures with low
temperature incubation, and studies with partially synchronized starting populations have considerably elucidated this cell killing potentiation effect.
These results are consistent with the interpretation that the observed potentiation is attributable partly to radiation-induced synchronization, and partly
to a sensitization process.

The early work with charged particles at several MeV/amu suggested a split-
dose potentiation[8,9]. These experiments were conducted with synchronized
hamster fibroblasts, and asynchronous human T-1 cells. This phenomenon, however, had not been further studied by these workers. Increased radiosensitivity following split doses of fast neutrons, and of x-irradiation has also been
reported in murine lymphoma cells[10]. A more profound effect was later observed
in a radiosensitive subline of murine lymphoma irradiated with x-rays by Yau
et al[11]. While the cell lines used differ in each of the two reports, their
interpretations for the potentiation are similar, namely, cell synchronization.
In this regard, our study is unique in that we were able to characterize the
potentiation effect as having two entirely distinct processes, sensitization
coupled with the development of cell synchronization. Radiation-induced cell
synchrony has been well documented. The interesting question is what is the
mechanism underlying the sensitization phenomenon. The work of Ward and Kuo[12]
suggests that there are potential DNA strand breaks which form strand break-
ages as a function of time post-x-irradiation by slow hydrolysis of damaged
sugar molecules. During the processes of deterioration of molecular integrity
critical for cell survival, damaged cells may tend to be more radiosensitive.
This may account for the sensitization following split-dose treatments.

An alternative mechanism for sensitization could be related to the processes involved in repairing DNA damaged sites. Perhaps some of these processes require a change in the tertiary structure of the macromolecules e.g.

regional unwinding of the superhelices, thereby increasing the radiosensitivity of the damaged cell.

Whatever the mechanism, it can not be ruled out a priori that sensitization may also take place after repeated low-LET or intermediate-LET irradiation. If this is indeed the case, the sensitization process would be competing with sub-lethal damage repair or Elkind-Sutton repair[13] associated with all radiation qualities.

Because of the simultaneous presence of repair and redistribution of cell-stage density in dose-fractionation experiments, it is not immediately clear whether the development of radiosensitization is unique to high-LET radiation or is a phenomenon equally applicable to low-LET. McNally and de Ronde[14] have shown that with stationary cultures of aerobic and hypoxic V79 hamster cells, repair of sublethal damage was not complete as anticipated by multifractiona-tion x-irradiation, although the "recovery" time was 6 hours between two con-secutive doses. The possibility that a conditioning dose of irradiation can render cells more radio-sensitive, as suggested here, may account for their ob-servation. It appears that the work by McNally and de Ronde[14] and the study by Yau et al[11] would support the hypothesis that the radiation-induced sensitiza-tion demonstrated here with heavy ions also exists with low-LET radiations under certain conditions.

We believe that in studies which involve protracted irradiation or irradia-tion at low dose rates, repair of sublethal damage and radiation-induced poten-tiation (sensitization plus synchronization) are equally important factors to be considered. Potentiation of cell killing is more biologically significant for intermediate- and high-LET radiation, where repair of sublethal damage is usually reduced. For example, the apparent absence of survival increase with fractionated exposures of fast neutrons[15,16,17], and of heavy ions[8,9] reported in the literature could be explained on the basis of a balanced competition be-tween the two processes.

Dose-fractionation factor

In the second part of this study, we investigated the dose-fractionation effects with a clinically-used particle beam. At each of the two selected depth positions (plateau and mid-peak), we have shown the extent to which the RBEs for V79 cells are changed due to fractionated irradiation compared to the RBEs after single-dose exposures. The differential change in RBE between these two depth positions can be attributed to the difference in radiation quality which influences the operation of sublethal damage repair and poten-tiation in the irradiated cells. In heavy-ion radiotherapy one aims to cover the tumor cells by the spread-out Bragg peak whereas cells of normal tissues are situated at the plateau and the exit regions of a particle beam. Assuming this is the case, the present data suggests there is a biological dose-fractionation gain factor with this particular heavy-ion beam, as a result of the changes in RBE.

To illustrate this point, one may define the biological dose fractionation factor (DFF) as

$$DFF = \frac{[RBE_{pk}/RBE_{pt}] \text{ fractionated}}{[RBE_{pk}/RBE_{pt}] \text{ single}}$$

Pertinent to the present discussion, we note that when DFF > 1, a biological advantage or gain factor is realized. Using the RBE data for the V79 cells, one obtains the following values of the split-dose gain factor at the various survival levels:

S/So	DFF (gain)
50%	1.72/1.48 = 1.16
10%	1.65/1.43 = 1.15
5%	1.64/1.42 = 1.15

These results imply that a fractionated-dose scheme is potentially more effective than a single-dose protocol, in favor of eradicating cells at the Bragg peak region and sparing cells at the plateau.

It should be remembered that in the treatment of deep-seated malignancies, there are likely other factors which may effect the outcome of DFF. These are, for example, potential heterogeneities in the tumor population which may differ in radiosensitivity, and in capacity for repair of radiation damage, or potentiation. There may also be different levels of oxygen tension in the tumor or in normal tissues. The importance of these radiobiological variations will depend on the individual therapeutic situation; its consideration is beyond the scope of this work.

ACKNOWLEDGEMENTS

The author is grateful to Drs. E.A. Blakely and C.A. Tobias for productive discussions and critical criticisms during the course of this investigation. Special thanks go to P. Chang, L. Lommel, O. Oleszko, and M. Yezzi for their technical help. Heavy-ion dosimetry was provided by Dr. T. Criswell and J. Howard. It is a pleasure to acknowledge Dr. J. Bartholomew of the Chemical Biodynamics Division who has provided generous assistance in the use of the Flow Microfluorometer and subsequent analyses of the histograms. Support of this study by Drs. J. Castro, J.Q. Lyman, E.J. Ainsworth, and E.L. Alpen is

266

recognized with appreciation. This investigation was supported by US National Cancer Institute Grant CA15184, and the US Department of Energy under contract No. W-7405-Eng-48.

REFERENCES

1. Blakely EA, Tobias CA, Yang TCH, Smith KC, Lyman JT (1979) Inactivation of human kidney cells by high-energy monoenergetic heavy-ion beams. Radiat Res 80:122-160.

2. Ngo FQH, Blakely EA, Tobias CA (1981) Sequential exposures of mammalian cells to low- and high-LET radiations. I. Lethal effects following x-ray and neon-ion irradiation. Radiat Res 87:59-78.

3. Lucke-Huhle C, Blakely CA, Chang PY, Tobias CA (1979) Drastic G_2 arrest in mammalian cells after irradiation with heavy-ion beams. Radiat Res 79:97-112.

4. Ngo FQH, Blakely EA, Yang TCH, Yezzi MJ, Tobias CA (1980) Cellular damage and repair following heavy-ion irradiation. In Pirruccello MC, Tobias CA (eds.), Biological and Medical Research with Accelerated Heavy Ions at the Bevalac. Lawrence Berkeley Laboratory Report 11220.

5. Elkind MM, Whitmore GF (1967) The Radiobiology of Cultured Mammalian Cells. New York: Gordon and Breach. pp 420-421.

6. Sinclair WK, Morton RA (1965) Survival and recovery in x-irradiated synchronized Chinese hamster cells. In Cellular Radiation Biology. Williams and Wilkins Co.

7. Whitmore GF, Gulyas S, Botond J (1965) Radiation sensitivity throughout the cell cycle and its relationship to recovery. In Cellular Radiation Biology. Williams and Wilkins Co.

8. Skarsgard LD, Kihlman BA, Parker L, Pujara CM, Richardson S (1967) Survival, chromosome abnormalities, and recovery in heavy-ion- and x-irradiated mammalian cells. Radiat Res Supplement 7:208-211.

9. Todd PW (1968) Fractionated heavy ion irradiation of cultured human cells. Radiat Res 34:378-389.

10. Caldwell WL, Lamerton LF, Bewley DK (1965) Increased sensitivity of in vitro murine leukaemia cells to fractionated x-rays and fast neutrons. Nature 208:168.

11. Yau TM, Kim SC, Gregg EC, Nygaard OF (1979) Inverse x-irradiation split-dose effect in a murine lymphoma cell line. Int J Radiat Biol 35:577-581.

12. Ward JF, Kuo I (1976) Strand breaks, base release and postirradiation changes in DNA γ-irradiated in dilute O_2-saturated aqueous solution. Radiat Res 66:485-498.

13. Elkind MM, Sutton H (1960) Radiation response of mammalian cells grown in culture. I. Repair of x-ray damage in surviving Chinese hamster cells. Radiat Res 13:556-593.

14. McNally NJ, de Ronde J (1976) The effect of repeated small doses of radiation on recovery from sublethal damage by Chinese hamster cells irradiated in the plateau phase of growth. Int J Radiat Biol 29:211-234.

15. Ngo FQH, Han A, Elkind MM (1977) On the repair of sublethal damage in V79 Chinese hamster cells resulting from irradiation with fast neutrons or fast neutrons combined with x-rays. Int J Radiat Biol 32:507-511.

16. Ngo FQH, Utsumi H, Han A, Elkind MM (1977) Comparative radiobiology of fast neutrons: relevance to radiotherapy and basic studies. Int J Radiat Oncology Biol Phys 3:187-193.

17. Ngo FQH, Utsumi H, Han A, Elkind MM (1979) Sublethal damage repair: Is it independent of radiation quality? Int J Radiat Biol 36:521-530 and references cited therein.

Published 1982 by Elsevier Science Publishing Co., Inc.
PION AND HEAVY ION RADIOTHERAPY:
Pre-Clinical and Clinical Studies
L. D. Skarsgard

RADIOBIOLOGICAL COMPARISON OF PIONS AND HEAVY IONS

M.R. Raju,
Life Sciences Division, Los Alamos National Laboratory,
Los Alamos, New Mexico.

INTRODUCTION

The rationale for pions and heavy ions in radiotherapy is in their combined characteristics of dose localization with high LET. The dose localization characteristics of pions and heavy ions are similar.[1] Heavy ions (Helium – Argon) cover a wide range of LET values. Neon and argon ions cover the LET values approximately comparable to fast-neutrons, and the LET range of carbon ions is similar to pions. Although the importance of dose localization in radiotherapy is well established, the potential advantage of high-LET compared to low-LET radiations such as X rays or protons is not established as yet. The radiobiological rationale of high-LET radiation in radiotherapy was based upon its increased effectiveness compared to X rays in inactivating hypoxic cells and cells in resistant phases of the cell cycle. However, it is not certain whether hypoxic tumor cells and tumor cells in resistant phases of the cell cycle are limiting factors in fractionated radiotherapy. Unfortunately, normal tissue tolerance was not emphasized adequately at the time when high-LET radiations were proposed in spite of a warning by Stone on neutron late effects.[2] The crucial question that needs to be answered is whether the effectiveness of high-LET radiations is more pronounced in tumor cells than in dose-limiting normal tissues. These differential effects on tumor cells compared to late effects in dose-limiting normal tissues for pions may be different from heavy ions because of their differences in LET distributions.

In this presentation, the physical and radiobiological differences between some aspects of pions and heavy-ions will be discussed, followed by a discussion of acute and late effects of high-LET radiations compared to low-LET radiations.

A. Physical Aspects

While the increase in LET for heavy-ions in the peak region due to Bragg ionization characteristics is radiobiologically very significant, it is insignificant in the case of pions (e.g., the LET value of 1 MeV pions is

270

about 6 KeV/m). The Bragg ionization characteristics of pions, however, do
contribute higher doses in the peak region compared to the beam entrance
(plateau) region, although to a somewhat lesser extent than protons.[3] The
high-LET contribution by pions in the peak region derives predominantly
from pion "stars" producing charged particles and fast neutrons. Charged
particles arising from pion stars are important in terms of percent dose contribution as well as in increasing LET when the stopping volumes are small
(∿30 cc or less). The contribution of fast neutrons in small stopping volumes is rather small when compared to charged particles. However, with increasing pion stopping-volume, fast neutrons become important. As shown in
Fig. 1 (a schematic representation), the total dose deposited by pions in
small and large volumes can be divided into three components: energy loss of
pions (low-LET), charged particles from pion stars, and fast neutrons from
pion stars. The decrease in high-LET components due to charged particles from
pion stars with increasing peak width of pions is partly compensated for by
the increase in contribution by fast neutrons from pion stars. While the LET
distribution of heavy-ions varies considerably with peak width, such variations for pions are smaller.

DOSE DEPOSITION BY PIONS

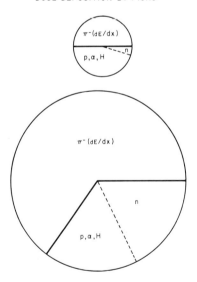

Fig. 1. Schematic representation
of doses deposited by pions in
small (∿0.2 Liter) and large
(∿1.5 Liter) volumes. The numbers
used in this figure are from
Monte-Carlo Calculations kindly
supplied by Dr. D.J. Brenner.

B. Radiobiological Aspects

The Bragg peaks of pions and heavy ions need to be modified to cover the treatment volume. The dose distribution across the treatment volume should be designed to produce uniform effect on tumor cells. Since the tumor effects can be considered as acute, it may be appropriate to choose systems that measure acute effects (such as inactivation of cultured cells) to verify the dose distribution for producing uniform effects. Figure 2 shows the depth-dose distribution of pion and heavy-ion beams of 14 cm peak width and cell-survival as a function of depth. These beams are being used in therapy. The cell-killing is uniform across the peak for both beams. However, one should expect larger differences in RBE for late effects between the distal region and proximal region. The dose variation from proximal- to distal-peak positions is larger for carbon ions than for pions. For a given dose, the cell survival is higher for pions than for carbon ions.

Figure 3 shows the RBE data for pions and carbon ions from intestinal crypt cell-survival measurements by Goldstein and his associates. While the RBE is independent of dose-per-fraction at the plateau position, the RBE at the peak position increases with decreasing dose-per-fraction for both pions and carbon

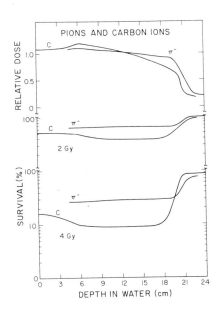

Fig. 2. Depth-dose and cell killing with depth of penetration of carbon ions and pions of peak width 14 cm. Cell-killing data are obtained by using the gel technique. Cultured human cells (T_1) were used in the carbon ion experiment and cultured Chinese hamster cells (V79) were used in the pion experiment. Cultured human cells are slightly more radiosensitive than are hamster cells. The comparison between pions and carbon ions may not be valid because of different cell lines used.

ions. The peak-to-plateau RBE ratio of pions and carbon ions is similar, but pions are less effective than carbon ions in both peak and plateau positions. While the radiobiological data of both carbon and neon ions indicate decreasing RBE with increasing peak width, such differences are found to be rather small for pions.[4]

Figure 4 shows the oxygen-gain factors (i.e., ratio of X ray OER to particle OER) for various heavy particles.[5] In this respect, pions are similar to carbon ions, while the heavier ions, neon and argon, are more neutron-like. Also OGF varies considerably with the peak width of heavy ions. The small variation of OGF values for pions of different peak width is comparable to that of fast neutrons of different energies currently being used for radiotherapy.

We have been measuring variation of radiosensitivity as a function of cell-cycle for pions and heavy-ions using CHO cells synchronized by combining mitotic selection and hydroxyurea techniques.[6,7] Figure 5 shows percent cell survival plotted as a function of time after release from hydroxyurea for pions, neon and argon ions, and for 250 kVp X rays. The positions of particle exposures correspond closely to the maximum LET for these particle beams (at the narrow peak for pions, the distal end of the 10 cm peak for neon ions, and the distal end of the 4 cm peak for argon ions). The reduction of variation in radiosensitivity as a function of cell-cycle position for pions is approximately 50%; no significant variation was observed for argon. No significant

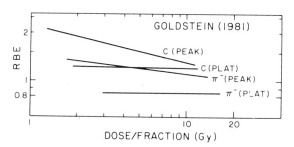

Fig. 3. RBE values plotted as a function of dose-per-fraction from intestinal crypt cell survival data of pions and heavy ions. (Kindly supplied by Dr. L. Goldstein) Reference radiation was ^{137}Cs gamma rays. The peak widths were 4 cm for carbon ions and 3.5 cm for pions. Peak exposures of mice were done at the peak center.

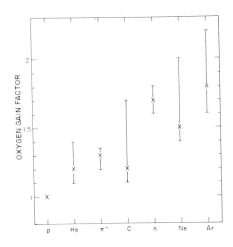

Fig. 4. Oxygen-gain factors for various particle beams.

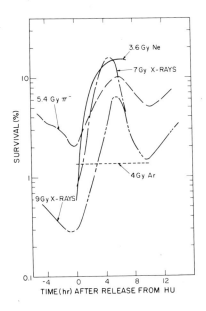

Fig. 5. Percent cell-survival plotted as a function of time after release from hydroxyurea.

reduction in variation was observed for neon ions, most likely due to the presence of nuclear secondaries in the neon beam used in this investigation (range 30 cms, peak width 10 cm). Thus, it appears that while LET values $\sim$ 30 KeV/μm could increase RBE, higher LET values ($\geq$ 70 KeV/μm) are required to reduce OER and still higher values may be required to reduce differences in radiosensitivity as a function of cell cycle position.

DISCUSSION

Instead of designating all radiations with LET greater than X rays as high-LET, it may be appropriate radiobiologically to consider: a) X rays and protons as low-LET; b) helium, carbon and pions as intermediate LET; and c) neon, silicon, argon, and fast-neutrons as high-LET. In the past, most of us (the author is no exception) have been comparing these particles using parameters that can be easily measured (RBE, OER, peak-to-plateau RBE ratio, age response, etc.), even if their relevance in clinical radiotherapy is somewhat questionable. We have been hoping that the role of high-LET in radiotherapy will be answered by the extensive, ongoing clinical investigations with fast neutrons around the world. In the absence of information which shows a definitive role for high-LET, the role of pions and heavy-ions in radiotherapy remains uncertain. The crucial question is whether changes in microscopic distribution of dose by pions and heavy-ions (relatively fewer, but densely ionizing tracks in a given area compared to X rays for comparable doses) will lead to higher therapeutic gain in radiotherapy.

Withers and his associates postulated that late effects of radiation could be a result of the death of slowly-proliferating cells instead of vascular injury.[8] The development of radiation effects in a tissue depends not only on the radiosensitivity of target cells, but also on their proliferation characteristics. Just as the early death of rapidly-proliferating cells causes acute effects, the late effects could be caused by the depletion of parenchymal cells by slow death. Withers et al. further postulated that the survival characteristics of "target cells" responsible for late effects in normal tissues are different from those for the "target cells" responsible for acute effects. The target cells responsible for late effects are able to accumulate more sublethal radiation injury, or repair a greater part of it than target cells for acute effects. Thus, when low-LET radiations are used, dose fractionation, especially at low doses per fraction ($\stackrel{\sim}{<}$ 2 Gy), shows a greater sparing for late-effects than for acute effects.

It appears, therefore, that the currently-used X-ray fractionation schemes of 2 Gy-per-fraction for 4 - 6 weeks provide the possibility for hypoxic tumor cells to reoxygenate, and the resistant stages of cell cycle to redistribute during the course of the treatment on one side, while, on the other side, protect against the late effects of radiation in dose-limiting normal tissues. For lack of information, more-or-less the same fractionation scheme (using approximately 2 Gy X-ray equivalent doses-per-fraction) is being used for particles as well. Since cell killing by high-LET radiations is less influenced by hypoxia and stage in the cell cycle, the sensitizing effect on tumor cells by fractionated treatment with high-LET particles may not be as large as for X rays. Also, since accumulation of sublethal damage is less important for high-LET radiations, no advantage is obtained in sparing normal tissues from late effects when conventional fractionation schemes are used, as indicated in the schematic presentation shown in Fig. 6. The difference in accumulation of sublethal damage in cells responsible for late- and acute-effects may be a more important consideration than hypoxic cells in fractionated high-LET radiotherapy.

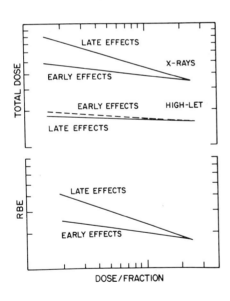

Fig. 6. Schematic representation of total dose and RBE plotted as a function of dose-per-fraction for low- and high-LET radiations. Adapted from Withers et al., 1980 (for illustration purposes only).

Breur and his associates studied the response of human lung metastases to neutrons and X rays.[9] Figure 7 shows a schematic representation of their tumor RBE data plotted as a function of tumor doubling time. The range of normal tissue RBE values for neutrons is also indicated in this figure. The RBE of fast neutrons in human lung metastases is found to increase with increasing doubling time. These results suggest that high-LET radiations could be useful only for slowly-growing (well-differentiated) tumors which comprise approximately 30% of the tumors currently being treated with fast neutrons. Classical histopathological observations supplemented with flow cytometry could be useful for the selection of tumors that would respond better to high-LET radiation. The concept developed for low-LET radiations in using low doses-per-fraction to spare normal tissues is not relevant for high-LET radiations. Lower doses-per-fraction of high-LET radiations in terms of producing late-effects may be similar to the situations experienced when higher doses-per-fraction of low-LET radiation are used in radiotherapy. Since the accumulation of sublethal damage is still important for intermediate-LET radiations, small doses-per-fraction may still be helpful to spare late effects, although not to the same extent as for X rays. If the tolerance limits of normal tissues require the survival of a minimum number of target cells, pions and heavy

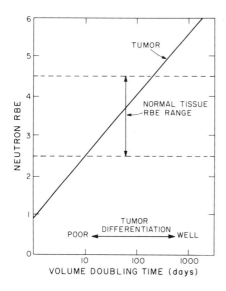

Fig. 7. Neutron RBE in human pulmonary metastases plotted as a function of tumor doubling-time from the data of Breur and his associates (Batterman, 1981). The range of normal tissue RBE is also shown in this figure.

ions will have some advantage over neutrons because of their improved dose-localization characteristics.

Higher doses-per-fraction are known to produce more severe late effects for a given early effect, even for X rays. This increase in late effects is even more pronounced for fast neutrons. The favorable dissociation of normal tissue late effects from acute effects seen for X rays at low doses-per-fraction cannot be expected for high-LET radiations and, hence, higher doses-per-fraction of high-LET radiations should not be viewed from X ray experience. While acute effects may be used to monitor low-LET radiation treatment at low doses-per-fraction ($\stackrel{\sim}{<}$ 200 rad) because of the possible sparing of normal tissues from late effects, the value of acute effects as a guide either at higher doses-per-fraction of X rays or $\sim$ 200 rad equivalent dose-per-fraction of high-LET could be disastrous. The dissociation between acute and late effects for high-LET radiations does not change significantly with increasing dose-per-fraction. Early effects could be a relatively safer guide for high-LET radiation at higher dose-per-fraction than at lower dose-per-fraction.

The clinical experience with protons in Uppsala does not seem to indicate the same degree of severity in late effects as is expected from conventional low-LET radiations when larger doses-per-fraction were used.[11] This suggests that improved dose localization of protons could have partially compensated for the increased late effects at higher doses-per-fraction. While the optimum dose-per-fraction for low-LET radiations could be $\overline{<}$ 2 Gy, it may be higher for high-LET. If the experimental data on animal systems suggest therapeutic gain at higher doses-per-fraction for high-LET radiations, it may be possible to use higher doses-per-fraction without exceeding normal tissue tolerance with pions or heavy ions because of their improved dose localization characteristics.

The technical complexities in using pions and heavy-ions have distracted us from obtaining critical radiobiological data. Our future radiobiological research should be shifted from easily-measurable parameters such as RBE, OER and single-dose RBE measurements of tissues to more clinically-relevant late-effects in various dose-limiting normal tissues such as the spinal cord, brain, lung, kidney, colon, etc., as a function of dose-per-fraction in addition to the acute effects on normal tissues and tumors, and studies that would help select tumors that are more responsive to high-LET radiations. In the absence of such radiobiological research, it is unrealistic to expect definitive

278

and valid answers regarding the role of pions and heavy-ions in radiotherapy only from the currently-planned clinical investigations using 200-rad X ray equivalent doses-per-fraction.

ACKNOWLEDGMENTS

This investigation was supported by Grant CA 17290 awarded by the U.S. National Cancer Institute, Department of Health, Eduction and Welfare, and D.O.E. The author is grateful to Dr. L. D. Skarsgard for his extensive and helpful comments for improvement of the manuscript and to Drs. R. A. Tobey, R. A. Walters, and A. J. van der Kogel for general suggestions for improvement of the manuscript.

REFERENCES

1. Raju MR, Amols HI, DiCello JF, Howard J, Lyman JT, Koehler AM, Grarus R, Smathers JB(1978a) A Heavy Particle Comparative Study. Part I. Depth-Dose Distributions. Br J Radiol 51:699-703.
2. Stone RS(1948) Neutron Therapy and Specific Ionization. Am J Roentgenol 59:771-785.
3. Raju MR(1980a) Radiobiological Properties of Pions and Heavy Ions. A Comparison. Canadian J Radiol 31:26-29.
4. Tokita N(1981) Effects of Pions on Normal Tissues. In Proceedings of the International Workshop on Pion and Heavy Ion Radiology: Preclinical and Clinical Studies. Elsevier, North Holland (in press).
5. Raju MR(1980b) Heavy Particle Radiotherapy. New York: Academic Press.
6. Raju MR, Amols HI, Tobey RA, Walters RA(1978b) Age Response for Line-CHO Chinese Hamster Cells Exposed to Peak Negative Pions. Rad Res 76:219-223.
7. Raju MR, Bain E, Carpenter SG, Jett J, Walters RA, Howard J, Powers-Risius P(1980) Effect of Argon Ions on Synchronized Chinese Hamster Cells. Rad Res 84:152-157.
8. Withers HR, Thames HE, Peters LJ, Fletcher GH(1980) Normal Tissue Radioresistance in Clinical Radiotherapy. In GH Fletcher, C Nervi and HR Withers (eds.), Biological Basis and Clinical Implications of Tumor Radioresistance, Proceedings of 2nd Rome International Symposium. Masson Publication Co., in press.
9. Batterman JJ(1981) Clinical Application of Fast Neutrons. The Amsterdam Experience (Thesis).
10. Withers HR, Flow BL, Huchton JI, Hussey DH, Jardine JH, Mason KA, Raulston GL, Smathers JB(1977) Effect of Dose Fractionation on Early and Late Skin Responses to Gamma Rays and Neutrons. Int J Radiat Oncol Biol Phy 3: 227-233.
11. Graffman S, Larsson B(1975) High Energy Protons for Radiotherapy—A Review of the Activities at the 185-MeV Synchrocyclotron in Uppsala. In Proceedings of an International Workshop on Particle Radiation Therapy, Key Biscayne, Florida, October. American College of Radiology, pp. 505-527.

RADIATION BIOLOGY IN VIVO

EXPERIENCES WITH SINGLE BEAM AND PIOTRON PIONS ON NORMAL AND EMBRYONIC TISSUES

KUDYADI RAMCHANDRA RAO, RUTH LANDOLT AND CHRISTIAN MICHEL
Radiobiological Institute of Zurich University
P.O. Box 64, CH-8029 Zurich, Switzerland

INTRODUCTION

For the application of pions in the radiotherapy of human cancers, detailed
radiobiological information on the following aspects may be of considerable
help in planning an effective treatment:

(a) The effect of pions on normal tissues (early and late effects)

(b) Relative biological effectiveness (RBE) of pions using test systems which
are sensitive to differences in linear energy transfer (LET) either in the
whole pion profile or size of the volume irradiated

(c) Whether it is at all possible to influence the biological effectiveness of
peak pions with radiosensitizing substances which are selective in their action,
or through drugs such as rutosides which are specific in their radioprotective
action, and with hyperthermia.

Therefore it was decided to investigate some of the above-stated topics with
three separate in vivo systems using single and multiport pion beams.

1. Small intestine of mouse: because the crypt cell survival assay is generally
used as an 'in vivo biological dosimeter' for intercomparison of the RBE values
of different high LET radiation beams.

2. Capillary system: because of the radiation induced pathological changes in
microvasculature of normal tissues which is important for clinical purposes.

3. Embryonic development: because it is extremely radiosensitive.

I. RESPONSE OF MOUSE SMALL INTESTINE TO SINGLE DOSE OF IRRADIATION

In the following study the mouse small intestine, a therapeutically relevant
normal tissue, was used to estimate the RBE of peak pions. Data on the initial
experiments with single doses of pions and X-rays are presented.

MATERIALS AND METHODS

Female NMRI mice weighing 25-30g were used. Unanesthetised animals restrained
in special ventilated phantoms were irradiated singly with graded doses of

either pions or X-rays. The isodose field of the pion beam was 22mm broad.
Therefore only the abdomen of the mouse was irradiated or animals were given
'whole body' treatment with two successive exposures to each half of the body.
At least 5 mice were used for each dose.

Pion sources were πE3 (single beam) or piotron (multiport) at the Swiss
Institute for Nuclear Research (SIN). Details of these pion sources and on dosimetry are already described elsewhere in these proceedings. The dose rates
used in the following experiments were 0.6 or 1.2 Gy/min. 200kVp X-rays (HVL
0.93mm Cu) were taken as reference radiation at corresponding dose rates. Irradiation procedures were uniform in all cases.

The estimation of jejunal crypt cell survival was based on the method described by Withers and Elkind [1]. From the data obtained for the test and
reference radiation, dose response curves were fitted by linear regression analysis.

RESULTS AND DISCUSSION

The crypt cell survival curves after irradiation of mice with a single dose
of peak pions and X-rays are presented in Figures 1 and 2. Figure 1 shows the
results obtained when radiation was delivered at 1.2 Gy/min to the abdominal
region of animals. For intercomparison of our data with other reports, the
second experiment (Fig. 2) was done by 'whole body' treatment. The pion dose
rate in this case was 0.6 Gy/min but there is some uncertainty regarding the
actual dose delivered because some of the momentum slit shutters were not
functioning properly. However the biological response observed did not differ
significantly from the previous experiment and the results are therefore taken
into consideration.

With the limited crypt cell data available at the moment, we can only estimate the RBE value of peak pions with reference to 200 kVp X-rays for single
exposure. And this was done by taking the radiation dose required to reduce
the surviving jejunal crypt cells to 20 per circumference as the criterion for
comparison. In the first experiment (Fig. 1) this isoeffect dose was 12.53 Gy
and 14.22 Gy for pions and X-rays respectively, which gives a RBE of 1.13 for
pions. The isoeffect doses in the second experiment were 13.24 Gy for X-rays
and 11.86 Gy for pions with a RBE of 1.12 for the latter.

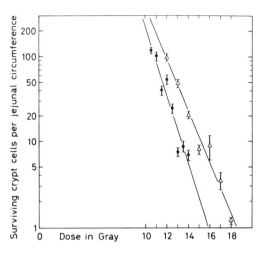

Fig.1. Dose response curves with standard errors for jejunal crypt cells in mice partial-body irradiated with pions (•) or X-rays (△).

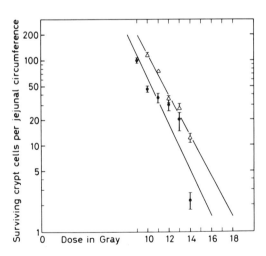

Fig. 2. Dose response curves for crypt cells in mice whole-body irradiated with pions (•) or X-rays (△).

Since the application of pions in radiobiological research using various in vitro and in vivo test systems, considerable information was gathered on the RBE values of pions. The earlier studies were done mostly with pions beams of low dose rate, which was not always suitable for assay systems requiring high doses of radiation. Thus in their studies with the single beam πE3 pions source (0.03-0.05 Gy/min) at SIN, Rao et al.[2] had to irradiate the Ehrlich ascites tumor (EAT) cells in vitro at 4°C because of the protracted exposure. When these EAT cells were subsequently tested for proliferation in vivo, peak pions had a RBE of 1.0 with reference to 140 kVp X-rays (HVL 0.96mm Cu) at 50% survival level and the RBE increased to about 1.2 at 10% survival. Using the same pion source but the mitotic inhibition in jejunal crypts and survival of EAT cells as the criteria, peak pions had a RBE of 1.4 compared to plateau pions[3]. Other data involving low dose rate pions are reviewed in detail by Skarsgard[4] and by Fritz-Niggli[5].

Using the high dose rate pions from the Los Alamos Meson Physics Facility, there have been some recent observations on the peak pion induced normal tissue injury in mice. Of particular interest here is the report of Peters et al.[6], where the experimental conditions were comparable with the present study except that Co^{60} gamma rays were taken as reference radiation. For single fraction of pions and using isoeffect of 20 surviving crypt cells per circumference, they estimated a RBE of 1.22 for pions. This is in general agreement with our values of 1.12 and 1.13 where 200 kVp X-rays served as standard radiation. For acute skin reaction the RBE of pions is reported to be 1.11 for single exposure[7]. Jordan et al.[8] have taken murine kidney injury as the biological end point and have derived a RBE value of 1.12 for single dose pion application. Thus the reported RBE values of single fraction of peak pions for mouse normal tissue injury lie within a narrow range between 1.11 and 1.22. The observed low RBE values of pions for normal tissues may indicate an advantage if the radiation has higher RBE ratios for tumor cells thereby increasing the therapeutic gain factor.

II. EFFECT OF SINGLE BEAM PIONS ON BRAIN CAPILLARIES IN NEONATAL RATS

Radiation can induce increased permeability of the capillary wall resulting in extravasation of blood into the brain or into other tissues visible as puncuate hemorrhages (petechiae).

The cerebral microvasculature of the neonatal rat and its radiation induced petechiae distributed over the surface of the brain is a convenient system for the radiobiological investigation of a normal tissue[9]. The vascular damage is assessed by a semiquantitative method (scores). Results are obtained within less than two weeks. Neither the fastidious histological nor the microscopic .work-up is needed. This assay allows the evaluation of effects induced by radiations of different qualities (e.g. low and high energy photons, high energy electrons and pions). It has been used for the estimation of the RBE and for the study of radioprotectors (rutosides). The well known increased radiosensitivity of developing tissues renders this system rather sensitive to irradiation as compared to the same vasculature in the adult rat. It even allowed irradiation with very low dose rates such as obtained from the πE3 channel at SIN.

METHODS·

The test system described earlier[9] is briefly outlined: Newborn Holtzman rats were irradiated to the head at the age of about 24 hours. During irradiation they were kept immobilized without anesthesia in a well areated and warmed plexiglass phantom molded to their body shape. One day following irradiation the rat brains were removed and fixed in formalin. One to two weeks later the extent of the hemorrhages was estimated by means of a scoring scale ranging from 0 to 5 according to the number and the size of the petechiae. Radiation conditions: πE3 pions of SIN, proton energy 590 MeV, target material beryllium, 10% electron contamination, field size 2.5cm in diameter at 85% isodose. Dose rates: peak 0.06 to 0.11 Gy/min, plateau 0.035 to 0.06 Gy/min. X-rays: 200 kVp. HVL in Cu: 0.7mm. Dose rates 0.035, 0.06 and 0.10 Gy/min.

RESULTS AND DISCUSSION

The results obtained by irradiation with peak and plateau pions are shown in figure 3. The response curves of peak and plateau pions are different in length. This is due to the limited number of beam hours which were available for the experiments at the πE3 channel.

286

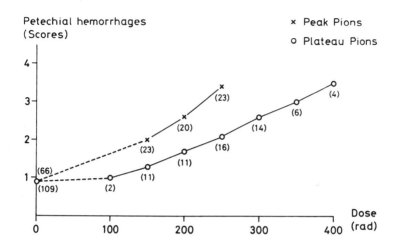

Fig. 3. Dose response curves for radiation induced cerebral hemorrhages in neonatal rats. Abscissa: dose in rad. Ordinate: effects in scores. Peak(x) and plateau(o) pions. The numbers in parenthesis indicate the number of animals used per dose group.

The values of the peak pion curve are significantly (Mann-Whitney U test) higher than those of the plateau curve. The peak/plateau ratio varied between 1.5 and 1.6 in regard to the effects and was even 1.8 in regard to the RBE. The RBE was estimated by comparing pions with 200 kVp X-rays. It was 1.1 and 0.6 in peak and plateau, respectively. The difference in effects between pions and X-rays was statistically significant in the plateau, but not in the peak. The RBE peak of 1.1 in the described system of cerebral microvasculature agrees well with that obtained for other normal tissues such as discussed in the previous paragraph about small intestine irradiation. A higher RBE of 1.7, however, was estimated for peak pions by Fike and Gillette [10] in another in vivo microvascular system (capillary proliferation in neovascularization of cornea). This might be due to various factors: different reference radiation (^{60}Co gamma rays), different endpoints, a questionable difference in interaction between pions and gamma rays with drugs (antibiotics and anaesthetics) in Fike's system. Such interactions of drugs and radiation can be studied by the described microvascular system. It has also been used to investigate the effects of rutosides as radioprotectors in irradiation with pions, but due to technical difficulties with the piotron the results can not be evaluated.

III. MODIFICATION OF RADIATION EFFECTS IN MOUSE EMBRYOS

Using the embryonic development in mammals as a reaction system, three problems of interest can be studied: 1) RBE differences in a normal cell system which has a metabolism partially similar to cancer cells. 2) Interaction with drugs and other factors and 3) Health risk aspects.

According to the BEIR III report [11] radiation induced developmental anomalies represent a high risk for human health and are therefore of greatest concern. In radiation embryology the biological end points of most importance are death, malformation, growth retardation, viability decrease and tumor induction. For the low dose level and for different radiation qualities the experimental data are still very limited. A further aspect that has been only scarcely touched on concerns combined effects of radiation and other environmental influences. Regarding risk estimations and radioprotection for human development both antagonisms and synergisms are of obvious significance.

MATERIALS AND METHODS

Our research program concentrates on the analysis of developmental anomalies after treatment of a sensitive stage of gestation in NMRI-mice (day 8 of pregnancy). Irradiations with pions were performed with a beryllium target at a dose rate of 0.008 to 0.01 Gy/min for the single beam and 0.6 Gy/min for piotron pions. X-irradiation was administered at 140 kVp and 200 kVp using the same dose rates as in pion experiments. The evaluation of fetuses occured at day 13 of gestation.

RESULTS AND DISCUSSION

Previous investigations using drugs which may interfere with the cellular energy metabolism and repair processes (iodoacetamide, tetracyclines, lucanthone) revealed an enhancement of radiation induced damage in rat and mouse embryos [12].

In our first experiments with the biomedical pion beam it was found that low doses of 0.01 Gy and 0.135 Gy produce significant effects in mouse fetuses compared to sham irradiated controls. With respect to 140 kVp X-rays the effectiveness of peak pions was increased by a factor of 1.7 and 1.3 for plateau pions. In studies on combined effects, lucanthone (a drug against schistosomiasis) was applied i.p. 30 min before whole-body irradiation. The substance showed a sensitizing action which was more pronounced at the higher dose levels used (Table 1).

TABLE 1

INCIDENCE OF IMPLANTED, DEAD AND ABNORMAL MOUSE FETUSES ON DAY 13 OF GESTATION. WHOLE-BODY IRRADIATION WITH PEAK PIONS ON DAY 8. LUCANTHONE (Luc) INJECTED I.P. 30 MIN BEFORE EXPOSURE.

Treatment		Total implants	Embryonic death	Growth retardation	Malformation
None		318	5.0%	8.3%	1.3%
Luc:	35 mg/kg	217	7.8%	7.5%	5.5%
	70 mg/kg	170	8.2%	16.0%	14.1%
0.01 Gy		181	6.1%	21.8%	4.7%
Luc + 0.01 Gy[a]		63	12.7%	21.8%	10.9%
0.135 Gy		108	5.6%	23.5%	4.9%
Luc + 0.135 Gy[b]		39	30.8%	40.7%	33.3%

[a]Lucanthone 35 mg/kg
[b]Lucanthone 70 mg/kg

Preliminary data obtained with piotron pions in the peak region indicate a potentiating effect in combination with the hypoxic cell radiosensitizer misonidazole (MISO). Till now only the following treatments could be performed: MISO + 50 rad and 100 rad without drug application (Figure 4). A dose effect curve will be produced to evaluate the quantitative and qualitative aspects of single or combined treatments.

At present it is interesting to note that the combination of MISO + 50 rad results in effects which exceed those found after exposure to 100 rad alone. Also in qualitative respects the incidence of severe and multiple damages was greater in the group that received both MISO plus pions than after irradiation alone.

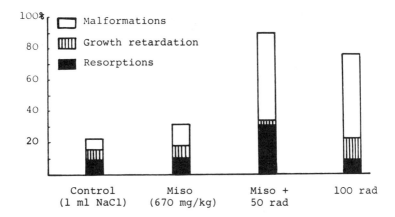

Fig.4. Preliminary data on frequencies of developmental
anomalies in mouse fetuses on day 13. Misonidazole
injected i.p. 30 min before exposure to Piotron
pions on day 8 of gestation.

Whether or not embryonic tissues are hypoxic or contain a component of
hypoxic cells at the time of treatment is not known. This question is important for elucidation of whether misonidazole enhances radiation effects
also in normal tissues.

CONCLUSIONS

   The RBE of peak pions observed for mouse jejunum (1.12) and brain vascular
injury (1.1) are in general agreement with other in vivo studies. For embryonic tissues, the tentative RBE was 1.7 and it was demonstrated that the biological effects of pions could be potentiated with certain drugs. The effectiveness of peak pions compared with that of plateau pions is between 1.4 and 1.6
for the three test systems used in this study.

ACKNOWLEDGEMENTS

   The authors are grateful to D. Arn, P. Binz, T. Busch, V. Gut and R. Venzin
for their skillful technical assistance. We thank H. Blattmann, I. Cordt and
K. Schäppi for dosimetry.

   We thank the Swiss National Foundation for Scientific Research for supporting
this project (grant No. 3.436.-0.78).

REFERENCES

1. Withers HR, Elkind MM (1970) Microcolony survival assay for cells of mouse intestinal mucosa exposed to radiation. Int J Radiat Biol 17:261-267
2. Rao KR, Blattmann H, Cordt I, Fritz-Niggli H (1979) Effect of negative pions, relative to 140 kV - 29 MeV photons and 20 MeV electrons, on proliferation of Ehrlich ascites carcinoma cells. Radiat and Environm Biophys 16:261-265.
3. Fritz-Niggli H, Blattmann H, Michel C, Rao KR, Schweizer P (1977) Preclinical experiments with the SIN negative pi-meson beam. RBE values for tumor and normal cell systems, and genetic damage studies in the beam peak and plateau regions. In Radiobiological Research and Radiotherapy. Vol.II. International Atomic Agency. Vienna.
4. Skarsgard LD (1979) The biological properties of pions. In Proceedings of the sixth International Congress of Radiation Research, Tokyo, May.
5. Fritz-Niggli H (1979) Radiobiological evaluation of the suitability of negative pions in tumor therapy: Facts and theories. Radiat Environm Biophys 17:47-65.
6. Peters LJ, Withers HR, Mason KA, DiCello JF (1980) Effect of fractionated doses of pions on normal tissues: Part II. Mouse jejunum. Int J Radiat Oncol Biol Phys 6:1667-1669.
7. Raju MR, Carpenter S, Tokita N, DiCello JF, Jackson D, Fröhlich EM, von Essen C (1980) Effect of fractionated doses of pions on normal tissues: Part I. Mouse skin. Int J Radiat Oncol Biol Phys 6:1663-1666.
8. Jordan SW, Juhas JM, Butler JLB, Kligerman MM (1981) Dependence of RBE on fraction size for negative pi-meson induced renal injury. Int J Radiat Oncol Biol Phys 7:223-227.
9. Landolt R, Arn D (1979) Effect of negative pi-mesons on vascular permeability of brain in neonatal rats. Rad and Environm Biophys 16:303-308.
10. Fike JR, Gillette EL (1978) ^{60}Co gamma and negative pi-meson irradiation of microvasculature. Int J Oncol Biol Phys 4:825-828.
11. BEIR III report (1980) National Research Council, Advisory Committee on the Biological Effects of Ionizing Radiation. The Effects on Populations of Exposure to Low Levels of Ionizing Radiation. National Academy of Sciences, Washington, D.C.
12. Michel C, Fritz-Niggli H (1978) Radiation-induced developmental anomalies in mammalian embryos by low doses and interaction with drugs, stress and genetic factors. In Late Biological Effects of Ionizing Radiation. Vol.II. International Atomic Agency. Vienna.

EFFECTS OF PIONS ON NORMAL TISSUES

N. Tokita
Life Sciences Division, Los Alamos National Laboratory,
Los Alamos, New Mexico, USA

INTRODUCTION

Pions, an intermediate-LET radiation, bear complex physical characteristics which depend on beam dimensions. For therapeutic application of pion beams, the Bragg peak must be spread out to encompass the treatment volume, and the range must be modulated to produce a uniform biological effect across the peak. The LET variation across the modulated peak must also be considered in terms of providing a uniform biological effect when fractionated schemes are employed. Verification of the uniform biological effectiveness of beams of various dimensions produced at LAMPF has been made using cultured mammalian cells[1] and mouse jejunum.[2] The latter is of more clinical relevance since fractionated doses of pions are used.

The contribution of charged particles and fast neutrons resulting from pion capture in tissue and the dependence of this contribution on pion treatment volume are another aspect to be considered[3] and are discussed in detail in this workshop.[4,5,6] The role of fast neutrons becomes significant for larger pion treatment volumes. The volume dependent RBE differences have been estimated by using cultured mammalian cells.[5,6] Our preliminary study using the mouse jejunum also indicates that fractionated treatment appears to result in a higher RBE value for large treatment volumes if the peak width remains the same.

In addition to the characterization of pion beams as a part of pretherapeutic radiobiology studies, RBE measurements in normal tissues, particularly for late effects, are of considerable importance since the normal tissue tolerance is often determined by its late effects.

In this paper, normal tissue radiobiology studies at LAMPF are reviewed with regard to: (1) biological beam characterization for the therapy program; and (2) the current status of acute and late effect studies using rodents.

A. Radiobiological Characterization of Pion Therapy Beams

(1) Verification of biological effectiveness at two different peak positions

Mice in a water phantom were exposed to four pion dose fractions (3 hr

292

intervals between fractions) at the proximal and distal peak positions of a
modulated 14 cm peak width beam (Fig. 1). Using the intestinal crypt survival
assay as described by Withers and Elkind,[7] the results plotted as a function
of the proximal peak dose indicated that the biological effects at both peak
positions were similar (Fig. 2). This study confirmed that the modulation of
the pion beam was appropriate.[2] It suggests that the RBE at the distal position is approximately 16% higher than at the proximal position.

(2) RBE variations for beams of small versus large peak width

A similar study was made to determine if variation in RBE exists for clinical beams of large (14 cm) or small (6 cm) peak width but having equal field
size of 11 cm x 14 cm. Mice were given four pion dose fractions (3 hr intervals between fractions) at the mid peak position of the beams (Fig. 3). The
intestinal crypt survival data showed no significant differences in biological
effects for these two beams as shown in Fig. 4.[2]

(3) Volume Effects

Two beams of an 8 cm peak width but of different field sizes, 7.5 cm x
7.5 cm or 20 cm x 20 cm (full width at half maximum), were tested using the
mouse jejunum for one and four pion dose fractions given at the mid peak
position.

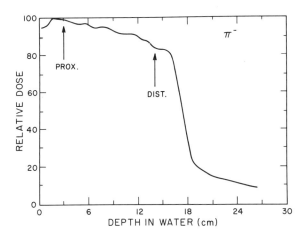

Fig. 1. Dose distribution curve of a 14 cm peak width beam in a water phantom. The beam size was 11 cm x 14 cm. The arrows indicate the positions at
which mice were exposed to pions. Note that the distal peak dose is approximately 16% less than the proximal dose (Figure modified from Ref. 2).

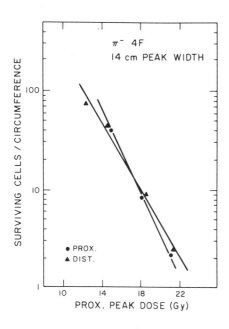

Fig. 2 The intestinal crypt cell survivals for 4 pion dose fractions expressed as a function of the <u>proximal</u> peak dose (Figure modified from Ref. 2).

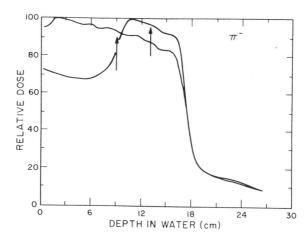

Fig. 3 Dose distribution curves of large (14 cm) and small (6 cm) peak beams with an equal field size, 11 cm x 14 cm. The arrows indicate the positions at which mice were exposed to pions (Figure modified from Ref. 2).

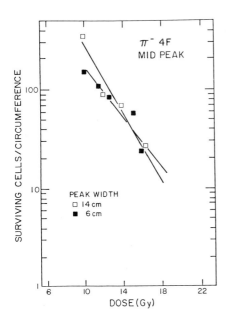

Fig. 4. The intestinal crypt cell survivals for 4 pion dose fractions expressed as a function of the dose for the two beams of different peak width which are described in Fig. 3 (Figure modified from Ref. 2).

The dose rate was 0.1–0.12 Gy/min for the large beam and 0.6 Gy/min for the small beam. Our preliminary data indicate that at four fractions the biological effect is greater for the large beam compared to the small beam despite the fact that the dose rate for the large beam is considerably lower than that for the small beam. No differences in biological effects, however, are observed at single fractions as shown in Fig. 5.

B. RBE Measurements

RBE measurements with pions for various normal tissues at LAMPF have, so far, been made using beams with narrow peak widths because of limited dose rate in the past. The RBE values of such beams may be different from beams used clinically due to differences in LET, thus limiting the use of such data for the clinical program. The RBE data available to date were compiled for acute effects on mouse skin,[8] mouse jejunum,[2,9,10] and for late effects on the mouse kidney,[11] rat spinal cord[12] and rat colon[13] as shown in Fig. 6 and Table 1. The RBE values are, in general, best-fitted by a power function when the RBE is plotted as a function of dose per fraction. The slopes for late

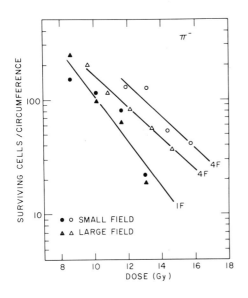

Fig. 5. Effect of beams of 8 cm peak width but different field sizes (7.5 cm x 7.5 cm and 20 cm x 20 cm) on survival of intestinal crypt cells following 1 and 4 pion dose fractions.

TABLE 1

PARAMETERS FOR RBE VALUES EXPRESSED AS A FUNCTION OF DOSE PER FRACTION

$$RBE = K D^{-S}$$

Tissues	Beam Size	K	S	Ref.
Skin	3 cm	1.97	0.20	(8)
Jejunum	3 cm	1.98	0.24	(9)
Jejunum	4 cm	1.43	0.12	(10)
Jejunum	14 cm	2.04	0.27	(2)
Kidney	3 cm	2.46	0.33	(11)
Spinal Cord	2 cm	3.69	0.33	(12)
Colon	2 cm	3.66	0.38	(13)

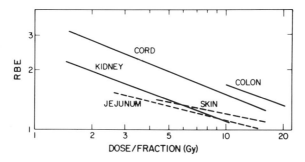

Fig. 6. RBE values plotted as a function of dose per fraction. Solid lines for late effects and dotted lines for acute effects. Sources: Skin,[8] Jejunum,[9] Kidney,[11] Spinal Cord,[12] and Colon.[13]

effects appear to be steeper compared to those for acute effects. For example, at clinically relevant dose fraction regions, the RBE value for the jejunum (acute effect) is considerably less than that for the spinal cord (late effect).

When the values for repair per dose fraction (fractional repair) were compared, the data suggest that the fractional repair is considerably less for pions compared to X rays regardless of tissue studied (Table 2). Further, the fractional repair ratios (pions/X rays) also appear to vary depending on tissue, fraction number as well as beam tune. At five fractions, this ratio for mouse skin, for example, is 0.65 ± 0.11 and that for jejunum is 0.37 ± 0.09. As the number of fractions increases, the fractional ratio for acute effects seems to decrease, whereas, that for the kidney late effect appears to increase.

DISCUSSION

Prelinical radiobiology studies required for the therapy program are designed to: (1) verify the uniformity of biological effect across the peak; (2) provide RBE data for beams of various dimensions; and (3) provide RBE data for acute and late effects of different normal tissues. For verification of large clinical beam tunes using fractionted schemes, the mouse jejunum may be the appropriate experimental system since the exposure area differences do not affect the final outcome.[7] Partial shielding of pion beams could change the quality of radiation. In addition, if collimation is required to shield part of the body of the animal, the effect of neutrons produced in the collimator must also be taken into consideration.

TABLE 2

COMPARISON OF FRACTIONAL REPAIR VALUES[a] FOR X RAYS AND PIONS

				Number of Fractions			
Tissues		2F	4F	5F	10F	15F	Ref.
Skin	X	0.59		0.57			(8)
	Pi	0.39		0.37			
Jejunum	X	0.45		0.52			(9)
	Pi	0.18		0.19			
Jejunum	X		0.30		0.44		(10)
	Pi		0.21		0.25		
Jejunum	X		0.42				(2)
	Pi		0.19				
Kidney	X	0.51		0.63		0.78	(11)
	Pi	0.25		0.37		0.52	
Spinal Cord	X			0.63		0.76	(12)
	Pi			0.25		0.30	
Colon	X	0.51					(13)
	Pi	0.19					

[a] Fractional repair is expressed as $((D_n - D_1)/(n-1))/(D_n/n)$, where n is the number of fractions; D_1 is the single fraction dose; and D_n is the total dose given in n fractions.

A comprehensive review of pion radiobiology has been reported previously.[14] In our studies of pion therapy beams, fractionated irradiation with pion beams modulated as shown in Fig. 1 seems to provide a uniform biological effect across the peak. Further, the volume effect appears present for fractionated doses although repeated experiments are required to confirm this phenomenon.

From the limited RBE studies to date, it appears that: (1) RBE values for late effects are greater than for acute effects; and (2) pion treatment with a small dose per fraction may not prevent the development of late effects, as suggested by the steeper slopes for late effects compared to acute effects. The latter is in contrast with X-ray experience in which a smaller dose per fraction treatment results in a lesser late tissue damage for a given total dose. These preliminary studies suggest that comprehensive RBE data on normal tissues, particularly for late effects, are required to obtain a better understanding of optimal pion fractionation schemes. Such efforts on the late effect studies of normal tissues (spinal cord, lung, kidney, liver, colon and lens in rodents) are in progress through collaborations at Los Alamos.

ACKNOWLEDGEMENTS

The author is grateful to Drs. L. D. Skarsgard, M. R. Raju, R. A. Tobey and A. J. van der Kogel for their comments and advice during the preparation of the text and to Marla Griffith for typing this manuscript.

This investigation was supported by the Grant CA17290 awarded by the U.S. National Cancer Institute, DHEW and by DOE.

REFERENCES

1. Raju MR, Butler JLB, Carpenter SG, Pierotti D, Smith A, Tokita, N(1981) Biological effects of pion therapy beams. I. Cultured cells. Int J Radiat Oncol Biol Phys (submitted).
2. Tokita N, Butler JLB, Pierotti D, Raju MR, Smith A(1981) Biological effects of pion therapy beams. II. Mouse jejunum. Int J Radiat Oncol Biol Phys (submitted).
3. Schillaci ME, Roeder DL(1973) Dose distribution due to neutrons and photons resulting from negative pion capture in tissue. Phy Med Biol 18: 821-829.
4. DiCello JF(1981) Radiation quality of pion beams. In Proceedings of the International Workshop on Pion and Heavy Ion Radiobiology: Preclinical and Clinical Studies. Elsevier, North Holland (in press).
5. Skarsgard LD(1981) RBE mapping in pion beams using the gel technique. In Proceedings of the International Workshop on Pion and Heavy Ion Radiobiology: Preclinical and Clinical Studies. Elsevier, North Holland (in press).
6. Raju MR(1981) Radiobiological comparison of pions and heavy ions. In Proceedings of the International Workshop on Pion and Heavy Ion Radiobiology: Preclinical and Clinical Studies. Elsevier, North Holland (in press).
7. Withers HR, Elkind MM(1970) Microcolony survival assay for cells of mouse intestinal mucosa exposed to radiation. Int J Radiat Biol 17:261-267.
8. Raju MR, Carpenter S, Tokita N, DiCello JF, Jackson D, Frohlich E, von Essen C(1980) Effect of fractionated pions on normal tissues: Part I. Mouse skin. Int J Radiat Oncol Biol Phys 6:1663-1666.
9. Peters LJ, Withers HR, Mason KA, DiCello JF(1980) Effect of fractionated pions on normal tissues: Part II. Mouse jejunum. Int J Radiat Oncol Biol Phys 6:1667-1669.
10. Goldstein L(1981) unpublished data.
11. Jordan SW, Yuhas JM, Butler JLB, Kligerman MM(1981) Dependence of RBE on fraction size for negative pi-meson induced renal injury. Int J Radiat Oncol Biol Phys 7:223-227.
12. Amols HI, Yuhas JM(1981) Induction of spinal cord paralysis by negative pi-mesons. Brit J Radiol 54:682-685.
13. Yuhas JM, Li A, Kligerman MM(1979) Present status of the proposed use of negative pi mesons in radiotherapy. Adv Radiat Biol 8:51-83.
14. Skarsgard LD(1979) The biological properties of pions. In Proceedings of the Sixth International Congress of Radiation Research, Tokyo, pp. 788-801.

PION BEAM STUDIES IN MICE AND IN PIGS

BRUCE G. DOUGLAS
Medical Biophysics Unit, B.C. Cancer Research Centre, 601 West 10th Avenue,
Vancouver, B.C. V5Z 1L3

INTRODUCTION

To date most of the in vivo work that has been carried out in the TRIUMF
project has been directed toward obtaining base line information on the effects
of x-rays in the systems to be employed for pion RBE studies. These x-ray
studies have given us a better understanding of the in vivo effects of
irradiation, and of some of the factors that influence the results. The studies
have examined the effects of some anaesthetic agents employed in experimental
animals, the effects of stress, as well as the effects of dose fractionation
factors including the time between doses of irradiation. Where we felt we
required large numbers of observations we have employed mice as experimental
animals, and where we believed it was important to mimic the set-up or physical
geometry to be employed with human subjects, we have employed pigs.

MOUSE SKIN STUDIES

Our baseline and x-ray control RBE studies in mice have been carried out
using the irradiation system originally developed by Douglas and Fowler[1] which
employs no anaesthesia. The baseline studies were done to obtain information
needed for the proper design of the RBE studies. These can be subdivided into
five general groups of experiments; first, fractionation experiments which
established an isoeffect relationship for mouse skin irradiation effects in vivo
(which also defined the shape of the in vivo cell survival curve); second, split
dose irradiation studies designed to determine the time course of sublethal
damage repair in vivo; third, fractionation studies carried out to determine the
time course of tissue repair (repopulation) during dose fractionation studies;
fourth, studies to examine the effects of stress on the results we might obtain
using the mouse foot system; and fifth, studies on the effects of lowering the
irradiation dose rate to 0.10 to 0.15 Gy per minute, the dose rate available at
TRIUMF for most of these studies. The initial thrust of these experiments was
to establish an isoeffect relationship (and incidently the shape of the cell
survival curve in vivo) for mouse skin. We found these could be well described
by cubic polynomial equations.[2,3] The isoeffect relationships which have been
established for mouse skin have facilitated the design of our experiments.

Sublethal Damage Repair Studies

These _in vivo_ studies of what is commonly referred to as Elkind & Sutton repair[4], have involved the use of two doses of radiation separated by short intervals of time. Figure 1 presents the results of an experiment where two x-ray doses of 13.5 Gy were separated by increasing time intervals. The scale

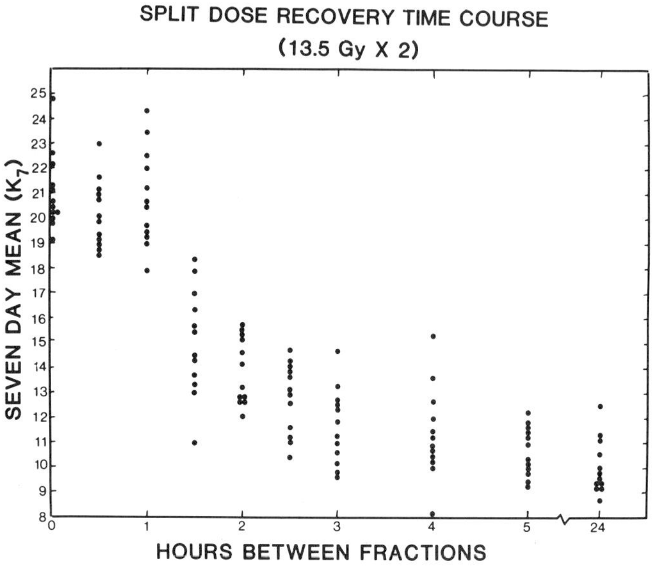

SPLIT DOSE RECOVERY TIME COURSE
(13.5 Gy X 2)

HOURS BETWEEN FRACTIONS

Fig. 1. Plot of average reaction versus time between doses for two doses of 13.5 Gy given at short time intervals. Low reactions reflect high cell survival. There is no suggestion of a decrease in reaction over the first hour.

employed is a ranked rather than an interval scale and has been previously published.[1,2] In this figure the severity of the reaction is plotted against the time between the start of the two dose fractions (exposure time: 10 min. approx.). Where the arbitrary visual scale has been transformed into an estimate of actual cell survival,[2,3] the data are presented in a more familiar form in figure 2. It can be seen that recovery _in vivo_ does not appear to be initiated for a period of about one hour after the start of the first radiation dose. The discovery of a repair free interval was unexpected, and we have not yet established whether it occurs after every dose of radiation or only after the first dose. Once repair has been initiated, recovery from sublethal injury occurs at a rate consistent with an exponential repair process with a half life

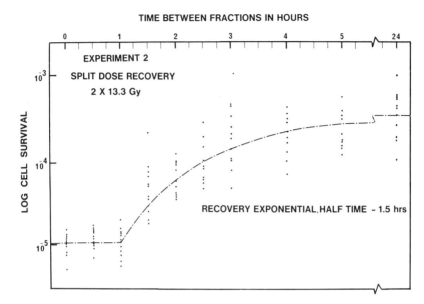

Fig. 2. Data from figure 1 with the K_7 value converted to estimates of real cell survival.[2,3] Sublethal damage repair[4] appears to be exponential with a half time of about 1.5 hours.

of about 1.5 hours. It is of interest in the interpretation of the early RBE studies reported below that at 6 hours repair is clearly incomplete, with between 10% and 20% of the sublethal injury remaining unrepaired.

Repopulation

Studies employing two and four dose fractions were also carried out to determine the time course of tissue recovery due to cell proliferation in this system. In the first experiment two fractions of 16.5 Gy were separated by time intervals varying from 24 hours to 21 days. Here we could find no evidence of a decrease in the severity of the reaction where a time period of less than 7 days had elapsed between the first and second doses of irradiation. Thus it appears that a dose of 16.5 Gy causes a cell proliferation delay of about 168 hours, or approximately 10 hours per Gray. The results of this experiment are presented in figure 3. Once proliferation is initiated, a cell cycle time of approximately 20 hours can be estimated from the data, a rate that is in agreement with published rates for similar conditions obtained using tritiated thymidine.[5] In a similar experiment, where four fractions of 11.25 Gy were

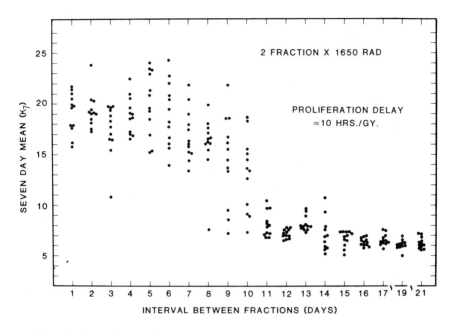

Fig. 3. Plot of average reaction versus time between doses for two doses of 16.5 Gy given at daily or longer intervals between doses. There is no significant reduction in the reaction for up to six days between doses, giving a cell proliferation delay of ∿ 10 hours per Gray.

delivered in up to 13.5 days (324 hours), no proliferation was evident; again indicating a cell proliferation delay of approximately 10 hours per gray for each of the first three dose fractions. This would suggest that the proliferation delay may have resulted from radiation-induced cell cycle delays that are proportional to dose. The most likely position in the cell cycle for these delays is probably G_0 or G_1. These results are consistent with our previously reported studies involving 8 and 64 dose fractions where we found no evidence of proliferation for these numbers of dose fractions in a 16 day overall time period[1], and with our results with 20 dose fractions where proliferation was evident in an experiment where the overall time period was 20 days.[2] This information has been useful to us in the planning of our experiments, as by an appropriate choice of overall time we can avoid repopulation during our studies.

Effects of Stress

For the majority of our studies we have employed male mice, with six mice being kept in each cage. The dimensions of the cages were 28 cm x 16 cm x 12 cm. In the early RBE experiments supervised by another investigator, mice for pion irradiations had been housed three per cage for convenience in handling, as only three mice can be irradiated at one time using our pion irradiation setup.[6] We noticed that the amount of fighting going on in the cages appeared to be greater in the cages housing six animals than in the cages housing three animals. As this could affect the wear and tear on the feet, an experiment was executed to determine if the number of animals housed per cage had any influence on the severity of the reactions resulting from a given dose of irradiation. In this experiment 120 mice were given a single dose of 26.5 Gy of 270 kv x-rays and then were split into two groups of 60 animals each. One group was then housed three animals per cage, and the second group was housed six per cage. The K_7 (seven day average reaction[2]) obtained for the animals housed three per cage was 17.9 ± 0.3, while the K_7 value obtained for the animals housed six per cage was 19.1 ± 0.3, indicating that the number of mice housed per cage did influence the results.

We also noticed that the animals became easier to handle as fractionation experiments proceeded. As we had found that prior handling was important in the swine irradiation experiments which are reported below, we felt that we should look to see if a series of sham irradiations given prior to the actual exposure would influence the results in the mouse foot studies. The results of this experiment are presented in figure 4. It can be seen that the reactions increase as the number of sham irradiations increase. We have yet to establish how many sham irradiations are necessary, but care in handling and sham irradiations do appear to be important. We assume that in the animals which do not receive sham irradiations, endogenously produced adrenaline causes a degree of hypoxia in the epithelium of the foot, but some other mechanism may be responsible. We anticipate that the elimination of this effect will reduce the cubic term in the isoeffect relationship for mouse skin.

Dose Rate

The final group of base line studies that we have carried out at TRIUMF have been studies on the effects of dose rate on the severity of the reactions that we observe in the mouse foot system. The dose rates that we have been employing to the present have been in the range of 0.12 to 0.15 Gy per minute, and as a result we have recently been carrying two control groups in our pion RBE studies, to determine both the "true RBE" (the RBE for the same dose rate

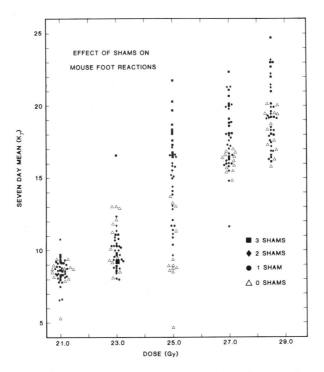

Fig. 4. Plot of average reaction for single doses versus the number of sham irradiations employed. Reactions increase as the number of sham irradiations increase.

x-rays), and the "practical RBE" (the RBE relative to x-rays at 1.5 Gy per minute), as we feel both are important. The "true RBE" will hopefully be relatively independent of dose rate, and these values should therefore be useful when higher or lower dose rates are used clinically, while the "practical RBE" has been useful in the choice of doses for the swine and human pion experiments that have been done to date.

It is of interest that these studies have given us an indication of the dose resolution that can be seen with the mouse foot system. Figure 5 shows the K_7 values obtained from a 10 and 20 fraction dose rate study. It can be seen that higher reactions are obtained with the high dose rate for the doses per fraction employed for the 10 fraction study, but not for the doses chosen for the 20 fraction study. It is also evident that the doses per fraction used for the high dose rate studies were lower than those used for the low dose rate ones.

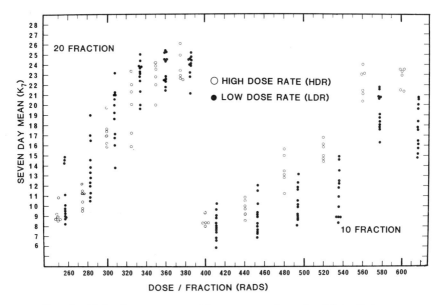

Fig. 5. Plot of average reactions versus dose for high (1.6 Gy per minute) and low (0.15 Gy per minute) dose rates for 10 and 20 dose fractions.

This was not the experimental design, but resulted from a dosimetry error of 3%. This was picked up because, when the data were first plotted assuming that the doses were the same, the low dose rate 20 fraction data had higher reactions than the high dose rate data. This could not be explained except through a dosimetry error of at least 3% with the low dose rate being the higher. Thus the biological system is capable, through multiple observations, of picking up dosimetry errors which are of the same order of magnitude as we are currently accepting in the determination of the physical radiation dose.

Mouse Skin RBE

To date seven mouse foot RBE experiments have been successfully completed at TRIUMF, and the results are listed below in Table 1. These experiments were completed before some of the baseline information detailed above was available and the experimental design was influenced both by the lack of some of this information and by constraints placed on the experimental design by the availability of the cyclotron. For doses between 3 and 5 Gy (10 and 20 dose fractions), the values obtained were between 1.4 and 1.6, but we anticipate that these values are underestimates of the true RBE for this system.

TABLE 1

MOUSE SKIN RBE

RBE values for peak pions relative to 270 KVP X-rays obtained at
TRIUMF using the mouse foot system

Experiment No.	No. of Fractions	Min. No. Hours between fract.	RBE	Reference X-ray dose in Gray
1	1	-	1.1	30
2	2	24	1.2	18
3	10	5	1.5	5
4	10	6	1.4	5
5A	16	5	1.4	4
5B	20	5	1.5	3
6	10	12	1.6	5
7	10	12	1.5	5

All irradiations at approximately 0.15 Gray per minute.

We have two reasons for believing that the RBE will ultimately prove to be
higher than the values given in Table 1. These are as follows. First, the
animals for these experiments were housed three per cage for the pion treated
animals and six per cage for the x-ray control animals. As mentioned above,
this will have yielded low reactions in the pion animals, and thus an error in
the RBE value which we would estimate should be about 7% higher than the values
obtained. The second reason relates to the time intervals employed between
doses for the majority of the multifraction experiments. Early in the in vivo
program, cyclotron limitations played a large part in experimental design. In
addition, the time course of repair of sublethal injury had not been accurately
defined when the experiments were carried out, and it was not appreciated that a
significant degree of sublethal injury remained unrepaired at the time interval
chosen for the time between fractions in these early experiments. While
sublethal injury will likely have affected both the pion studies and their x-ray
controls, we anticipate that double event cell killing will be less important
with pion irradiation. Thus incomplete repair will have affected the x-ray
control animals more, causing the reactions to be relatively higher than they
would otherwise have been, again causing the experiment to yield an
underestimate of the true RBE. While we do not know how large an error the
incomplete repair will have caused, we feel from the two experiments that have
been done using a 12 hour interval that the values for the RBE may be low by a

further 3 to 7%. Thus we feel that the effect of these two experimental design problems was to yield an overall underestimate of the RBE of between 10 and 15 percent. Further experiments are needed and are planned.

PIG SKIN STUDIES

With pig skin, as with mouse foot, a large number of control experiments have been carried out in order to examine several aspects of the pig skin irradiation system, including the following: first, the time course and dose response of irradiation induced skin reactions in the pig; second, the effects of various anaesthetic agents administered during irradiation exposure on the severity of the reactions generated; third, fractionation studies to determine the variation in dose required when the number of fractions is altered, and fourth, RBE studies.

Pig skin radiation reaction time course

Some of the investigators who have previously employed pig skin for irradiation studies have reported seeing two waves in the skin radiation reaction of pigs.[7] We, too, have noted two waves, an early reaction (which is not seen consistently for small numbers of fractions) which occurs between 15 and 40 days from the start of the irradiation, and a later wave, which we refer to as the medium term reaction, which we tend to see between day 40 and day 180. Figure 6, which is taken from an RBE study which will be further discussed

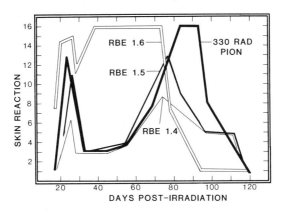

Fig. 6. Time course plot of pig skin radiation reactions from a Pion RBE study. Early and medium wave reactions are clearly evident. X-ray doses were 4.63, 4.95 and 5.29 Gy per fraction for 10 fractions, corresponding to possible RBE values of 1.4, 1.5 and 1.6.

below, shows some examples of the time course of the skin reactions seen. The scale employed used visual criteria for defining the severity of the reactions and is a ranked scale rather than an interval scale. On this scale numbers over 6 indicate that increasing proportions of the areas are ulcerated, while lower numbers indicate degrees of erythema and dry desquamation. Where a ranked scale is employed one can only say that reaction A is greater or less than reaction B, and means, standard deviations, and other mathematical manipulations that can be used with interval data cannot be legitimately employed. It can be seen that three of the areas whose reactions are plotted show clearly defined early and medium term reactions, centered on days 25 and 80 to 90 respectively. The fourth curve (x-rays, RBE 1.6) is different from the other three. We have found that where the early wave reaction is very severe, such as occurred for the 1.6 RBE x-ray curve, the reaction tends to progress directly into the medium wave without full healing, and while the duration of the medium term reaction tends to be longer under these circumstances, the reactions do tend to heal much earlier than if the early wave ulceration does heal. We feel that the early wave reaction is almost certainly based on the loss of the epithelial layer, while the medium wave appears to be vascular in origin. Where the early wave is small or absent, the medium term reaction wave is occasionally preceeded by a purplish discoloration similar to a bruise. This discoloration is deep to the epidermis, and proceeds to ulcerate through the epidermis over the week to 10 days that follow the initial appearance of the discoloration. We feel that because of this, the medium term reaction is likely vascular in origin, with the discoloration being a bruise, and of more general relevance to "tissue tolerance" than the early reaction. For low doses there may be no medium term reaction seen.

The Effects of Anaesthetic Agents Administered During Irradiation

When we first started doing experiments with pigs we employed an anaesthetic system similar to those used by previous investigators.[8] Initially we employed premedication with atravet (a phenothiazine) and morphine; induction with pentothal (pentobarbital sodium) and maintenance with nitrous oxide (68 to 69%), fluothane (halothane, 1 to 2%), and 30% oxygen. While we obtained reasonably consistent dose response curves for fraction numbers four or higher, we found an extreme variability in our responses for single doses and for two fractions. We interpreted these findings as indicating that we had variable degrees of hypoxia in the skin when we did our irradiations, and a series of experiments were done to investigate the effects of the various anaesthetic agents that we were using. The first frame of figure 7 shows a plot of the medium wave reactions we

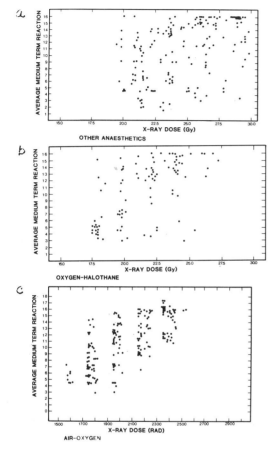

Fig. 7. Plot of average medium wave reactions versus dose for (a) animals irradiated using a variety of anaesthetic agents in addition to oxygen and halothane (b) animals irradiated with oxygen and halothane anaesthesia (c) animals irradiated without anaesthesia.

obtained as a function of dose of irradiation for single doses when we were using our initial anaesthetic system and while we were doing the studies on the various anaesthetic agents themselves. It can be seen that no consistent dose response is present. For a period of time we felt that it might be possible to use an anaesthetic system employing only oxygen and halothane, and the reactions we obtained with these agents are presented in the second frame of this figure. It can be seen that while a dose response is now evident, a significant number of low reaction scores are still present for some of the higher doses employed.

Finally we decided that we could not use any anaesthetic agents, and we developed a method of restraining the animals such that we could irradiate them without either upsetting them unduly or resorting to the use of pharmacological tranquilizing agents. The responses we obtained without anaesthesia are presented in the last frame of figure 7. A dose response is now evident in the data, and reactions are generated with radiation doses that are lower than those we had previously found necessary.

We also noted that animals that were very upset tended to have reactions that were lower than those for animals which were more settled. As adrenaline (a pharmacological agent produced endogenously in response to stress) tends to constrict cutaneous blood vessels, we felt that irradiating the animals while they were in a new and stressfull environment, without the chance to become accustomed to it and realize that they were not going to be hurt, might also generate hypoxia related artifacts in our results. To test the importance of this effect we did an experiment to look at the effect of sham irradiations on the severity of the reactions generated, and again we found that at least three sham irradiations were necessary if we wished to minimize the effects of stress in our results.

Fractionation

In order to facilitate the design of RBE studies, we have done several fractionation studies using unanaesthetized animals. The results of one such experiment are presented in figure 8. The 2 to 16 fraction data from this experiment were used to generate an F_e plot[1] (plot of inverse of total dose versus dose per fraction) in figure 9, from which we were able to calculate a value for β/α : the value obtained was 3.5×10^{-3} rad^{-1}. This value is higher than that obtainable for both mouse (0.96×10^{-3} rad^{-1}), and man (2.9×10^{-3} rad^{-1}). It is of interest, however, that mouse and pig skin β/α values bracket the value for human skin.

Pig Skin RBE

The pig skin RBE studies that have been carried out and are planned have been designed, because of the limitations of a ranked reaction scoring system, to determine a narrow range within which the RBE for pig skin falls. As mentioned above, on a given animal all that can be said is that one reaction is greater or less than another. Because of this we have designed our experiments using one pion irradiation area per animal, and three different x-ray doses, with the x-ray doses being chosen to determine if the RBE is greater or less than 1.4, 1.5 and 1.6. This permitted the treatment of each animal as an experiment as

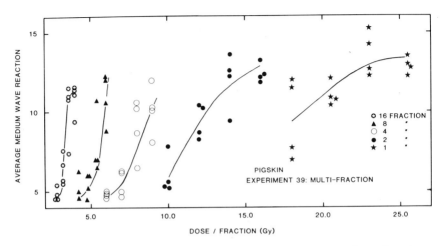

Fig. 8. Plot of average medium wave reaction versus dose for a fractionation study employing 1, 2, 4, 8 and 16 dose fractions.

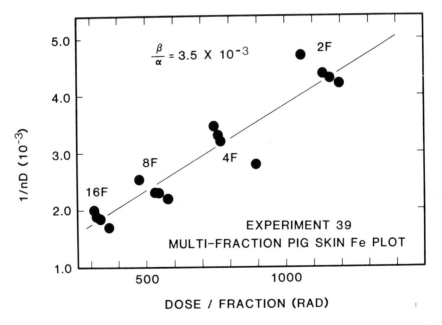

Fig. 9. Fe Plot (1) taken from the data from figure 9. The β/α value that can be calculated here is 3.5×10^{-3} rad^{-1}.

312

well as the pooling of the data from all animals in a given experiment. The
positions of the irradiated areas are indicated schematically in figure 10. One

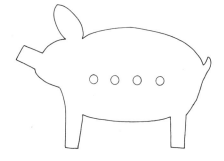

Fig. 10. Schematic representation of
the areas irradiated in the pion pig
skin RBE studies. The positions pion
and x-ray doses were systematically
altered in any given experiment to
eliminate the chance of position
depends on the severity of the
reactions.

area was irradiated using pi-mesons, while the other three were irradiated using
three different doses of x-rays chosen as mentioned above. To date we have only
succeeded in completing the irradiations and readings of two ten dose fraction
pig skin RBE studies. The first of these studies employed two different pion
doses per fraction (2.9 and 3.3 pion Gy) and purebred Yorkshire pigs. The x-ray
doses were chosen to cover the RBE range of 1.4 to 1.6, and six animals were
employed in the experiment. As an example, the results for one of the three
animals given 3.3 pion Gy were presented in figure 6. It is of interest that
the early wave RBE that can be determined from this data is less than the medium
wave RBE; from figure 11a the early wave RBE can be seen to be approximately
1.4, in keeping with the RBE values obtained for both mouse and human early
(epithelial) reactions. However it appears that the situation may be different
for the medium term reaction (see Figure 12a). Here the RBE obtained for the
low reaction generated by 290 pion rad is again about 1.4, but the value
observed for the more severe reaction generated by the 330 pion rad is much
higher: over 1.6 for the pooled data. The results from the individual animals
were the same: for two animals the RBE was over 1.6, and for the third
approximately equal to 1.6. The second pig skin RBE study could not be carried
out using Yorkshire pigs for logistic reasons. This experiment employed animals
from the UBC Swine Unit which are not of a uniform genetic background. These
animals are primarily a mixture of Yorkshire and Landrace strains. The early
wave RBE values are similar to our previous results (see figure 11b) but the
medium wave results may be different from those of our first experiment. A
distinct separate second wave has not as yet been seen with all of these
animals, and the preliminary results to six months, which are currently

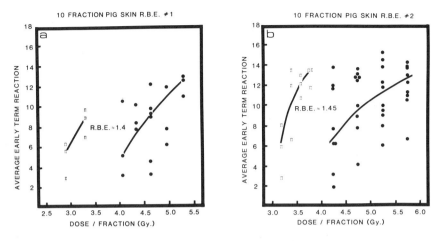

Fig. 11. Plot of average early reaction versus dose for the first (a) and second (b) pig skin RBE experiments. The RBE values for early reactions are about 1.4 for both experiments. Curves are fitted by eye through the median reactions as the data and scale are ranked rather than interval in nature.

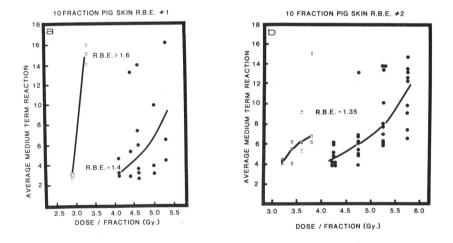

Fig. 12. Plot of average medium wave reaction versus dose for the first (a) and second (b) pig skin RBE experiments. In the first experiment the RBE for the 2.9 pion Gy dose is ∿ 1.4, but for 3.3 pion Gy it is greater than 1.6. Final data are not as yet available for the second experiment, but the available data to six months (b) do not show a high RBE. Curves are fitted by eye through the estimated median reaction values as the data and scale are ranked rather than interval in nature.

314

available, do not show the high RBE for high dose pions (see figure 12b).
These results, while inconclusive to date, suggest two things of concern to the
Radiation Oncologist; first that the late RBE may be higher than the early RBE,
making it risky to use the familiar early reaction as an estimate of what
reactions may be seen later, and that there may be a threshold tissue damage
level for severe late term effects. If these observations are supported in
further experiments, it will be necessary to be very cautious in the
introduction of pions to clinical use.

CONCLUSIONS

RBE studies completed in vivo to date at TRIUMF indicate that the dose rate
corrected RBE will be in the vicinity of 1.6, with a working RBE for dose rates
of 0.15 Gy per minute of about 1.4 for epithelial (early wave) reactions. The
RBE for "tolerance" may be significantly higher, and a threshold for severe
reactions may be present.

REFERENCES

1. Douglas BG, Fowler JF (1976) The effect of multiple small doses of x-rays on
   skin reactions in the mouse and a basic interpretation. Radiat. Res.
   66:401-426.
2. Douglas BG, Henkelman RM, Lam GKY, Fowler JF, Gregory CJ (1979) Practical and
   theoretical considerations in the use of the mouse foot system to derive
   epithelial stem cell survival parameters. Radiat Res 77:453-471.
3. Lam GKY, Henkelman RM, Douglas BG, Gregory CJ (1979) Method of analysis to
   derive cell survival from observation of tissue damage following fractionated
   radiation. Radiat Res 77:440-452.
4. Elkind MM, Sutton H (1960) Radiation response of mammalian cells grown in
   culture. 1. Repair of x-ray damage in surviving chinese hamster cells. Radiat
   Res 13:556-593.
5. Denekamp J, Stewart FA, Douglas BG (1976) Changes in the proliferation rate
   of mouse epidermis after irradiation: continuous labelling studies. Cell
   Tissue Kinet 9:19-29.
6. Skarsgard LD, Henkelman RM, Eaves CJ (1980) Pions for radiotherapy at TRIUMF.
   J Can Assoc Radiol 31:3-12.
7. Fowler JF, Morgan RL, Silvester JA, Bewley DK, Turner BA (1963) Experiments
   with fractionated x-ray treatment of the skin of pigs. 1. Fractionation up to
   28 days. Br J Radiol 36:188-196.
8. Fowler JF, Hill DW, Morgan RL, Nunn JF, Weaver B, Woolmer RF (1962)
   Anaesthesia for the irradiated pig: a study in remote control. Br J Anaesth
   34:327-331.

Published 1982 by Elsevier Science Publishing Co., Inc.
PION AND HEAVY ION RADIOTHERAPY:
Pre-Clinical and Clinical Studies
L. D. Skarsgard

IN VIVO RADIOBIOLOGY WITH HEAVY IONS

S. B. Curtis[+] and L. S. Goldstein[++]
[+]Lawrence Berkeley Laboratory, Berkeley, California 94720, [++]Department of
Radiation Oncology and Laboratory of Radiobiology, University of California,
San Francisco, California 94143

INTRODUCTION

In reviewing the data as it exists at present in the area of in vivo heavy
ion radiobiology, it becomes evident that compromises must be made between
completeness and conciseness. The present analysis will rely on results that
were selected primarily for two reasons: (1) several beams and beam configurations (i.e., ion ranges and ridge filter thicknesses) were employed with
a single animal system and end point and (2) the data are of relatively recent
origin. A review of earlier work has been published[1], and a comprehensive
article reviewing much of the more recent work is presently in preparation[2].

The motivation behind the present approach stems from a desire to evaluate the relative merits of the various charged particle beams. Other attempts
at such an evaluation have been made[3,4,5,6], but most of the data used were
from in vitro cell survival studies and none explicitly took into account
the ability of cells or tissues to recover after fractionated doses. The
present treatment borrows freely from several of the concepts already defined
and adds to them consideration of recovery effects after dose fractionation.

QUANTITATION OF THREE POSSIBLE ADVANTAGES OF HIGH-LET CHARGED PARTICLE RADIATION

In the evaluation of a given radiation beam for clinical use, three factors have been mentioned as being possibly advantageous for charged particle
beams with high LET components in their stopping regions: (1) the increased
dose and RBE in the target (or tumor) region over that in the plateau or normal tissue region, (2) the decreased repair capacity in the tumor region over
that in the plateau region, and (3) the decreased oxygen effect in the tumor
region over that from photon radiation, thus increasing the probability of
killing any radioresistant hypoxic cells that might be present in the tumor.
The first two are a result of the difference in LET in the peak relative to
the plateau region and the third is a result of the increased LET of the
radiation over that of photons.

We now define three factors reflecting each of the above three characteristics.

1. The Biological Dose Factor (BDF)

The product of the RBE for a given biological effect and the absorbed dose gives a measure of the efficiency of a given irradiation to produce the effect. For a chosen beam of radiation, the efficiency to produce any effect will be a function of depth within the absorbing medium. If the dose and the RBE vary with depth, so will the biological efficiency. Thus, we define the biological dose factor (BDF) as a ratio of the product of the absorbed dose and RBE in the target or peak region to the product of the absorbed dose and RBE in the plateau or entrance region:

$$BDF = \frac{RBE_{peak} \cdot D_{peak}}{RBE_{plateau} \cdot D_{plateau}} \tag{1}$$

This is the same quantity defined in the "vector representation" of therapy modalities by Blakely et al.[3] The ideal situation would be to use the absorbed dose and RBE for tumor cure in the target region in the numerator of equation (1) and the absorbed dose in the critical normal tissue along with the RBE for the most critical effect in that tissue in the denominator. Eventually, enough data may be gathered so that it will become possible to evaluate certain tumor sites in this manner. Presently, however, not enough is known about either the RBE values for human tumor cure and regression or the RBE values for the critical normal tissues surrounding the tumors to proceed in this way. Therefore, the following analysis will be made using RBE values in both the peak and plateau regions for the same end point. This will also be the case for the other two factors defined below.

2. Relative Non-Recovery Factor (RNF)

It is well known that repair is less evident in cells irradiated with high LET radiation. A quantity, D_r, known as the average recovered dose per interval is defined as:

$$D_r = \frac{(D_n - D_s)}{(n-1)} \tag{2}$$

where D_n is the total dose given in n fractions to produce a given biological effect, D_s is the single dose necessary to produce the same biological effect, and (n-1) is the number of intervals in the fractionated schedule. If D_r

is divided by the dose per fraction, D_n/n, we have the fraction (F) of dose recovered on the average per interval:

$$F = \frac{D_r}{D_n/n} = \frac{(D_n - D_s)/(n-1)}{D_n/n} = \frac{(D_n - D_s)n}{D_n(n-1)} \tag{3}$$

The fraction of dose not recovered, i.e., 1-F, is then a measure of the inability of this tissue to recover. Thus, we define the relative non-recovery factor (RNF):

$$RNF = \frac{(1-F)_{peak}}{(1-F)_{plateau}} \tag{4}$$

where all doses are chosen to obtain the same biological effect.

3. Oxygen Gain Factor (OGF)

The suggestion has been made that the presence of surviving hypoxic cells after photon radiation may be a cause for the lack of local tumor control for some human tumors[7].

High LET radiation decreases the difference between hypoxic and oxygenated cell radiosensitivity. Thus, it appears reasonable that high LET radiation might increase local control of some tumors that have large hypoxic fractions or for which reoxygenation is lacking or diminished. The oxygen enhancement ratio (OER) is defined as the ratio of dose producing a given effect in hypoxic cells to that producing the same effect in oxygenated cells. The value of OER is generally between 2.5 and 3.0 for x- or γ-radiation and decreases as the LET of the radiation increases. Thus, a measure of the decrease of the effect of oxygen on radiosensitivity is given by the ratio of the OER for x-rays to the OER for the radiation in question. This ratio, called the oxygen gain factor (OGF) is defined:

$$OGF = \frac{OER_{x-rays}}{OER_{heavy\ ion}} \tag{5}$$

The independence of the factors

Although all three factors depend on the LET of the beam in question, it is not necessary that the cellular characteristics or processes affected be related or that the probability for the events leading to the final end point have the same dependence on LET. The oxygen effect and its decrease with increasing LET appear to have a different dependence on LET than the RBE for cell killing; the OER does not change appreciably in the intermediate LET range where RBE is already increasing significantly. Also, there is evidence that for some cell lines, no repair is evident for neutron radiation even though a shoulder exists on the single dose survival curve[8]. There is, in addition, evidence that sublethal damage may occur even in situations where the survival curve is exponential[9]. This implies that the RBE for cell killing and for repair may, in fact, be decoupled to some extent.

COMBINATION OF THE FACTORS: THE THERAPEUTIC MERIT FACTOR (TMF)

The assumption is made that the three factors can be combined in an independent way into an overall therapeutic merit factor (TMF). Following the general concept of the vector representation of radiation modalities[3], a generalized vector in a three-dimensional space can be defined. The three orthogonal axes define all possible values for the BDF, RNF, and OGF factors. A vector can be defined in this space; its absolute magnitude is given by:

$$|V| = \left[BDF^2 + RNF^2 + OGF^2 \right]^{\frac{1}{2}} \tag{6}$$

For a photon beam, each of these factors equals unity if we ignore any drop in the dose versus depth curve. Thus, we normalize the magnitude to unity for a photon beam with a flat dose versus depth curve by introducing appropriate weighting factors and call this the therapeutic merit factor (TMF):

$$TMF = \left[w_1 \cdot BDF^2 + w_2 \cdot RNF^2 + w_3 \cdot OGF^2 \right]^{\frac{1}{2}} \tag{7}$$

The weighting factors determine the relative importance of each term. If other considerations are found to be important, it is easy to generalize still further by increasing the dimensionality and adding the squares of other factors, suitably weighted. In general, then:

$$TMF = \left[w_1 \cdot BDF^2 + w_2 \cdot RNF^2 + w_3 \cdot OGF^2 + \ldots \right]^{\frac{1}{2}} \tag{8}$$

where $\Sigma w_i = 1$, is summed over the numbers of factors.

At present, there is no consensus on the most appropriate weighting factors. It is reasonable that the weighting of each term may depend on tumor type and site. In the following discussion we will restrict ourselves to three dimensions and assume equal weighting for the three terms ($w_1 = w_2 = w_3 = 1/3$).

The biological systems

For the subsequent analysis, the animal (and cellular) systems chosen were those that yield values of the three factors at various depths being studied with carbon, neon and argon ion beams at the Berkeley Bevalac.

In no single animal system are data available to obtain all three factors. The most complete set of data comes from the studies with the jejunal crypt cell system in the mouse[10,11]. Both BDF and RNF values for several beams, ranges, and ridge filter depths can be calculated from the results obtained with this system. Values of BDF can also be obtained for the jejunal crypt cell system[12], the mouse testes system[13], the rat rhabdomyosarcoma system[14], the 9-L gliosarcoma[5], and the EMT6 tumor cell system in mice[10]. The values for BDF for these systems are summarized in Table 1. Also included for comparison are in vitro BDF values for cell survival of R2D2 rat tumor cells[6]. The end points used for each system are given in the footnotes to the table. We note a wide range of values for the carbon and neon ion beams; in general, they yield higher values than for the argon ion beam. Also, the shorter range neon beam (425 MeV/amu, range: 14-15 cm) gives higher values than the longer range neon beam (557 MeV/amu, range: 24-25 cm).

TABLE 1
BIOLOGICAL DOSE FACTOR (BDF) FOR IN VIVO SYSTEMS $BDF = (Dose_{pk} \cdot RBE_{pk})/(Dose_{pl} \cdot RBE_{pl})$

Ion	Carbon		Neon				Argon	
Energy	400 MeV/amu		425 MeV/amu		557 MeV/amu		570 MeV/amu	
Ridge Filter	4 cm	10 cm	4 cm	10 cm	4 cm	10 cm	4 cm	10 cm
Proximal peak	1.5^g	1.00^a	1.7^g	1.2^e		0.85^a	1.2^f	0.86^a
	1.7^f	1.2^e	1.7^f			1.0^e	0.86^g	1.1^e
Midpeak	1.53^b		1.55^b				1.08^b	
	1.33^a	1.13^a	1.275^a	1.0^e	1.04^a	0.91^a	0.77^d	0.95^a
		1.1^e						
	$1.4-1.5^e$		$1.8-1.9^e$			1.0^e	$1.3-0.9^e$	0.9^e
Distal peak	2.1^c		1.6^c				1.0^c	
	1.3^f	1.23^a	1.1^f			1.04^a	0.71^f	0.92^a
	1.3^g	1.2^e	1.1^g	1.0^e		0.9^e	0.59^g	0.6^e

[a]End point: 10 surviving crypt cells per circumference in jejunal crypt cells in mice (Goldstein et al., 1981b).
[b]End point: 1% survival of EMT6 tumor cells irradiated in vivo in mice (Goldstein et al., 1981a).
[c]End point: 50-day growth delay of R-1 tumors irradiated in rats (Tenforde et al., 1981).
[d]End point: 10 surviving crypt cells per circumference in jejunal crypt cells in mice (Goldstein et al., 1981a).
[e]Range of values from in vitro cell data at 10% survival (R2D2 tumor cells) (Curtis et al., in press).
[f]End point: 10% survival of clonogenic crypt cells (Alpen et al., 1980).
[g]End point: Ratio of D_0 values for mouse spermatogonial cell killing (Alpen et al., in press).

The factors measuring recovery (RNF) in the various beams are summarized in Table 2. Here fewer data exist: the jejunal crypt cell data of Goldstein et al.[11], and the rat spinal cord data of Leith et al.[15] Here both carbon and neon ion beams yield higher values than the argon beam and both the carbon and neon ion beams appear to be comparable in producing relatively less net recovery in the peak as compared to the plateau region.

TABLE 2
RELATIVE NONRECOVERY FACTOR (RNF) FOR IN VIVO SYSTEMS $RNF = (1-F)pk/(1-F)pl$ where $F = \dfrac{(D_n - D_s)}{(n-1)} \cdot \dfrac{n}{D_n}$

Ion		Carbon		Neon				Argon	
Energy		400 MeV/amu		425 MeV/amu		557 MeV/amu		570 MeV/amu	
Ridge Filter		4 cm	10 cm	4 cm	10 cm	4 cm	10 cm	4 cm	10 cm
Proximal peak	2Fx	-	0.98^a	-	-	-	-	-	0.88^a
	5Fx	-	1.03^a	-	-	-	1.41^a	-	-
	10Fx	-	1.21^a	-	-	-	1.24^a	-	-
Midpeak	2Fx	1.45^a	1.12^a	1.38^a	-	-	-	-	0.91^a
	4Fx	2.0^b	-	1.08^b	-	-	-	-	-
	5Fx	1.86^a	0.98^a	1.36^a	-	1.37^a	1.32^a	-	-
	10Fx	1.72^a	1.36^a	-	-	1.62^a	1.25^a	-	-
Distal peak	2Fx	-	1.21^a	-	-	-	-	-	0.95^a
	5Fx	-	1.21^a	-	-	-	1.42^a	-	-
	10Fx	-	1.58^a	-	-	-	1.35^a	-	-

[a]End point: 10 surviving crypt cells per circumference in jejunal crypt cells in mice (Goldstein et al., 1981b).
[b]End point: 50% paralysis in rats (Leith et al., 1980)

There are very few in vivo animal data available for obtaining OGF values. Table 3 summarizes the data presently available. The majority come from in vitro T-1 and R2D2 cell survival studies[3,6]. The only two animal systems yielding data are the 9-L rat gliosarcoma system[5], in which there is no measurable hypoxic fraction in the tumors in air-breathing animals, and the rat rhabdomyosarcoma[14], in which an hypoxic fraction of 35% was measured and a correction was made in the air-breathing animal cell survival data to obtain a calculated survival curve for oxygenated cells. From Table 3 we see that argon ions clearly yield the highest values, with neon ions, in general, yielding values higher than carbon ions.

TABLE 3

OXYGEN GAIN FACTOR (OGF) FOR IN VIVO SYSTEMS $\quad$ OGF = $OER_{x-rays}/OER_{heavy\ ions}$

Ion	Carbon		Neon				Argon	
Energy	400 MeV/amu		425 MeV/amu		557 MeV/amu		570 MeV/amu	
Ridge filter	4 cm	10 cm	4 cm	10 cm	4 cm	10 cm	4 cm	10 cm
Proximal peak	1.6^b	$1.0-1.5^b$	$1.4-1.5^b$	$1.1-1.3^b$	-	$1.2-1.3^b$	$1.9-2.1^b$	1.9^b
Midpeak	1.27^c	$1.1-1.3^b$	1.4^c 1.4^b	$1.3-1.6^b$	-	$1.3-1.4^b$	2.2^b	1.9^b
Distal peak	1.2^a 1.5^b	$1.4-1.5^b$	1.3^a $1.7-1.8^b$	$1.7-1.9^b$	-	1.7^b	2.2^b	2.1^b

[a]End point: 10% cell survival in R2D2 rat rhabdomyosarcoma tumors; oxygenated curve calculated from air breathing curve and an assumed hypoxic fraction of 35% (Tenforde et al., 1980).
[b]Range of values at 10% survival in T-1 and R2D2 cells in vitro (Curtis et al., in press; Blakely et al., 1980).
[c]End point: 10% cell survival in 9-L gliosarcoma tumor in the rat (Wheeler et al., 1979).

Values for the therapeutic merit factors

Averaging the values for the proximal, mid, and distal peak regions, we can calculate the therapeutic merit factors from equation (7), with $w_1 = w_2 = w_3 = 1/3$. The values for 24-cm-range carbon and neon ion beams, both with a 10-cm ridge filter, are compared in Table 4. The available values for 14-cm range neon and argon beams with a 4-cm ridge filter are also given in the table. Unfortunately, the TMF value for the argon ion beam cannot be calculated because repair data for this beam are lacking.

TABLE 4

THERAPEUTIC MERIT FACTOR (TMF) $\qquad$ TMF = $\left[1/3\ BDF^2 + 1/3\ RNF^2 + 1/3\ OGF^2 \right]^{\frac{1}{2}}$

Range, Ridge filter	Ion	Average Values of the Factors in Midpeak			
		BDF	RNF	OGF[a]	TMF
24-cm, 10-cm spread peak	Carbon	1.12	1.15	1.3	1.19
	Neon	0.93	1.29	1.4	1.22
14-cm, 4-cm spread peak	Neon	1.43	1.27	1.5	1.40
	Argon	0.89	-	2.2	-

[a]Data from R-1 tumor cells and T-1 human cells in vitro.

CONCLUSIONS

From Table 4 we see that there is little difference in the therapeutic
merit factor between the long range (24 cm) carbon and neon ion beams (1.19
for carbon ions as compared with 1.22 for neon ions). Data are not available
to compare the neon and argon ion beams even at the shorter range. However,
with an estimate of RNF for argon ions as low as 0.9, the TMF for argon ions
would exceed that for neon ions. It appears likely that an ion with mass
and charge intermediate between those of neon and argon might yield values
as high or higher than the neon or carbon ion beams at long range. Thus,
it is important to pursue ongoing studies with silicon ions, a beam with such
intermediate charge and mass values. Data necessary to obtain TMF values
for comparison with the above values must be gathered. Finally, we conclude
that for the heavy ion beams for which adequate data are available for analysis, the short range (14 cm) neon beam has the best overall characteristics
for clinical application, taking depth-dose, relative RBE, the oxygen effect,
and relative recovery capabilities into account.

ACKNOWLEDGEMENTS

It is a pleasure to acknowledge the able editorial assistance of M.C.
Pirruccello in the preparation of this paper. This research was supported
by the National Cancer Institute (Grants CA-17227 and CA-17411), the Office
of Health and Environmental Research (U.S. Department of Energy under Contract
W-7405-Eng-48), and the Laboratory of Radiobiology and Environmental Health
(U.S. Department of Energy under Contract DE-AM03-76-SF01012).

REFERENCES

1. Raju MR (1980) Heavy Particle Radiotherapy. New York: Academic Press.
2. Leith JT, Ainsworth EJ, Alpen EL Radiation biology of heavy ions: effects
   on normal tissues. In Leith J (ed.) Advances in Radiation Biology. New
   York: Academic Press, in press.
3. Blakely EA, Tobias CA, Ngo FQH, Curtis SB (1980) Physical and cellular
   radiobiological properties of heavy ions in relation to cancer therapy
   applications. In Pirruccello MC, Tobias CA (eds), Biological and Medical
   Research with Accelerated Heavy Ions at the Bevalac, 1977-1980, pp. 73-
   86. Lawrence Berkeley Laboratory Report LBL-11220.
4. Raju MR, Amols HI, DiCello JF, Howard J, Lyman JT, Koehler AM, Graves R,
   Smothers JB (1978) A heavy particle comparative study. Part I. Depth-dose
   distributions. Br J Radiol 51:699.
5. Wheeler KT, Deen DF, Leith JT, Norton KL (1979). Cellular response of a
   rat brain tumor to a therapeutic carbon ion beam. Radiology 133:757-760.
6. Curtis SB, Schilling WA, Tenforde TS, Crabtree KE, Tenforde SD, Howard J
   Survival of oxygenated and hypoxic tumor cells in the extended peak regions of heavy charged particle beams. Radiat Res, in press.

7. Thomlinson RH, Gray LH (1955). The histological structure of some human lung cancers and the possible implications for radiotherapy. Br J Cancer 9:539-549.
8. Ngo FQH, Han A, Utsumi H, Elkind MM (1977) Comparative radiobiology of fast neutrons. Relevance to radiotherapy and basic studies. Int J Radiat Oncol Biol Phys 3:187-193.
9. Ngo FQH, Blakely EA, Tobias CA (1981) Sequential exposures of mammalian cells to low- and high-LET radiation. I. Lethal effects following x-ray and neon-ion irradiation. Radiat Res 87:59-78.
10. Goldstein LS, Phillips TL, Fu KK, Ross GY, Kane LJ (1981a) Biological effects of accelerated heavy ions. I. Single doses in normal tissue, tumors and cells in vitro. Radiat Res 86:529-541.
11. Goldstein LS, Phillips TL, Ross GY (1981b) Biological effects of accelerated heavy ions. I. Fractionated irradiation of intestinal crypt cells. Radiat Res 86:542-558.
12. Alpen EL, Powers-Risius P, McDonald M (1981) Survival of intestinal crypt cells after exposure to high Z, high LET charged particles. Radiat Res 83:677-687.
13. Alpen L, Powers-Risius P The relative biological effect of high Z, high LET charged particles for spermatogonal killing. Radiat Res, in press.
14. Tenforde TS, Curtis SB, Crabtree KE, Tenforde, SD, Schilling WA, Howard J, Lyman JT (1980) In vivo cell survival and volume response characteristics of rat rhabdomyosarcoma tumors irradiated in the extended peak region of carbon- and neon-ion beam. Radiat Res 83:42-56.
15. Leith JT, McDonald M, Powers-Risius P, Bliven SF, Walton RE, Woodruff KH, Howard J (1980) Response of rat spinal cord to single and fractionated doses of accelerated heavy ions. In Pirruccello MC, Tobias CA (eds.), Biological and Medical Research with Accelerated Heavy Ions at the Bevalac, 1977-1980, pp. 237-245. Lawrence Berkeley Laboratory Report LBL-11220.

COMPARISON OF THE EFFECTS OF PION AND HEAVY ION BEAMS IN A MOUSE TUMOR SYSTEM

K. SAKAMOTO[1], S. OKADA[2], G.K.Y. LAM[3] AND J. HOWARD[4]
[1]Department of Radiation Research, Tohoku University School of Medicine, 2-1 Seiryocho, Sendai 980, Japan; [2]Department of Radiation Biophysics, Faculty of Medicine, University of Tokyo; [3]TRIUMF, University of British Columbia, Vancouver; [4]Lawrence Berkeley Laboratory, Berkeley.

INTRODUCTION

Negative pi-mesons and heavy ions are being evaluated for their potential to enhance the therapeutic ratio in tumor radiotherapy. Since 1976 we have conducted biological studies of these particle radiations using the same materials and the same assay methods. In the present paper relative biological effectiveness (RBE), oxygen enhancement ratio (OER) and PLD repair of murine epithelioma cells exposed to negative pi-mesons and neon ions are reported in comparison to results obtained from X-irradiation.

MATERIALS AND METHODS

Mice and tumor. Male or female mice of strain WHT/Ht were used as tumor hosts in the TD50 experiments. The tumor was a transplantable keratinizing squamous carcinoma which arose spontaneously in a WHT/Ht mouse and has since been maintained by serial passage as a subcutaneous tumor.

Irradiation. X rays were generated using a therapy machine operated at 250 kV and 20 mA with filtration of 0.5 mm Cu and 1.0 mm Al. The exposure dose rate was 0.56 Gy/min.

Negative pi-mesons were produced by bombarding a beryllium target with 500 MeV protons extracted from an isochronous cyclotron at TRIUMF, Canada.[1] The dose rate at the pion peak was 0.15 - 0.20 Gy/min. The tumors were irradiated with pions at four different depths along the axis of the beam as shown in Figure 1. The peak was spread out to 4 cm and the pion beam field size was approximately 4 x 4 cm.

Neon ions were obtained from the Bevalac, which is a high energy heavy ion accelerator combining the SuperHILAC (a heavy ion linear accelerator) with the Bevatron (a proton synchrotron) at Lawrence Berkeley Laboratory, U.S.A. The neon ions were accelerated to an extraction energy of 577 MeV/amu and were fully stripped when reaching the target. The dose rate was 4.0 Gy/min. The tumors were irradiated with neon ions at three different depths along the axis of the beam as shown in Figure 2. The peak was spread out to 4 cm and neon ion beam field size was 5.6 x 5.6 cm.

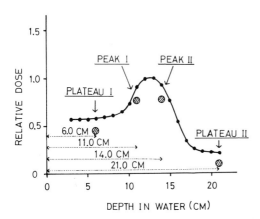

Fig. 1. Depth-dose distribution of pion beam in a water phantom. Tumors are located at the depths indicated by shaded circles.

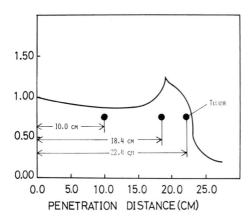

Fig. 2. Depth-dose distribution of neon ion beam. Tumors are located at the positions indicated by circles.

Survival of tumor cells. Irradiated mice bore subcutaneous tumors in the hind legs produced by an innoculum of 100,000 tumor cells injected 10-12 days previously; tumors measured 0.6-0.7 cm in diameter at the time of exposure. Single-cell suspensions of tumor cells were prepared from the tumors by a method described previously.[2] Transplantation assays of counted suspensions were performed by the technique described by Hewitt et al.[3] using the same tumor. The TD50 (number of cells required for successful transplantation to half of a group of injected sites) and 95% confidence limits were calculated from the results by the method of Lichfield and Wilcoxon.[3]

RESULTS

Effects of pions on murine epithelioma.

Distal peak pions: The single-dose survival curve of squamous carcinoma cells irradiated with the pion beam is shown as the solid line in Figure 3.[4] The curve drawn through the closed circles appears to bend slightly at a dose of 2-3 Gy. The D_o of the

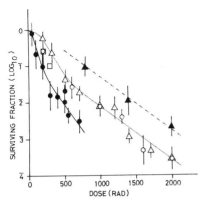

Fig. 3. Survival of clonogenic squamous carcinoma cells after irradiation in mice breathing air or under hypoxic conditions.

● = Pion beam
O = Cobalt-60 gamma rays
△ = 250 kVp x-rays
▲ = 250 kVp x-irradiation in nitrogen-killed mice
□ = Pion irradiation under hypoxic conditions

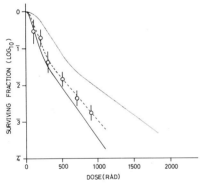

Fig. 4. Survival of clonogenic epithelioma cells exposed to negative Ⅱ-mesons at proximal peak (peak I). The solid and the dotted lines are survival curves of cells irradiated with pions at the distal peak (peak II) and 250 kVp x-rays, respectively. The dashed curve is a two-component linear regression fit for the data points.

first component is 0.73 ± 0.08 Gy and that of the second segment is 1.3 ± 0.21 Gy.

Proximal peak pions: The single dose survival measurements for squamous carcinoma cells irradiated with pions at the proximal peak are shown in Figure 4[5] together with the survival measurements at the distal peak and with 250 kV x-rays reported previously for comparison. The curve drawn through the data points at the proximal peak also appears to bend slightly at about 2 to 3 Gray. When fitted by the method of least squares, the D_o of the first component is 0.92 ± 0.1 Gy and that of second component is 1.84 ± 0.17 Gy.

Plateau pions: The survival measurements of the tumor cells exposed to pions in the plateau regions before and after the peak region are shown in Figure 5.[5] The plateau measurements appear to be in good agreement with the 250 kV x-ray data which have been estimated previously to have a D_o of 1.15 ± 0.09 Gy for the first and 2.76 ± 0.75 Gy for the second component.

328

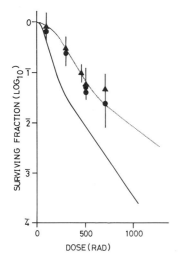

Fig. 5. Survival of clonogenic epithelioma cells irradiated with pions at prepeak plateau (plateau I) or at postpeak plateau regions (plateau II). The solid and the dotted lines are the same as in Fig. 4.

● = surviving fraction of cells at prepeak plateau

▲ = surviving fraction of cells at postpeak plateau

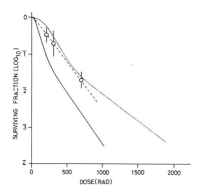

Fig. 6. Survival curve of epithelioma cells exposed to pions at distal peak (peak I) under hypoxic conditions. The dashed line is a linearregression fit to the data points. The solid and the dotted lines are the same as in Fig. 4.

Anoxic cell survival at distal peak: To estimate the oxygen enhancement ratio of pions, tumor bearing mice were sacrificed by cervical dislocation and then irradiated with pions at the distal peak position. The results are shown in Figure 6.[5] The curve drawn through the data points seems to have the same slope as the second component of the aerobic distal peak pion survival curve with a D_o value of 1.30 ± 0.27 Gy.

PLD repair at distal peak: Tumor bearing mice were exposed to 2.5 Gy, 5.0 Gy and 8.0 Gy of pions at the distal peak position or to 10 Gy of 250 kV x-rays.

The survival of tumor cells was assayed at various times after irradiation to study the repair of potentially lethal damage of the tumor cells. The repair ratios (the surviving fraction at 8 hours/the surviving fraction at 0 hour) are 1.9 for 2.5 Gy, 2.5 for 5.0 Gy, and 3.9 for 8.0 Gy of pion irradiation. The repair ratio is 9.8 for 10 Gy x-ray irradiation, significantly larger than for pions.

RBE and OER of pions: The RBE values obtained from the present study are summarized in Table 1. They have been calculated from the ratio of the D_o values as well as from the doses which give equivalent survival values. The RBE values of pions at the proximal peak relative to 250 kV x rays are 1.6 ± 0.2 and 1.4 ± 0.1 at surviving fractions of 0.1 and 0.01 respectively. The RBE at the proximal peak determined from the D_o values is 1.3 ± 0.2 for the first component (aerobic cells) and 1.5 ± 0.2 for the second component (hypoxic cells). These values are significantly lower than the corresponding RBE values measured at the distal peak. The OER of pions at the distal peak is estimated to be 1.8 ± 0.5 from the data in Figure 6 compared to the OER value of 2.4 for x rays. Thus, the oxygen gain factor is calculated to be 1.3.

TABLE 1

PION RBE VALUES RELATIVE TO 250 kVp X RAYS FOR MURINE EPITHELIOMA CELLS

	$(D_o)_x$ / $(D_o)_{pi}$		Actual ratio of S.F.	
	Aerobic 1st component	Hypoxic 2nd component	At S = 0.1	At S = 0.01
At Distal Peak	1.6 ± 0.3	2.1 ± 0.5	2.2 ± 0.3	2.0 ± 0.2
At Proximal Peak	1.3 ± 0.2	1.5 ± 0.3	1.6 ± 0.2	1.4 ± 0.1

Effects of neon ions on murine epithelioma

Distal peak neon ions: The single dose survival curve of murine epithelioma cells irradiated with distal peak neon ions is the solid line in Figure 7, which was fitted by the method of least squares. The dotted line in Figure 7 shows the survival curve of cells exposed to distal peak pions. The curve drawn through the open circles appears to bend slightly at a dose of 2-3 Gy. The D_o of the first component is 0.74 ± 0.11 Gy and that of the second component is 1.39 ± 0.27 Gy, for the neon curve.

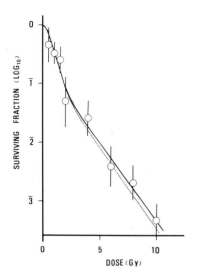

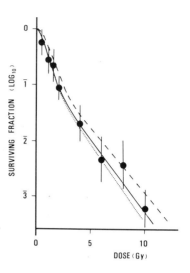

Fig. 7. Survival of clonogenic cells exposed to neon ions at the distal peak. The dotted line is the survival curve of tumor cells irradiated with pions at the distal peak (from Fig. 3).

Fig. 8. The closed circles show survival of clonogenic epithelioma cells exposed to neon ions at the proximal peak. The dotted line is the same as in Fig. 7 and the dashed line demonstrates the survival curve of epithelioma cells irradiated with pions at the proximal peak (from Fig. 4).

Proximal peak neon ions: In Figure 8 survival of the murine squamous carcinoma cells exposed to proximal peak neon ions is shown. The closed circles show the surviving fraction of cells irradiated with neon ions at each dose level, and these surviving fractions are fitted by the solid line. The D_o values of the first and second segments of the survival curve are almost the same as those obtained in Figure 7. This means that there is little difference between the distal and proximal peak in cell killing effect. The dotted line in Figure 8 is the same as in Figure 7.

Plateau neon ions: The survival of tumor cells irradiated with neon ions in the plateau region before the peak is shown in Figure 9 by the closed circles, and the data have been fitted by the solid line. The dotted line is the survival curve of the same tumor cells exposed to negative pi-mesons at the pre-peak plateau position. The solid curve appears to bend slightly at a dose of around

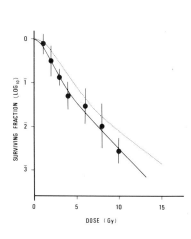

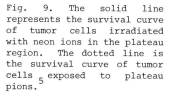

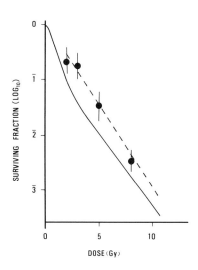

Fig. 9. The solid line represents the survival curve of tumor cells irradiated with neon ions in the plateau region. The dotted line is the survival curve of tumor cells exposed to plateau pions.[5]

Fig. 10. Closed circles represent the survival of epithelioma cells exposed to neon ions at the distal peak under hypoxic conditions. The solid curve is for aerobic conditions (from Fig. 7).

5 Gy, and the D_o values are calculated as 1.07 ± 0.13 Gy for the first component and 2.09 ± 0.31 Gy for the second component. These values of D_o are smaller than those of the dotted line, which were 1.15 ± 0.9 Gy for the first segment and 2.76 ± 0.25 Gy for the second segment.

Anoxic cell survival at distal peak: To estimate the OER of neon ions, tumor-bearing mice were sacrificed by cervical dislocation just before irradiation. Figure 10 shows the survival of epithelioma cells irradiated with neon ions at the distal peak under hypoxic conditions. The solid line is for aerobic cells, and is taken from fig. 7. The D_o value of the dashed line is 1.31 ± 0.21 Gy.

PLD repair at distal peak: The PLD repair of murine epithelioma cells exposed to neon ions at the distal peak was investigated as for pions. The PLD repair of cells reached a maximum at 6 hours after 8.0 Gy irradiation and the repair ratio was calculated to be 3.2.

RBE and OER of neon ions: In Table 2 the RBE values obtained from the present study are shown. They have been calculated from the ratio of the D_o values, as well as from the doses which give equivalent survival values. At surviving fractions of 0.1 and 0.01, the RBE values of peak neon ions (distal and proximal positions) relative to 250 kVp x rays, are 2.2 ± 0.4 and 2.0 ± 0.3 respectively. The RBE determined from the D_o values is 1.6 ± 0.4 for the first component and 2.0 ± 0.3 for the second component in the survival curve of cells irradiated with neon ions at the distal and proximal peaks. On the other hand, RBE values for neon ions at the plateau are 1.4 ± 0.3 and 1.2 ± 0.2 for surviving fractions of 0.1 and 0.01, respectively. The RBE determined from the D_o values is 1.1 ± 0.2 for the first component, and 1.3 ± 0.4 for the second component. The OER of neon ions at the distal peak is calculated to be 1.8 ± 0.6. This is the ratio of the D_o for the first component of fig. 7 and the D_o of the hypoxic response of fig. 10 (dashed curve). Therefore, the oxygen gain factor is calculated to be 1.3, the same as for distal peak pions.

TABLE 2

NEON ION RBE VALUES RELATIVE TO 250 kVp X-RAYS FOR MURINE EPITHELIOMA CELLS

	$(D_o)_x / (D_o)_{neon}$		Actual ratio of S.F.	
	1st component	2nd component	At S = 0.1	At S = 0.01
Peak Region	1.6 ± 0.4	2.0 ± 0.3	2.2 ± 0.4	2.0 ± 0.3
Plateau Region	1.1 ± 0.2	1.3 ± 0.4	1.4 ± 0.3	1.2 ± 0.2

DISCUSSION

The data presented here were obtained from experimental results using the same materials and the same assay method. However, RBE or OER values for these particle radiations have been shown to have different values depending on the system used, the endpoint measured, the irradiation method (single or fractionated doses) and the beam energy. In addition, pi-mesons and neon ions, demonstrate different RBE and OER values depending on the width of the spread out stopping peak as summarized by Curtis[6] and Skarsgard.[7] Therefore, it is very difficult to give absolute or universal values for the RBE and OER of these particle radiations. Nevertheless, it is clear that in the stopping region, both pions and neon ions have higher RBE's and lower OER's than conventional radiations. Using epithelioma cell survival _in vivo_ as the end point and stopping peaks 4 cm wide, the RBE's for distal and proximal peak pions were 1.6 - 2.3 and 1.3 - 1.6 respectively, while neon ions yielded an RBE of 1.6 - 2.3 for both proximal and distal positions. In the entrance plateau region, however, the RBE was 1.0 for pions and 1.1 - 1.4 for neon ions.

Concerning PLD repair, the repair ratio obtained from the present study of pion and neon ion irradiations was smaller than the repair ratio for x-ray exposure. For pions, repair ratios were 1.9, 2.5 and 3.9 for distal peak doses of 2.5 Gy, 5.0 Gy and 8.0 Gy respectively, while for distal peak neon ions the repair ratio for 8.0 Gy was 3.2. These ratios are significantly lower than the repair ratio of 11.2 observed for an x-ray dose of 10 Gy. As you might expect, the repair ratio decreases with decreasing dose (pion data) since there is less damage to be repaired. Raju et al. detected no PLD repair when CHO cells were exposed _in vitro_ to Polonium alpha particles[8], an observation which is consistent with the results described here.

REFERENCES

1. Henkelman RM, Skarsgard LD, Lam GKY (1977) Recent developments at the pi-meson radiotherapy facility at TRIUMF. Int J Radiat Oncol Biol Phys 2: 123-127.
2. Hewitt HB (1966) The effect on cell survival of inhalation of oxygen under high pressure during irradiation in vivo of a solid mouse sarcoma. Br J Radiol 39:19-24.
3. Hewitt HB, Chan DP, Blake ER (1967) Survival curves for clonogenic cells of a murine keratinizing squamous carcinoma irradiated in vivo or under hypoxic conditions. Int J Radiat Biol 12:535-549.
4. Sakamoto K, Okada S, Lam GKY, Henkelman RM, Skarsgard LD (1979) The comparative survival of clonogenic cells of a murine epithelioma irradiated in vivo with 250 kVp X rays, ^{60}Co gamma rays, or negative pions produced by the cyclotron at TRIUMF. Radiology 133:501-505.
5. Sakamoto K, Takai Y, Lam GKY (1981) Survival of murine epithelioma cells exposed at various positions to pions produced by the cyclotron at TRIUMF. Radiat. Res. 87:159-165.
6. Curtis SB (1979) The biological properties of high-energy heavy charged particles. In Okada S, Imamura M, Terasima T, Yamaguchi H. (ed.), Radiation Research (Proceedings of the Sixth International Congress of Radiation Research, May 13-19, 1979, Tokyo) Tokyo: JARR, 780-787.
7. Skarsgard LD (1979) The biological properties of pions. In Okada S, Imamura M, Terasima T, Yamaguchi H. (ed.), Radiation Research (Proceedings of the Sixth International Congress of Radiation Research, May 13-19, 1979, Tokyo) Tokyo: JARR, 789-801.
8. Raju MR, Frank JP, Bain E, Trujillo TT, Tobey RA (1977) Repair of potentially lethal damage in Chinese hamster cells X and α irradiation. Radiat Res 71: 614-621.

HARDERIAN GLAND CARCINOGENESIS FROM HIGH LET, HIGH Z, CHARGED PARTICLES

EDWARD L. ALPEN, P. POWERS-RISIUS, R.J.M. FRY[1] AND E.J. AINSWORTH
Donner Laboratory and Lawrence Berkeley Laboratory, University of California,
Berkeley
[1]Oak Ridge National Laboratory, Oak Ridge, Tennessee

INTRODUCTION

As part of a large program at Berkeley, the aim of which is the evaluation of the clinical utility of charged particle beams, we have been evaluating the carcinogenic potential of these beams. The choice of the Harderian gland system previously reported upon by Fry and coworkers[1] was made based on several special properties of this sytem. (1) The tumors that are induced in this gland by radiation are epithelial in origin: adenomata and carcinomata. (2) For the strain of mice used by Fry the natural incidence is low, less than 3% for the lifetime. (3) In unirradiated mice the tumors which are seen are benign and appear late in life. (4) Fry has discovered that by the implantation of pituitary isografts there is a large increase in tumor incidence and a shortening of the latent period without concomitant large increases for the control mice. (5) Finally, there is a large body of data, both published and unpublished, carried out at the Argonne National Laboratory with neutrons from the JANUS reactor, and at the National Accelerator Laboratory for neutrons produced by their accelerator.

All of the above properties might improve the liklihood that we would be able to develop statistically reliable data for increased tumor incidence at low doses. The experimental objectives of the program are to establish the LET dependence of the carcinogenic potential of charged heavy particles and to examine the shape of the dose-response relationship at low doses.

METHODS AND PROCEDURES

In order to make our data as comparable as possible with that done previously at the Argonne National Laboratory we chose to use the same hybrid mouse which was developed at the laboratory. We are, of course, especially indebted to the management of that Laboratory for their kind cooperation in making animals available.

The female B_6Cf_1/ANL mice were received at less than eight weeks of age. Mice were isografted with two pituitary glands before they were twelve weeks old. Two pituitaries were removed from syngeneic donor mice, usually older than the recipients, and, under metofane (methoxyflurane) anesthesia these pituitaries were implanted beneath the capsule of the spleen. For early experiments regular vaginal smear examination was done to demonstrate the abnormal activity of the implants, but it was quickly observed that much more reliable assessment of the viability of the implant could be made at ultimate sacrifice. At that time an assessment of hypertrophy of the mammary glands and evidence of ovarian stimulation are used to demonstrate pituitary hyperactivity. More recently the availability of a procedure for radioimmunoassay of mouse prolactin levels has permitted us to measure blood levels of prolactin in the implanted animals.

In theory, an ectopic pituitary, outside the influence of the hypothalamus, produces pituitary hormones continuously because the hypothalamic inhibiting factors do not reach the general circulation in sufficient quantities to control the secretory activity of the pituitary implants. Which of the pituitary hormones is responsible for the special tumor promoting activity on the Harderian gland is only a matter for speculation at this time. We believe that, because of histologic homologies, it is likely that prolactin is the relevant hormone.

The animals were irradiated generally about two weeks after implant surgery. Irradiation was done with the appropriate ion beam at the Berkeley Bevalac for all ions except helium, and irradiations with that ion were done on the 184" Berkeley synchrocyclotron. Dosimetry and beam arrangements have been described in great detail for both machines[2].

Animals were irradiated in a partial body mode using a 3x5 cm beam collimator which was placed in such a fashion that all of the mouse caudal of the xyphoid was in the beam. The beam axis in this fashion was centered on the head. We chose to use partial body irradiation to reduce the liklihood of tumors arising in other sites that might confuse the analysis. The Bragg curves for the beams used are shown in Figure 1. The position of the front (ventral surface) of the mouse's head is shown by an arrow. The thickness of the head is 1 cm or less. We used, as shown, the distal portion of the 10 cm spread out Bragg peak for Helium, Carbon, and Neon; and the distal portion of the 4 cm spread out Bragg peak for Argon. Since beam intensities for the Iron beam are low, usually less than 5 rad per minute, the plateau region of the Iron beam was used, with no modification of the Bragg peak. The beam was

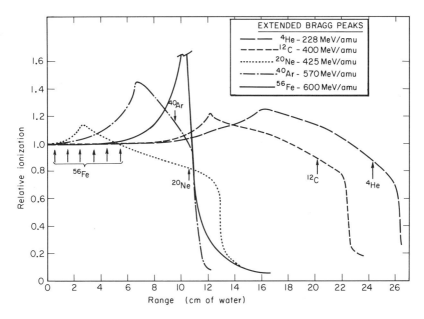

Fig. 1. Depth-dose profiles of the modified Bragg curves used for heavy-ion irradiation. The position of the front of the mouse heads in the spread Bragg peak regions of ionization is indicated by the arrows.

passed through the heads of six mice aligned on the beam axis. A 1 cm circular field centered in the head was used for the Iron beam.

For all ions except Iron the dose rate was adjusted such that the exposure was always accomplished in thirty to sixty seconds.

The number of mice exposed for each ion and dose level is shown in Figure 2. Approximately 3500 pituitary-implanted mice have been irradiated, of which we have completed sacrifice and analysis on about 2600. The goal is ultimately to have approximately 200 mice at each dose point for each ion. It may be necessary to have 400 or more at dose levels at and below 10 rad.

In any experiment such as the one being described here it is possible to accumulate the data either as a census of total tumors seen in the irradiated population throughout life, usually expressed as percentage <u>incidence</u>; or one may terminate the experiment by sacrifice at a time determined before the start of the experiment. In this case the data is expressed as accumulated number of animals with tumors up to the time of sacrifice, usually expressed as percentage <u>prevalence</u>. Many arguements exist for both approaches. A bad

338

NUMBER OF MICE COMMITTED TO STUDY GROUPS

| | Dose (rad) | | | | | | | | |
	5	10	15	20	40	80	160	320	700
^{60}Co	—	—	—	—	—	130	180	181	90
Helium	—	—	—	—	201	203	200	210	40
Carbon	143	100	—	—	194	112	109	63	—
Neon	226	191	97	195	121	77	48	65	—
Argon	—	—	—	—	102	74	74	—	—
Iron	6	24	—	24	25	—	—	—	—

Unirradiated implant controls: 100

Fig. 2 The number of mice for each dose level for the radiations used to induce Harderian gland tumors in mice.

choice of time for experiment termination may cause one to miss a large number of late developing tumors, yielding a prevalence value which grossly distorts the true picture. Life time studies leading to life-time incidence are plagued by intercurrent disease and the fact that animals are at risk for variable periods.

Analytical instruments exist for both approaches, but we chose to examine our data in terms of prevalence at sixteen months after irradiation. Animals were sacrificed at that time and complete autopsies done on each animal. We routinely collected Harderian glands, ovaries, spleen with its implant, lung, mammary glands, and any tissue in which there was gross evidence of abnormality.

Final diagnosis of the existence of an Harderian gland tumor was made only on the basis of histologic examination. The final prevalence ratio was determined by taking the ratio of the number of mice with proved tumors to the number of mice at risk. The latter was determined from the survival of the animal to time of sacrifice and proof that an active pituitary isograft existed at time of sacrifice. It is important to note that rarely did mice succumb with a Harderian gland tumor before the 16 month sacrifice date, and very rarely did an animal have two Harderian gland tumors.

RESULTS

In Figure 3 are shown prevalence values as determined for mice sacrificed to date. The ordinate represents the prevalence at 16 months of microscopically proved Harderian gland tumors among all mice in that dose group having histologically proved pituitary isografts.

The data shown for ^{60}Co gamma radiation are still low at doses up to 160 rad, and rise more or less linearly after that. The data are quite similar to those reported for gamma radiation by the Argonne group[3]. Somewhat surprising to us is the increased incidence with helium ions. This is essentially a low LET radiation at about 1-2 keV/μm, but the prevalence values are appreciably higher than for ^{60}Co gamma at 160 rad. We are not convinced that this is more than sample variability, and we are awaiting the outcome of the sacrifice of further helium irradiated animals for confirmation.

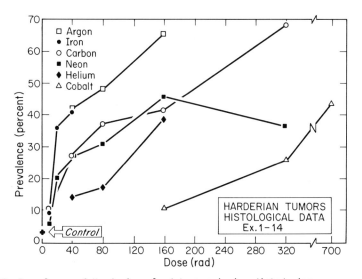

Fig. 3. Prevalence of Harderian gland tumors in irradiated mice.

Carbon and Neon ions are quite similar in prevalence ratios, in spite of quite large differences in the LET for these two beams, 78 keV/μm for Carbon and 150 keV/μm for Neon. The decreased prevalence for Neon at higher dose may be due to cell killing, and certainly we would predict that this ion is more efficient for cell killing than are Carbon ion beams.

The LET for the Argon beams is high, of the order of 650 keV/μm, yet prevalence is not higher than for Iron at 200 keV/μm. Analysis of all of these data must await further data collection, particularly at low doses.

DISCUSSION

It is possible to estimate the RBE values for several ions at several prevalence levels. We have done so, where possible, for prevalence levels of 10, 20 and 30%. The helium doses are so arranged that it is not possible to construct an RBE at the 10% prevalence level. Argon also is out of the 10% range.

At the 10% level, Carbon, Neon and Iron all yield an RBE value of 15. The RBE appears to increase slightly at higher prevalence levels, but the values

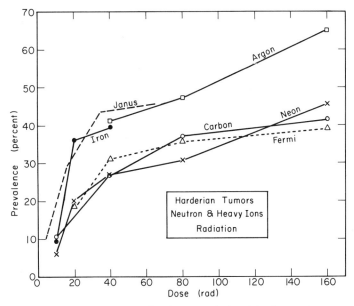

Fig. 4. Comparison of Harderian gland tumors induced by heavy ion or neutron radiation.

still fall in the range of 15–19, probably not significantly different from the value of 15 at 10% prevalence.

When we have evaluated the lower dose (5 rad) levels for Neon and Carbon we will be able to provide RBE values at lower prevalence levels.

Finally we can compare our data with that from Fermilab neutrons and Janus neutrons. This comparison is made in Figure 4. The Fermilab data are quite similar to our data for Carbon and Neon ions, even though the Fermilab exposures were whole body.

Comparison with Janus data are less relevant, since these latter data are lifetime incidence studies. However they fall remarkably close to our data for the higher LET beams, where they would be expected to fall.

ACKNOWLEDGMENTS

This work was supported by the Director, Office of Energy Research, Office of Health and Environmental Research of the U.S. Dept. of Energy under Contract #DE-AC03-76SF00098.

REFERENCES

1. Fry, R.J.M., Garcia, A.G., Allen, K.H., Sallese, A., Staffeldt, E., Tahmisian, T.N., Devine, R.L., Lombard, L.S., Ainsworth, E.J. (1975) Effect of pituitary isografts on radiation carcinogenesis in mammary and harderian glands of mice.   Biological Effects of Low-Level Radiation Pertinent to Protection of Man and His Environment. Vienna, IAEA 1: 213–227.
2. Curtis, S.B., Tenforde, T.S., Parks, D., Schilling, W.A., Lyman, J.T. (1978) Response of a rat rhabdomyosarcoma to neon and helium ion irradiation. Radiat. Res. 74: 274–288.
3. Fry, R.J.M. (1977) Radiation carcinogenesis. Int. J. Radiat. Oncology Biol. Phys. 3: 219–226.

CLINICAL STUDIES -- NEUTRONS, PROTONS, HEAVY IONS

NEUTRON BEAM EXPERIENCE IN EDINBURGH AND OTHER CENTRES IN EUROPE

WILLIAM DUNCAN
University of Edinburgh, MRC Cyclotron Unit, Western General Hospital,
Edinburgh, Scotland. EH4 2XU

The cyclotron facility in Edinburgh is situated next to the Radiation Oncology Department within the grounds of the teaching hospital. It houses a CS30 cyclotron from which is obtained a 15 MeV deuteron beam. The deuterons are directed on to a thick beryllium target to produce the neutron beam which has a penetration similar to that from a 250 kV X ray machine. The physical and biological properties of the neutron beam are virtually identical to that from the Hammersmith cyclotron in London. The cyclotron is normally run at about 70% of maximum beam current which provides a dose rate of about 30 cGy per minute at 125 cm FSD for a 10 x 10 cm field. The reliability of the facility has been excellent since it was commissioned in 1977. The facility is provided with two treatment rooms, one with a fixed horizontal beam, the other with a well designed isocentric treatment head.

TABLE 1

EDINBURGH CYCLOTRON FACILITY

MARCH 1977 - MARCH 1981

Study Group	Number of Patients
Preliminary neutrons	243
Preliminary mixed schedule	22
Controlled trials (neutrons)	333
Controlled trials (mixed schedule)	12
Controlled trials (+ surgery)	31
Total	641

Table 1 shows the numbers of patients recruited into the clinical studies in Edinburgh since the beam came on line in March 1977. Preliminary studies are concerned with the assessment of patients who have been accepted for elective neutron therapy, in distinction to those admitted to randomly controlled trials. However over 80% of patients now referred to the neutron clinic are entered into one of our randomly controlled trials. It is our prime objective to include as many patients as possible into these controlled studies.

The principal tumour sites of interest are given in Table 2.

TABLE 2

EDINBURGH CYCLOTRON FACILITY

Principal Tumour Sites	Number of Patients
Brain	84
Head and Neck	122
Bladder	101
Oesophagus	57
Rectum	50

Our first commitment was to undertake a controlled trial of patients with squamous cell carcinoma of the head and neck region similar to the Hammersmith trial.[2] This is the only trial which claims a significant improvement in local tumour control after treatment with neutrons compared with X rays. It is important to note that the statistical difference of significance occurred only in the group of patients with oral cavity and oropharyngeal cancers.[3] The response rate after neutrons was about 75% which is said to be close to the definitive control rate. By comparison, the control rate was only 19% after X ray therapy. The recurrence rate following neutron therapy was only 2%. These results have encouraged further laboratory and clinical research and an increased financial investment in neutron therapy facilities around the world. Clearly it was important that this single experiment be repeated.

We were able to take advantage of the clinical experience at Hammersmith and further radiobiological understanding in the design of the study in Edinburgh. The trial consists of patients with squamous cell carcinoma in four major sites in the head and neck region: oral cavity and oropharynx, larynx and hypopharynx. All T & N stage's of disease are included with the following exceptions. In the oral cavity and oropharynx T1 N0, and also T2 N0 cancers of the tongue are excluded when suitable for radionuclide implant. In the larynx T1 N0 and T2 N0 glottic tumours are excluded since results are so good with current photon therapy.

TABLE 3

EDINBURGH CYCLOTRON FACILITY

"HEAD AND NECK" TRIAL

Site	Neutrons	Photons
Oral Cavity and Oropharynx	30	29
Larynx and Hypopharynx	20	23
Total	50	52

Table 3 gives the numbers of patients randomised in this study. Some very preliminary data of the results are given below but it must be stressed that a formal report will not be published until greater numbers of patients have been followed-up for at least 12 months. No conclusion can be made at present about the final outcome of this trial.

The primary objective of the Edinburgh study was to ensure that the radiation morbidity was similar on both sides of the trial. About two years was spent in determining the optimum dose schedule for photons with which the neutron regime (with same number of fractions and overall time) would be compared. Table 4 gives the morbidity in the trial when last assessed and which is similar after neutrons and photons. Further follow-up is required for the incidence of late morbidity may increase disproportionately in the neutron treated group. There is no evidence at present that this possibility will be realised, but it has to be appreciated that morbidity and recurrence rates will increase with time.

TABLE 4

EDINBURGH CYCLOTRON FACILITY

"HEAD AND NECK" TRIAL

Morbidity	Neutrons	Photons
Early - fatal	1	1
Late - fatal	3	0
Severe	8	6
Total	12	7

Table 5 gives the local control rates in the Edinburgh study and there is no real difference between the two groups.

TABLE 5

EDINBURGH CYCLOTRON FACILITY

"HEAD AND NECK" TRIAL

Tumour Response	Neutrons	Photons
Cumulative complete regression assessed at 6 months	74.8%	74.6%
Later recurrence	32.4%	34.3%
Local tumour control	42.4%	40.3%

They are very similar to that reported after neutron therapy in the Hammersmith trial. It should be understood that the patients in the Edinburgh trial have less advanced disease. For example, the proportion of patients with metastatic cervical nodes is 50% compared to 70% in the Hammersmith study. A striking difference between the two trials is the recurrence rates - about 33% in Edinburgh compared with 2% after neutron and 60% after photon therapy at Hammersmith. The neutron dose used in Edinburgh was chosen to be about 5% less than that prescribed at Hammersmith. The dose-response curve may be so steep

that the difference in dose may largely explain the difference in tumour control
and morbidity. Unfortunately the morbidity in the Hammersmith trial was higher
after neutrons than after X rays, and there is no evidence that the therapeutic
ratio for neutrons was greater than for photon therapy. The number of patients
who have undergone surgery after radical radiotherapy in Edinburgh has been
similar in both groups. No increase in operative difficulties or morbidity has
been recorded. At present there is no difference in the overall survival rates
between the two treatment groups. When the results of patients with oral cavity
and oropharyngeal cancers are examined there is no significant difference in
local control rates although the neutron treated group is slightly higher. Again
larger numbers of patients and longer follow-up are required before a definite
conclusion may be reached. Morbidity is also a little higher in the neutron
treated group and so any difference may be due to a higher biologically effective dose. The crucial issue is to demonstrate a difference in tumour control
rates when the normal tissue morbidity is similar in the neutron and photon
treated groups. That essential question has to be answered and so in all trials
equal attention must be paid to the observation and measurement of early and
late normal tissue reactions and to the assessment of local tumour control.

It is important that in addition to good quality control of absorbed dose,
the target volume should be similar in both treatments. This is a relatively
simple matter in the head and neck trials and also when treating cerebral
gliomas, although an extra field may be necessary with low energy neutrons when
compared with megavoltage X rays.

A small trial has been carried out on patients with poorly differentiated
gliomas. The current assessment is given in Table 6.

TABLE 6

EDINBURGH CYCLOTRON FACILITY

GLIOMA TRIAL

	Neutrons	Photons
Total patients	18	16
Tumour related death	16	12
Autopsies	9	6
Abnormal white matter changes	2	0
Median survival (months)	7	10

In the 18 patients treated with neutrons, 16 were considered to have died
from recurrent tumour. In the 16 patients treated with photons, 12 deaths were
considered to be due to recurrent tumour. The mean survival was 7 and 10 months

respectively for neutron and photon treated patients. The short survival makes accurate assessment of radiation morbidity in the central nervous system diffi- cult, even at autopsy. We did find two patients with abnormal white matter changes considered to be related to neutron irradiation. No such changes were seen in the photon group. The dose of neutron irradiation was chosen to be about 10% lower than the lowest absorbed doses previously given to the brain in trials in Seattle[6] and Hammersmith.[4] They have reported a syndrome of progress- ive cerebral degeneration, refractory to dexamethasone, after neutron therapy to high doses. We have seen this syndrome in one patient. It is now understood that the RBE for normal brain is much higher for fractionated neutron therapy than previously recognised.[5] In our experience residual glioblastoma is present at neutron dose levels which produce abnormal white matter changes and it is unlikely that an advantageous therapeutic ratio for brain tumours can be found with fast neutrons alone.

Another tumour type that has been assessed is the transitional cell carcinoma of the bladder. The radiation technique employs small fields 11 x 11 cm. Using megavoltage X rays three fields are required compared to a six field arrange- ment with 15 MeV(d+Be) neutrons. Since the patient has to turn over for the sixth field, neutron treatment planning (and simulation) is much more complex and time-consuming than the simple megavoltage X ray technique. A satisfactory dose distribution can be obtained in patients whose girth does not exceed 1 metre. Fatter patients have to be excluded from the trial. Treatment times on our isocentric neutron facility are about 35 minutes, a period which patients find acceptable and does not cause any great discomfort.

TABLE 7

EDINBURGH CYCLOTRON FACILITY

BLADDER TRIAL

Stage & Tumour Grade	Neutrons	Photons
T1 & T2 (all grades)	6	9
T3 (GI & II)	9	9
T3 (GIII)	11	10
T4 (all grades)	7	6
Total	33	34
Local control at 6 months	60.6%	64.7%

Table 7 gives the preliminary results for the group of patients who have been followed-up for at least six months. All patients are assessed by a collabora- tive urological team before treatment, and cystoscopy and EUAs are carried out at regular intervals after treatment. The stage distribution and local tumour

control rates are similar in the neutron and photon treated groups. The morbidity rates are also similar in both groups but the pelvic fibrosis is much
greater in those treated by fast neutrons. This can make pelvic assessment
difficult after neutron therapy and salvage cystectomy, if necessary, is much
more difficult and hazardous. This problem of fibrosis does increase with time
after neutron therapy.

We have also been interested to evaluate the response of rectal adenocarcinoma to neutron irradiation compared to photons. Patients are eligible for
this study if they have either inoperable rectal cancer or assessable post-
operative recurrence provided there is no evidence of gross metastatic disease.
Recruitment has been slow to this study as the majority of these patients do
have widespread disease; we exclude patients, for example, with moderate elevation of CEA, above 75 ng/ml. The results following assessment at 12 months after
treatment are given in Table 8. The control rates are not significantly
different at this time. The radiation morbidity does appear again to be greater
in the neutron treated group.

TABLE 8

EDINBURGH CYCLOTRON FACILITY

RECTAL CANCER TRIAL

	Neutrons	Photons
Number of patients	14	18
Complete tumour regression	35.7%	22.2%
Radiation morbidity	3	1

The technique of irradiation for the rectal cancer trial is the same as that
used in the bladder cancer study. This has given us a greater experience of a
single technique of pelvic irradiation than we would have acquired otherwise.
Also the given doses are different on the six fields and so valuable information
may also be obtained on the RBE for late skin and subcutaneous tissue reactions.

It has been reported that tumours of the salivary glands have been found to
respond particularly well to fast neutron therapy. However this claim has not
been substantiated by the data in the RTOG registry and a multi-centre randomly
controlled study is in progress. Large numbers of patients will be required
because of the range of histological types of tumour arising in the salivary
glands, each with a characteristic natural history. Some, like the adenoid
cystic carcinoma, have a long natural history and so prolonged follow-up is also
important. Quite different response rates have been reported (Table 9) but this
is not surprising in relation to the different types of tumours evaluated and
the different neutron dose levels explored. Radiobiological studies on lung
metastases have shown that the RBE for fractionated neutron irradiation of

adenoid cystic carcinoma may be one of the highest for human tumours.[1] The
scientific evaluation of the clinical response of this type of cancer is therefore of great interest and may provide a rational basis for elective neutron
therapy. If an improved response of these tumours to neutrons is confirmed it
is likely to be due to their cell population kinetics rather than the presence
of a hypoxic sub-population.

TABLE 9

SALIVARY GLAND TUMOURS

Centre	Patients	Tumour Control
Amsterdam	25	18 (72%)
Edinburgh	16	9 (57%)
London	40	33 (82%)

    Soft tissue sarcomas are also a heterogenous group of tumours with a wide
range of local invasiveness, growth rates and proclivity to spread widely. At
a recent meeting in Europe the results of neutron therapy were reported from
Amsterdam, Edinburgh, Essen, Heidelberg and London. These tumours were inoperable or recurrent after operation in sites where measurement of regression was
possible.

TABLE 10

SOFT TISSUE SARCOMAS

INOPERABLE OR P/O RECURRENT

	Patients	Tumour Control	Morbidity
Amsterdam	22	8 (36%)	6 (27%)
Edinburgh	18	7 (39%)	3 (16%)
Essen	20	7 (35%)	3 (15%)
Heidelberg	13	4 (31%)	-
London	28	21 (75%)	9 (32%)

    It is clear that the local tumour control of these tumours is about 35% with
the exception of the London results. There may be differences in the distribution of the histological types of these tumours but the variation in response
rates may largely be dependent on a difference in absorbed neutron dose. This
is reflected in the differences in the rates of normal tissue morbidity recorded
in each centre. It has earlier been observed that relatively small changes in
neutron dose may be associated with large differences in tumour and normal
tissue responses. The dose-response curves are very steep indeed. This fact
places high demands for great accuracy in treatment planning and dose application in neutron therapy. Apparently large improvements in local tumour control
may be observed simply as a result of increased neutron dose although no real
improvement in therapeutic ratio has been achieved.

The assessment of therapeutic ratio depends on the reliable measurement of the late normal tissue effects on radiotherapy. Much greater recognition has to be given to the importance of improving our understanding of the pathogenesis of late normal tissue damage. Improved systems of scoring late radiation morbidity have also to be developed and evaluated. Much greater research efforts have to be made on normal tissue morbidity both in the laboratory and in the clinic if the results of controlled clinical trials of new radiation techniques are to be more meaningfully evaluated.

All clinical trials must be designed to produce the same acceptable level of morbidity with either neutrons or photons. Physical differences in the quality of the beams may make this difficult at some sites. When normal tissue morbidity is similar we do not, in our studies in Edinburgh, observe any appreciable improvement in tumour control following neutron compared to photon irradiation. However the evaluation of fast neutron therapy is not complete. It is essential that the qualitative differences known to exist between the response of mammalian cells and tissues to neutrons and photons are precisely assessed and documented in clinical trials. Since the introduction of clinical facilities for high LET therapy over 7000 patients have been treated with fast neutrons. It is to be regretted that less than 10% of these patients have been the subject of controlled studies, which alone can contribute to a definitive evaluation of neutron therapy.

REFERENCES

1. Battermann JJ (1981) Clinical applications of fast neutrons. The Amsterdam experience. Thesis, University of Amsterdam.

2. Catterall Mary, Sutherland I, Bewley DK (1975) First results of a randomised clinical trial of fast neutrons compared with X or gamma rays in treatment of advanced tumours of the head and neck. Report to the Medical Research Council. Br Med J 2:653-656.

3. Catterall Mary (1977) First randomised clinical trial of fast neutrons compared with photons in advanced carcinoma of the head and neck. Clin Otolaryngology 2:359-372.

4. Catterall Mary, Bloom HJG, Ash DV, Walsh L. Richardson A, Uttley D, Gowing NFC, Lewis P, Chaucer B (1980) Fast neutrons compared with megavoltage X rays in the treatment of patients with supratentorial glioblastoma: a controlled pilot study. Int J Radiat Oncol Biol Phys 6:261-266.

5. Hornsey Shirley, Morris Caroline C, Myers R, White Ann (1981) Relative biological effectiveness for damage to the central nervous system by neutrons. Int J Radiat Oncol Biol Phys 7:185-189.

6. Laramore G, Griffin TW, Gerdes AJ, Parker RG (1978) Fast neutron and mixed (neutron/photon) beam teletherapy for grades III and IV astrocytoma. Cancer 42:96-103.

FAST NEUTRON RADIOTHERAPY IN THE UNITED STATES WITH EMPHASIS ON THE UNIVERSITY
OF WASHINGTON EXPERIENCE AND RTOG RANDOMIZED STUDIES

GEORGE E. LARAMORE, and THOMAS W. GRIFFIN,
Department of Radiation Oncology, University of Washington
Seattle, Washington 98195

INTRODUCTION

Fast neutron radiotherapy in the United States dates back to the 1940's when
Stone and coworkers[10] used a neutron beam to treat patients having various advanced malignancies. Almost all of the long-term survivors had severe radiation
sequelae in the normal tissue surrounding the tumor sites. This was initially
interpreted as due to an increased relative biological effectiveness (RBE) for
late effects as compared to acute effects and this deterred further clinical investigation for approximately 20 years. In the 1950's, mammalian cell culture
techniques were developed and it became apparent that the shapes of post irradiation cell survival curves were very different for high energy photons and
fast neutrons. This meant that the clinically-used neutron fraction sizes
corresponded to much higher RBE's than were extrapolated from the large-dose
increment animal model studies prior to Stone's clinical work. Hence, nearly
all of Stone's patients with serious radiation sequelae had inadvertently received extremely high radiation doses as reflected by calculated nominal standard doses (Ellis NSD formula) of 2000-3200 rets[3].

Clinical trials were first resumed at Hammersmith Hospital, London, England
in the 1960's. After several hundred patients with extensive cancers were
treated, it was concluded that fast neutron radiotherapy was well tolerated and
that many advanced malignancies responded amazingly well to fast neutron irradiation[4]. Based upon these very optimistic results, various centers throughout
the world began clinical trials with fast neutrons.

In the United States, patient treatments were started in 1972 at the M.D.
Anderson Hospital utilizing the Texas A & M University variable energy cyclotron
(50 MeV d → Be reaction). Clinical trials were next instituted at the University of Washington utilizing a fixed energy cyclotron (22 MeV d → Be reaction)
in 1973. Significant numbers of patients have also received neutron radiotherapy at the MANTA facility (35 MeV d → Be reaction) centered at George Washington University in Washington, D.C., at the GLANTA facility (25 MeV d → Be
reaction) in Cleveland, Ohio, and at the Fermi Laboratory facility (66 MeV p →

Be reaction) in Batavia, Illinois. Initially, Phase I clinical trials were carried out utilizing patients with advanced tumors who were felt to have less than a 10% 5-year survival with conventional forms of treatment. This work yielded considerable information about the RBE's for different tissues and about the variation of the neutron RBE's from facility to facility. More recently, the majority of patients receiving fast neutron radiotherapy have been entered into randomized, prospective clinical trials designed to compare neutron irradiation with the best available photon control arm for a given tumor histology and site. Approximately 2500 patients have been treated in all re-sulting in a fairly extensive patient data base. A comprehensive report on this data base is obviously outside the scope of the present conference manuscript and so we will confine our discussion to three main areas; (1) squamous cell carcinomas of the head and neck region, (2) high grade gliomas of the brain, and (3) transitional cell carcinomas of the bladder. In areas (1) and (2) we will begin our discussion with the phase I clinical trials - drawing heavily on the University of Washington experience - and proceed from there to the most recent results of the RTOG randomized studies. In area (3) we will discuss the results of a recently completed RTOG non-randomized study. It should be emphasized that the results of the RTOG studies are only preliminary at this time and may change significantly when the final study reports are prepared.

CLINICAL RESULTS

Squamous Cell Carcinomas of the Head and Neck Region. From 1973 through 1977 a total of 100 patients with histologically-proven, advanced squamous cell car-cinomas of the head and neck region were treated with curative intent at the University of Washington using either "neutrons only" or neutrons as part of a "mixed beam" regime. Treating with "neutrons only" means that the primary tumor site and any region of clinically-involved cervical adenopathy received between 17-22 $Gy_{n\gamma}$ according to one of the following three fractionation schemes: (a) 1.5 $Gy_{n\gamma}$ on Mondays and Fridays, (b) 1.0 $Gy_{n\gamma}$ on Mondays - Wednesdays - Fridays, or (c) 0.75 $Gy_{n\gamma}$ on Mondays - Tuesdays - Thursdays - Fridays. The term "$Gy_{n\gamma}$" refers to the total measured radiation dose and in-cludes the gamma ray contaminant produced by neutron-nucleii interactions ($\leq$ 10% at a depth of 10 cm). These three treatment schemes were "normalized" to deliver 3.0 $Gy_{n\gamma}$ per week. At the time these clinical trials took place, an RBE = 3 was chosen to relate neutron dosages to megavoltage photon dosages but it now appears that a value of RBE = 3.3 is more appropriate for most tissues. In this work and for other sites as well, there appears to be no difference among these three fractionation schemes either in terms of tumor control or attendant morbidity. The "mixed beam" treatment consists of delivering combined neutron and photon irradiation according to the following scheme: 0.6 $Gy_{n\gamma}$ on Mondays - Fridays and 1.8 Gy_{γ} on Tuesdays - Wednesdays - Thursdays. Assuming an RBE =3 this corresponded to 9 Gy equivalent per week as did the "neutrons only" forms of treatment. The "mixed beam" patients received between 65-70 Gy equivalent to the primary site and any region of clinically involved cervical adenopathy. In the "neutrons only" form of treatment, the spinal cord dose was limited to 15 $Gy_{n\gamma}$ and in the "mixed beam" form of treatment the spinal cord dose was limited to 45 Gy equivalent.

In many cases, the primary tumors were quite extensive and involved more than one anatomical site. Nevertheless, Table I summarizes the sites of origin for the patients in this study according to the clinical judgment of the examining physicians.

TABLE I

LOCATION OF PRIMARY TUMOR SITE

Location	Mixed Beam	Neutrons Only
Nasopharynx	4	5
Oral Cavity	6	15*
Oropharynx	21	28
Hypopharynx	6	10*
Supraglottic Larynx	1	5
	38	63

* Includes one patient with two simultaneous primaries - T_2 oral cavity, T_3 hypopharynx.

The patients were all staged according to the most recent recommendations of the American Joint Committee for Cancer Staging and End Result Reporting. The two groups of patients had approximately the same T-stage distribution but the "neutron only" patients had a somewhat more advanced N-stage distribution: "mixed beam" T_1-2, T_2-10, T_3-17, T_4-9, N_0-13, N_1-7, N_2-3, N_3-15; "neutrons only" T_1-1, T_2-6, T_3-30, T_4-26, N_0-9, N_1-12, N_2-8, N_3-34. This asymmetry between the two groups of patients is an unfortunate consequence of all non-randomized, phase I pilot studies.

Figure 1 shows a graphical display of the local control rates at the primary site for the two groups of patients using the actuarial method to maximize the information obtained from a spectrum of follow-up times.

356

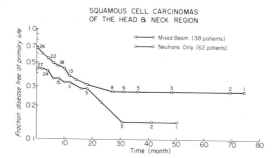

Fig. 1. Actuarial curves showing fraction of patients with squamous cell carcinomas of the head and neck region who are disease free at the primary site as
a function of time after completing therapy. The numbers indicate the patients
at risk at the indicated data points.

No patient was considered to have achieved a complete remission until either
examination revealed no clinical evidence of disease or until biopsy of a questionable area was shown to be negative. In cases where the patient died before
the suspicious area had declared itself, the patient was assumed to be a local
failure unless an autopsy was performed which yielded a negative result. The
overall initial complete remission rates were 68% for the "mixed beam" group
and 44% for the "neutron only" group. Comparing the initial complete remission
rates as a function of stage, we find, respectively, for the "mixed beam" vs.
the "neutron only" groups: 80% (8/10) vs. 86% (6/7) for T_2 lesions, 70% (12/17)
vs. 48% (14/29) for T_3 lesions, and 44% (4/9) vs. 30% (8/26) for T_4 lesions.
The overall local control rate at the cervical neck nodes for those patients
with pretreatment cervical adenopathy was 63% for the "mixed beam" group and
53% for the "neutron only" group. Using our strict criteria for assigning an
initial complete remission, no patient who was felt to have achieved an initial
local control subsequently relapsed in the cervical nodes. There was no significant difference between the two groups of patients in regards to a stage-by-
stage breakdown of the nodal control rates.

Table II compares our local control rates and survival rates at two years
with the results for comparable groups of patients treated with fast neutrons
at other institutions. The reader is referred to the appropriate references for
a more complete discussion of these various studies.

TABLE II

TWO YEAR LOCAL CONTROL RATES AT THE PRIMARY SITE AND ACTUARIAL SURVIVAL RATES
FOR PATIENTS WITH ADVANCED HEAD AND NECK CANCERS TREATED WITH FAST NEUTRON
TELETHERAPY

	Local Control of Primary (2 year actuarial)	Survival (2 year actuarial)
University of Washington		
Mixed Beam (38 patients)	30%	40%
Neutron Only (62 patients)	20%	10%
Catterall et. al.[5]		
Neutrons only (70 patients)	76%	28%
*Maor et. al.[9]		
Pilot Neutrons Only (49 patients)	43%	20%
Pilot Mixed Beam (25 patients)	35%	25%
**Batterman and Breur[1]		
Neutrons Only (59 patients)	61%	17%

* Pilot Neutron only includes 7 patients with salivary gland tumors, pilot
mixed beam includes 2 patients with salivary gland tumors.
** Includes 11 patients with salivary gland tumors.

In our series, there was a noticeable difference between the treatment-related complication rates of the "mixed beam" and "neutron only" groups - both
in terms of acute and late effects. Five patients in the "neutron only" group
developed a severe skin desquamation requiring a break in treatment. No such
skin reaction occurred for the "mixed beam" group. Significant pharyngeal wall
edema occurred in six patients in the "neutron only" group compared with only
one patient in the "mixed beam" group. Seven patients in the "neutron only"
group developed significant treatment-related neurological complications -
either cranial nerve damage or cervical myelitis - and no such problems occurred
in the "mixed beam" group. Moreover, the complications of salvage surgery were
much more severe in the "neutron only" group (6/10) than in the "mixed beam"
group (2/6). Significant morbidity associated with high dose neutron radiation
therapy for head and neck cancers has also been reported by Catterall et.al.,[5]
Griffin et.al.,[7] and Maor et.al.[9] The basic conclusion from the head and neck
pilot studies conducted in the United States was that the "mixed beam" form of
treatment yielded at least as high of local control rate as did treatments with
"neutrons only" and moreover was associated with a substantially lower complication rate. This conclusion greatly affected patient accrual to the on-
going RTOG study (76-10) for head and neck cancer.

RTOG study 76-10 is a randomized prospective study which was activated September, 1976, for patients with squamous cell carcinomas of the head and neck

region who were to be treated with radiation alone. It was originally designed
to have three treatment arms - photons, "mixed beam", and "neutrons only" - but
with the maturation of the phase I pilot studies, the majority of facilities only
randomized patients to either the photon or "mixed beam" arms. This effectively
converted the protocol into a two-armed study. Eligible patients had biopsy-
proven squamous cell carcinoma of the oral cavity, oropharynx, hypopharynx, or
supraglottic larynx staged T_{2-4} N_{0-3} M_0. The protocol requires delivering between 66-74 Gy equivalent to the primary site over 7-8 weeks with the radiotherapist having the option of doing an interstitial implant at 50 Gy equivalent.
Preliminary results thus far indicate no major differences between the two forms
of treatment. Case accession is continuing and an analysis on a site-by-site
basis will eventually be made.

High Grade Gliomas of the Brain. High grade gliomas are a particularly vir-
ulent form of brain tumors that if untreated result in a median survival of
approximately 26 weeks from the time of diagnosis. Conventional photon irradiation prolongs survival somewhat but almost invariably the patient dies of progressing disease. The initial studies[6,8] involved giving whole brain irradiation either with "neutrons only" to 15.5-18.5 $Gy_{n\gamma}$ or "mixed beam" irradiation
to 6.0-6.6 $Gy_{n\gamma}$ and 28-32 Gy_γ followed by a boost to the primary target volume
of between 1.2-1.8 $Gy_{n\gamma}$ and 5-10 Gy_γ. The basic conclusion from these studies
was that fast neutrons had the ability to erradicate this type of tumor, but
that the side effects of the neutron treatments were almost invariably fatal to
the patient. The pathological picture was that of a coagulation necrosis re-
placing the original tumor mass and an intense demyelination reaction often
extending far from the original tumor volume.

As a first step in compensating for this, the RTOG developed a protocol
(RTOG 76-11) which restricted the neutron irradiation to the primary tumor
volume as determined by radionuclide brain scans and/or CT scans. The patients
were to receive 50 Gy_γ whole brain photon irradiation over 5-5 1/2 weeks and
then were randomly assigned either photon boost field irradiation or neutron
boost field irradiation (15 Gy equivalent over 1 1/2-2 weeks). This study was
activated October, 1976, and closed September, 1980, after accruing 160 evaluable patients - 81 on the neutron boost arm and 79 on the photon boost arm.
The pathology is in the process of being reviewed now and the histologies are
being classified as either "anaplastic astrocytoma" or "glioblastoma multiforme."
Figure 2 shows a preliminary analysis of the survival data according to mode
of treatment for 116 patients thus far having had their tumor classified as
"glioblastoma multiforme".

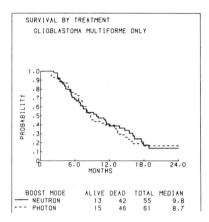

Fig. 2 Actuarially calculated survival curves for patients with glioblastoma multiforme treated according to RTOG protocol 76-11. The solid curve represents the neutron boost group and the dotted curve represents the photon boost group.

Figure 3 shows a corresponding analysis for 16 patients thus far having had their tumor classified as "anaplastic astrocytoma". Note that for these patients having the better prognostic histology, the neutron boost group had a substantially lower median survival than the photon boost patients.

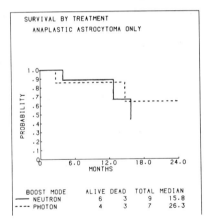

Fig. 3. Actuarially calculated survival curves for patients with anaplastic astrocytomas treated according to protocol 76-11. The solid curve represents the neutron boost group and the dotted curve represents the photon boost group.

The other patients in the study are in the process of having their tumor pathology reviewed and updated survival curves will be presented in the final report. Preliminary results seem to indicate that the neutron boost patients are dying without progressing tumor and have the same pathologic picture as described above while the photon boost patients are dying of progressing tumor.

Clinical data seems to indicate that for brain tissue the neutron RBE is of the order of 4.5-5 which is approximately 35%-50% greater than the RBE for muscle tissue. This was originally thought to be due in large part to the particular energy deposition mechanism of fast neutrons which should be more efficient in neural tissue with its high hydrogen content. However, detailed estimates[2] show that this can account for only about a 7% increase in RBE. Thus there appears to be something unique in the way neural tissue responds to high LET irradiation and this may be important for heavy ions and pi-mesons as well as for fast neutrons.

Currently, the neutron treatment centers in the United States have embarked upon a dose searching study (RTOG 80-07) for high grade gliomas in an effort to determine whether or not there is a "therapeutic window" for treatment with fast neutrons that will allow for tumor control without an unacceptable amount of normal brain tissue morbidity. This study differs from the previous one in that the neutron boost field irradiation is given along with the photon irradiation instead of at the end of it.

Transitional Cell Carcinomas of the Urinary Bladder. The RTOG has recently completed a non-randomized phase I study (RTOG 77-05) on the efficacy of fast neutron irradiation for transitional cell carcinomas of the bladder. The study was originally designed to have three arms: (1) "mixed beam" plus surgery for operable patients, (2) "mixed beam" alone, and (3) neutrons alone. The "mixed beam" plus surgery arm consisted of 50 Gy equivalents to the pelvis over approximately five weeks followed by a cystectomy at six weeks thereafter and accrued 15 cases - only nine of which have adequate follow-up at the present time. The definitive "mixed beam" and neutrons alone arms consisted of 50 Gy equivalent to the pelvis over approximately five to six weeks followed by a 15-20 Gy equivalent bladder boost over approximately 1 1/2-2 weeks. The "mixed beam" alone arm accrued 23 patients with 17 of these having adequate follow-up for evaluation at the present time. The neutrons alone arm accrued 5 patients with only 2 of these having adequate follow-up and so will not be considered further at this time. Preliminary results for the other two arms are shown in Table III.

Two things are of particular interest: (1) the preoperative "mixed beam" irradiation shows a very high rate of tumor clearance at the time of surgery and (2) in spite of the fact that the group of patients treated with radiation alone had a more advanced set of tumors, their median survival surpasses that of the group of patients treated with a combination of radiation and surgery. These results are very encouraging and a final report will await longer follow-up times. Currently, this study has been replaced by a randomized, prospective study, RTOG (81-10), which compared preoperative photon and mixed beam irradiation to 50 Gy equivalent followed by a cystectomy in 5-6 weeks.

TABLE III

RTOG 77-05: PRELIMINARY RESULTS ACCORDING TO TREATMENT FOR CASES WITH ADEQUATE FOLLOW-UP

	Mixed Beam and Surgery	Mixed Beam Alone
Number of Cases	9	17
Clearance of Tumor	6*	10
Median Survival (months)	8.6	13.2

* Negative cystectomy specimen.

FUTURE WORK

Of all the high LET particles of possible utility for clinical radiotherapy, the most experience thus far is with fast neutrons. The results for only a few of the tumor sites under study have been presented here. Currently, there are plans for four hospital-based clinical neutron radiotherapy units. Three of these units will be cyclotrons and these will be located at M.D. Anderson Hospital, Houston, Texas, The University of Washington in Seattle, Washington, and at the Wadsworth Veterans Administration Hospital (UCLA affiliated) in Los Angeles, California. A unit based upon a d-T neutron generator will be located at the University of Pennsylvania Hospital, Philadelphia, Pennsylvania. These units will in general have neutron beams with better depth-dose properties than the existing facilities and moreover will have rotating gantries with isocentric treatment capabilities. This should ensure that adequate clinical studies are carried out which will define the role of fast neutron radiotherapy in the treatment of cancer. This work will compliment the heavy ion and pi-meson work in that it provides a way of seperating the high LET properties from the better depth-dose properties of the charged particle modalities.

ACKNOWLEDGMENTS

This work was supported in part by the United States National Cancer Institute under Grants Ca-12441 and Ca-21661.

REFERENCES

1. Batterman JJ, Breur K (in press) Results of fast neutron teletherapy for locally advanced head and neck tumors. Int J Radiat Oncol Biol Phys.
2. Bewley DK (1970) Fast neutron beams for therapy. Curr Top Radiat Res VI: 251-292.
3. Brennan JT, Phillips TL (1971) Evaluation of past experience with fast neutron teletherapy and its implications for future applications. Europ J Cancer 7:219-225.
4. Catterall M (1974) The treatment of advanced cancer by fast neutrons from the medical research council's cyclotron at Hammersmith Hospital, London. Europ J Cancer 10:343-347.
5. Catterall M, Bewley DK, Sutherland J (1977) Second report on a randomized clinical trial of fast neutrons compared with x or gamma rays in treatment of advanced cancers of head and neck. Br Med J 1:1942.
6. Catterall M, Bloom HJG, Ash DU, Walsh L, Richardson A, Utley D, Gowing NFC, Lewis P, Chaucer B (1980) Fast neutrons compared with megavoltage x-rays in the treatment of patients with supratenturial glioblastoma: a controlled pilot study. Int J Rad Onc Biol Phys 6:261-266.
7. Griffin TW, Weisberger EC, Laramore GE, Tong D, Blasko JC (1979) Complications of combined surgery and neutron radiation therapy in patients with advanced carcinoma of the head and neck. Radiology 132:177-178.
8. Laramore GE, Griffin TW, Gerdes AJ, Groudine MT and Parker RG (1978) Fast neutron and mixed (neutron/photon) beam teletherapy for grades III and IV astrocytomas. Cancer 42:96-103.
9. Maor MH, Hussey DH, Fletcher GH, Jesse RH (1981) Fast neutron therapy for locally advanced head and neck tumors. Int J Radiat Oncol Biol Phys 7:155-163.
10. Stone RS (1948) Neutron therapy and specific ionization. Amer J Roentgenol. 59:771-785.

PROTON THERAPY AT HARVARD

JOHN E. MUNZENRIDER
Dept. of Radiation Medicine, Massachusetts General Hospital, Boston MA 02114

INTRODUCTION

That favorable dose distributions are potentially achievable with protons in human radiotherapy can be inferred from the comparative depth dose curves shown in Figure 1. The narrow width of the unmodulated 160 MeV proton beam Bragg peak (7 mm at the 80% level) is of limited use in clinical radiotherapy. However, the illustrated spread-out Bragg Peak (SOBP) gives a region of uniform ionization at depth 7.5 cm in width. The 10 MeV x-ray beam presented for comparison delivers maximum dose proximally in the entrance region and falls from 72% to 52% of the maximum dose in traversing the region treated uniformly by the SOBP proton beam.

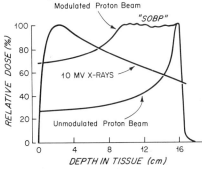

Fig. 1. The depth dose curve for a 10 MeV x-ray beam, a non-modulated 160 MeV proton beam, and a spread-out Bragg peak proton beam. Reproduced by permission of JAMA.[12]

The main rationale for the use of the SOBP proton beam in clinical radiotherapy is that improved dose distributions are potentially possible because of the physical characteristics of the beam. Essentially no dose is deposited beyond the end of range of the protons, which is 16 cm in tissue for a 160 MeV beam and 26 cm for a 200 MeV beam. Lateral fall-off is also quite sharp: distances between the 90% and the 50% isodose lines are 1.5 and 4.5 mm at depths of 1 and 10 cm, respectively, while the distance between the 50% and the 20% isodose lines is 1 and 4 mm at those depths. The potential gain in human radiotherapy with the proton beam is that a greater dose can be given to a defined tumor volume than would be possible with conventional techniques, since more precise control of the radiation dose distribution would allow better sparing of adjacent normal tissues. Constraints on the use of protons in clinical radiotherapy are several. Generally, skin dose with the SOBP is greater than with supervoltage x-rays (Fig. 1). Normal structures in the entrance region get a significant percentage of the dose, if not the same dose, which the target itself receives. Inhomogeneities in the entrance region and in the target volume itself can significantly alter dose distributions.[2,19] Precise tumor or normal tissue localization is required to avoid excess irradiation of distal normal structures or insufficient treatment of the target volume, which situations could occur if the target volume is improperly localized relative to the proximal and distal edges of the SOBP employed. Unconventional patient treatment positions are mandated by fixed (horizontal or vertical) beams designed specifically for physics research; decubitus, seated, and standing treatment positions must be employed, as well as the more usual supine and prone positions. Special immobilization devices are needed to reproducibly orient patients to the beam. CT scans in the treatment position in the immobilization device employed for treatment are essential for adequate treatment planning and compensation to be achieved. Lucite compensating boluses can be made by computer controlled milling machines from CT scan data to contour the beam at depth. Proton treatment planning considerations and techniques have been described in detail.[19]

HUMAN PROTON RADIOTHERAPY

Pituitary and arteriovenous malformations

In 1958, Tobias, Lawrence and associates[17] published a preliminary report on pituitary irradiation with high energy protons at the University of California Cyclotron in Berkeley. The Berkeley experience in this area has been recently reviewed.[11] Pituitary-related problems have been treated with single fraction proton beam irradiation at the Harvard Cyclotron by Kjellberg, Koehler and associates for approximately two decades with 961 patients having been treated at the time of the most recent report.[9] Arteriovenous malformations are also treated with single fraction proton therapy[8] using a stereo-tactic technique similar to that employed in the pituitary-related lesions. A recent monograph on heavy particle radiotherapy includes an excellent chapter on protons.[11] Human proton radiotherapy has recently been reviewed.[10]

Fractionated radiation therapy

Uppsala experience. Pioneering fractionated radiotherapy studies of human malignancies have employed the 185 MeV proton beam of the synchrocyclotron at the Gustaf Werner Institute in Uppsala, Sweden.[4] The Uppsala experience with 69 patients treated between 1957 and 1967 was recently summarized.[3] One Stage II cervical cancer patient was surviving without evident disease 16 years after treatment, and one child treated for a midbrain tumor was alive and well 8 years after proton therapy. A "good response" was observed in 75% of nasopharyngeal patients; 5-year survival rate in that group was 27%. Earlier conclusions concerning human proton radiotherapy were reaffirmed: protons were qualitatively and quantitatively similar to other low LET radiations, and acute and chronic radiation reactions were consistent with the dose and fractionation pattern employed. An RBE for protons for human radiotherapy in the range of 1.0 ± 0.2 was thought appropriate for future clinical use. The Uppsala Cyclotron has been inactive for several years and is being upgraded to deliver a 200 MeV proton beam for clinical radiotherapy with a range in tissue of 26 cm.

Harvard-Mass. General-Mass. Eye & Ear experience. The Harvard Cyclotron was completed in 1948, and animal experiments were first conducted there in 1959. A medical annex was completed in 1963, and was used primarily for single fraction pituitary-related irradiations until 1973 when the Department of Radiation Medicine at Massachusetts General Hospital (MGH) began a fractionated radiation therapy program. A second treatment room and additional clinical facilities were added in 1978. Each treatment room has a fixed horizontal beam delivery system. In one, portals up to 5 cm in diameter can be treated with dose rates in the range of 8.0 - 10 Gy/min. In the other, fields up to 30 cm in diameter can be treated with dose rates in the range of 0.8 - 1.5 Gy/min.

Precise patient set-up relative to circular and to X, Y and Z coordinates is possible at the sub-millimeter level in both rooms by radiographic visualization of fiducial points (clips, skeletal landmarks, etc.) in three dimensions relative to beam axis.[18,19] For treatment planning, an EMI-7070 CT scanner, dedicated to the fractionated radiotherapy project, is physically located at MGH. The scanning ring can rotate 90° from its usual vertical position for scanning in vertical, horizontal, or intermediate planes, depending on the desired position of the patient for treatment. Treatment planning from CT data is performed on a VAX 780 computer connected to a dedicated raster scan graphics display unit.

An RBE of 1.1 is used for clinical radiation therapy[13,19] and doses are defined in terms of Cobalt Gy equivalents (CGE), the RBE of 1.1 multiplied by the proton dose in Gy. Any portion of the treatment given with [60]Cobalt or x-rays is delivered at the rate of 1.8 - 2.0 Gy per fraction, 5 fractions per week. Proton treatment is given in 2.1 CGE fractions, 4 times a week, since the beam is used for the single-fraction pituitary and AVM treatments on the fifth day. Patients with uveal melanomas have generally received 5 treatments of 14 or 18 CGE per fraction over a period of 7-9 days, while a small number of non-uveal melanoma patients have received 6-10 fractions of 4-6 CGE each, with treatment being given twice per week.

Clinical experience has been described[13,14,15,16] and published results recently summarized.[10,19] A total of 272 patients were treated through June 1981. Number of patients in each category and distribution of proton and x-ray doses are shown in Table 1. Significant clinical experience and follow-up have been accumulated in patients with uveal melanomas, prostate carcinoma and para-CNS sarcomas. Techniques and results in these categories will be discussed.

TABLE 1

PATIENT POPULATION* - FRACTIONATED PROTON THERAPY

Category	#	Proton component of total dose		
		< 50%	≥ 50%	100%
Melanoma				
Uveal	101			101
Non-uveal	5		2	3
Prostate	65	65		
Sarcoma	42	26	14	2
Head & neck	21	15	6	
Ano-rectal	13	13		
Central nervous system	11	7	3	1
Miscellaneous & metastatic	14	7	3	4
Total patients	272	133	28	111
Percentage		49%	10%	41%

*1974 through June, 1981.

Prostate carcinoma. The prostate boost volume is within range of a peri-neal proton beam and presents no inhomogeneity problems. Technique and pre-liminary results have been described.[12] A retrospective analysis[1] has compared local control, survival and complication rates in 65 patients receiving proton boost with similar parameters in 118 patients treated concurrently with con-ventional techniques. Sixty-five proton boost patients ranged in age from 52 to 79 years (mean, 67 years); the control group was comparable in both age range and mean age. Sixty-five percent of the proton group had well or mod-erately differentiated histology, while 55% of the control group had poorly differentiated carcinoma. Patients in both groups received 50.4 Gy to the pelvis with 10 or 25 MeV x-rays. The prostate was boosted to a total dose of 73.5 CGE in the proton group, and 68.5 Gy in control patients. No difference in rectal or GU morbidity was seen between the two groups. Leg, penile, and scrotal edema were observed with equal frequency (13%) in both groups; all patients with that complication had undergone staging lymphadenectomy prior to radiotherapy. Local control was present in 61/65 (94%) proton patients and in 103/116 (89%) of the control group, with min. follow-up of 18 and 24 mo., respectively. There was no difference in actuarial survival between the two groups.

Proton boost therapy for prostatic carcinoma has been shown to be feasible, allowing increases of 7.5% and 28% in the total and the boost dose, respectively. Morbidity was similar in both groups while local control was slightly better in the proton group. A prospective randomized trial will be implemented to compare x-ray therapy only to x-rays plus proton boost in patients with prostatic cancer.

Uveal melanomas. Melanomas arising in the uveal tract of the eye are accurately diagnosed by clinical examination, indirect ophthalmoscopy, fluorescein angiography, ocular ultrasound and ^{32}P uptake studies. Ocular tumors are within range of a proton beam with a maximum energy in the 60-70 MeV range since the diameter of the globe itself rarely exceeds 23 mm. No inhomogeneities are present which would require compensation since the electron density of the eye is uniform across the globe. An anterior proton beam with the eyelids retracted from the beam path represents an ideal way to deliver a uniform dose to such tumors while severely limiting dose delivered to uninvolved ocular structures, as shown in Figure 2.

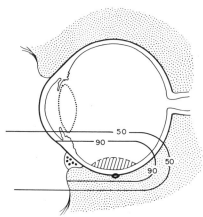

Fig. 2. Typical dose distribution for proton beam treatment of uveal melanoma. Tumor is inferior cross-hatched area, and a localizing clip on sclera is shown. Note sparing of lens and retina. Twenty percent isodose line is 2 mm beyond 50% line shown. Reproduced by permission of the Journal of the Canadian Association of Radiologists.[13]

Localization and treatment techniques have been described.[5,6,7] Coordinates of tantalum rings sutured to the sclera around the base of the tumor relative to beam axis, as well as tumor height and globe diameter determined by ultrasound, are incorporated into a treatment planning program which treats the eye as a sphere.[6] This program displays critical ocular structures (optic nerve, macula, and lens) as well as clip position and three-dimensional contour lines representing the tumor. The "eye" can be manipulated on the display screen in real time to determine optimal direction of gaze in which the beam will circumscribe the tumor and avoid to the greatest extent possible normal ocular structures. After initial radiographic set-up, patients are monitored during treatment with a video camera to assure that voluntary fixation on the predetermined point is maintained.

Between July 1975 and June 1981, 101 patients (52 male, 49 female, age range 25-83 yrs) received proton beam treatment for uveal tract melanomas. Six patients had treatment to their only eye, the other eye having been removed because of melanoma in 4 and following trauma in 2. Six patients had bilateral melanoma: 4 had had enucleation, 1 received bilateral proton irradiation, and the 6th had been treated with a [60]Cobalt plaque two years prior to proton radiotherapy. Seven lesions were small, 43 medium and 52 were large. Doses ranged from 46 to 100 CGE in five fractions over 6-15 days (only one eye received each extreme dose). Seventy-three percent received 70 CGE over 7-8 days. Patients with lesions less than 15 mm in greatest diameter and less than 5 mm in height randomly receive 70 or 90 CGE if the tumor is away from the optic nerve or the macula. Eleven percent were randomized to the higher dose level.

Minimum follow-up of 12 months is available for 61 eyes, of 24 months for 35 eyes, of 36 months for 21 eyes, and of 48 months for 10 eyes. In 60 patients with follow-up periods ranging between 12 and 72 months, 54 (90%) are alive without evident disease. No tumor growth has been observed in any treated eye. Six deaths have occurred: three from documented metastatic disease 17, 23 and 34 months after treatment, and one 4 months after radiation of pneumonia (brain and bone scans positive, bone and liver biopsies negative, autopsy not obtained). Two patients died of heart disease 11 and 21 months after treatment. Treatment complications have been associated with decreased visual acuity in 12 of the 76 treated eyes (16%) with minimum 6-month follow-up. Cataracts developed in 6 eyes and retinopathy in 3. Three eyes were enucleated following proton beam irradiation. Two were totally blind, one from progression of initially present retinal detachment and another from acute glaucoma. The third patient had enucleation elsewhere following progression of initially present retinal detachment, although significant vision was still present. Two of the tumors were significantly smaller than they had been prior to treatment while the third was unchanged from its initial size. Based on historical survival rates after enucleation as a function of tumor size, 7 or 8 metastatic deaths would have been expected in this population[7] had enucleation been done in all. Thus, it is highly encouraging that only three such deaths have been observed.

Tumor regrowth has not been observed within or at the margins of the irradiated volume, verifying assumptions made in the treatment planning program, and adequacy of voluntary patient fixation during treatment to retain the tumor within the irradiated volume. Survival has not been compromised, and complications have been acceptable. Proton beam radiation appears to be the treatment of choice for medium and large melanomas and offers the potential to retain vision in most treated patients.

Para-CNS sarcomas. Sarcomas arising in the base of the skull, vertebral bodies, and the paravertebral soft tissue represent a most challenging treatment planning problem because of their proximity to vital normal structures (brain stem, spinal cord, and optic nerve and chiasm). Twenty-two such patients have received proton therapy. Fourteen bone sarcomas included 7 chordomas, 4 chondrosarcomas, and 1 osteosarcoma involving the base of the skull, and 2 chordomas arising in the second cervical vertebral body. Six paravertebral soft tissue sarcomas arose in the dorsal region, 1 in the cervical area, and another in the upper lumbar region. The population and dose distributions achieved have been described.[14] Dose distribution achieved in a patient with a chordoma in C-2 is shown in Fig. 3.

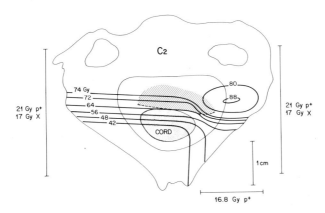

Fig. 3. Dose distribution at C-2 level for chordoma arising there and compressing spinal cord posteriorly. Cross-hatched area represents tumor within vertebral canal as determined from metrizamide CT scan. Doses ranged up to 88 Gy, with lateral portals and posterior portal receiving 10 MeV x-ray (X) and proton (P+) doses as shown. Note dose gradient across cord, and "hot spot" (80-88 Gy) in region of "overshoot" of posterior proton portal into bone.

Doses ranged from 57.8 to 80.1 CGE; between 33% and 100% of the dose was given with protons. Eighty-six percent and 59% received tumor doses greater than 68 and 70 CGE, respectively. Partial spinal cord or brain stem dose approached or exceeded 64 CGE in many patients. All patients presented challenging treatment planning problems with irregular entrance contours, bone, air and soft tissue inhomogeneities within the entrance region, and tumor adjacent to or abutting critical normal structures. Doses of this magnitude would not have been delivered in the Department of Radiation Medicine at MGH. Thirteen patients were treated 12 to 87 months ago (median time since treatment 27 months): 12 are alive without evident recurrence or neurological injury. One died of distant metastases with marginal recurrence 10 months after treatment.

Randomized trials are not planned in these patients: their rarity makes the patient population volume too low to achieve significant numbers, and it would be difficult if not impossible to design an adequate control arm for conventional treatment.

SUMMARY AND CONCLUSIONS

Observations on 272 patients treated with fractionated proton therapy at the Harvard Cyclotron through July 1981 confirm conclusions reached in the pioneering Uppsala studies[3,4] that human proton beam therapy can be carried out without unexpected acute or chronic normal tissue reactions. Tumor and normal tissue reactions observed are consistent with an RBE of 1.1 for protons relative to ^{60}Cobalt gamma rays. Proton beam therapy appears to be an ideal treatment for medium and large uveal melanomas and for bone and soft tissue sarcomas abutting critical CNS structures. Improved dose distributions achievable with protons have allowed greater doses to be delivered than would have been given with conventional techniques in several categories of patients. Continued feasibility studies are planned in patients with head and neck squamous cell carcinomas, para-aortic node metastasis, ano-rectal cancer, nonuveal head and neck melanomas, thyroid and salivary gland tumors, and retroperitoneal sarcomas. The full potential impact of proton beam therapy in treatment of human malignancies will only be realized if hospital based accelerators become more widely distributed so that the benefits of proton therapy are made conveniently available to a significant proportion of the cancer population.

ACKNOWLEDGEMENTS

Sincere and grateful appreciation is expressed to Michele Girolamo, Joan Horgan and Barbara Grzybek for their assistance in preparation of this paper, and to Patricia McNulty, R.N., B.A. for obtaining patient follow-up data. Appreciation is also expressed to Andreas M. Koehler and the Harvard Cyclotron Laboratory staff for their enduring cooperation and support, to Drs. Herman Suit, Michael Goitein, Lynn Verhey, and Marcia Urie and to Mr. Richard Gentry for their advice and assistance. The role of Dr. Evangelos Gragoudas in the primary management of the uveal melanoma patients is acknowledged with sincere appreciation. Supported in part by NIH Grant CA21239.

REFERENCES

1. Duttenhaver JR, Shipley WU, Perrone T, Verhey LJ, Munzenrider JE, Goitein M, Prout GR, Suit HD (1982) Protons vs. megavoltage x-rays as boost therapy for patients with localized prostatic carcinoma. Cancer (In Press).

2. Goitein M (1978) Compensation for inhomogeneities in charged particle radiotherapy using computed tomography. Int J Rad Oncol Biol Phys 4:499-508.

3. Graffman S (1979) Clinical experience of tumor therapy with high energy protons. Proc First Int Seminar on Uses of Proton Beams in Radiation Therapy, Atomic Press, Moscow, 3:119-24.

4. Graffman S, Jung B (1970) Clinical trials in radiotherapy and the merits of high energy protons. Acta Radiol Ther Phys Biol 9:1-23.

5. Gragoudas ES, Goitein M, Koehler AM, Verhey LJ, Tepper JE, Suit HD, Brockhurst R, Constable I (1977) Proton irradiation of small choroidal malignant melanomas. Am J Ophthalmol 83:665-73.

6. Gragoudas ES, Goitein M, Verhey LJ, Munzenrider JE, Suit HD, Koehler AM (1980) Proton beam irradiation: an alternative to enucleation for intraocular melanomas. Ophthalmol 87:571-81.

7. Gragoudas ES, Goitein M, Verhey LJ, Munzenrider JE, Urie M, Suit HD, Koehler A (1982) Proton beam irradiation of uveal melanomas: results of a 5½-year study. Arch Ophthalmol (In Press).

8. Kjellberg RN (1979) Bragg Peak proton radiosurgery for arteriovenous malformations of the brain. Proc First Int Seminar on Uses of Proton Beams in Radiation Therapy, Atomic Press, Moscow, 3:12-22.

9. Kjellberg RN, Kliman B (1979) Lifetime effectiveness--A system of therapy for pituitary adenomas, emphasizing proton hypophysectomy. In Linfoot JA (ed.), Recent Advances in the Diagnosis and Treatment of Pituitary Tumors, New York: Raven Press.

10. Munzenrider JE, Shipley WU, Verhey LJ (1981) Future prospects of radiation therapy with protons. Seminars in Oncology 8(1):110-24.

11. Raju MR (1980) Heavy Particle Radiotherapy. New York: Academic Press.

12. Shipley WU, Tepper JE, Prout GR, Verhey LJ, Mendiondo OA, Goitein M, Koehler AM, Suit HD (1979) Proton radiation as boost therapy for localized prostatic carcinoma. JAMA 241:1912-15.

13. Suit, HD, Goitein M, Munzenrider JE, Verhey LJ, Gragoudas E, Koehler AM, Urano M, Shipley WU, Linggood RM, Friedberg C, Wagner M (1980) Clinical experience with proton beam radiation therapy. J Can Assoc Radiol 31:35-39.

14. Suit HD, Goitein M, Munzenrider JE, Verhey LJ, Davis KR, Koehler AM, Linggood RM, Ojemann RG (1982) Definitive radiation therapy for chordoma and chondrosarcoma of base of skull and cervical spine. J Neurosurg (In Press).

15. Suit HD, Goitein M, Tepper JE, Koehler AM, Schmidt RA, Schneider R (1975) Exploratory study of proton radiation therapy using large field techniques and fractionated dose schedules. Cancer 35:1646-57.

16. Suit HD, Goitein M, Tepper JE, Verhey LJ, Koehler AM, Schneider R (1977) Clinical experience and expectations with protons and heavy ions. Int J Rad Oncol Biol Phys 3:115-25.

17. Tobias CA, Lawrence JH, Born JL, McCombs RK, Roberts JE, Anger HO, Low-Beer BVA, Huggins CB (1958) Pituitary irradiation with high-energy proton beams: A preliminary report. Cancer Res 18:121-34.

18. Verhey LJ, Goitein M, McNulty P, Munzenrider JE, Suit HD (1981) Precision positioning of immobilized patients using daily pre-treatment radiographic alignment. Int J Rad Oncol Biol Phys (In Press).

19. Verhey LJ, Munzenrider JE (1982) Proton Beam Therapy, Ann Rev Biophys Bioeng (In Press).

CLINICAL EXPERIENCE WITH HELIUM ION RADIOTHERAPY
AT THE LAWRENCE BERKELEY LABORATORY

W.M. Saunders, J.R. Castro, J.M. Quivey, G.T.Y. Chen, J.T. Lyman, and
J.M. Collier, University of California Lawrence Berkeley Laboratory
and University of California San Francisco School of Medicine

INTRODUCTION

The recurrence or persistence of a malignant tumor in its original location
is unfortunately a common cause of treatment failure. Suit[1] has estimated that
one patient in three dying from cancer has active tumor at the primary site.

Radiotherapists have discovered that they can decrease this local failure
rate in many of the tumors that they treat by increasing the radiation dose
delivered to the tumor. However, the maximum dose that can safely be given is
often severely limited by the necessity of keeping the dose to nearby critical
structures at acceptably low levels. In this circumstance, any different treatment technique or radiation modality which permits a higher dose to be delivered
to the tumor with the same or lower dose given to the critical structure should
give superior tumor control with the same or lower rate of damage to normal
tissue. Perhaps the best example of improved tumor control with improved radiation quality is to be found in the progressively improved cure rate for
Hodgkin's disease as kilovoltage techniques were replaced by orthovoltage and
megavoltage techniques.[2] Similar data exist for several other tumor sites.[3]
These improved results are due to many factors, but the improved dose distribution possible with each improvement in radiation quality is thought to be of
major importance.

Superb localization of dose is possible with the helium ion beam from the
Lawrence Berkeley Laboratory 184-inch synchrocyclotron because of the well
defined range of the beam, with most of its energy deposited at the end of this
range in the Bragg peak. The dose localization can also be enhanced by the very
sharp edges that can be obtained with these beams.

The helium beam offers very little biologic advantage relative to conventional radiation modalities.[4,5] Its primary advantage lies in its superior localization of physical dose. We would therefore expect to see an advantage with
this treatment modality in situations where critical tissues near the tumor

preclude delivery of tumoricidal doses with photons or electrons, and the sharp lateral edges and distal falloff of the helium beams permit higher doses to be delivered to the tumor. An increase in dose of 10-20 percent delivered to the tumor may be accompanied by a significant increase in local control because of the steep response curve.

The basic question being tested in these helium ion radiotherapy trials is whether or not the excellent dose localization properties of this beam when compared to beams of photons or electrons will be reflected in superior tumor control rates and a low incidence of significant damage to normal tissues.

Clinical trials to assess the clinical efficacy of helium ion radiotherapy of human cancers began at the Lawrence Berkeley Laboratory in July of 1975. Since that time, 257 patients have been treated with the helium beam or a combination of helium and photons. Two hundred three of these patients were treated with helium beam radiotherapy alone (Table 1).

TABLE 1

Helium Ion Radiotherapy - Summary to Date

Number of Patients	Site or Tumor Treated	Local Control Rate
75	Pancreas	14 percent
42	Ocular Melanoma	86 percent*
32	Esophagus	33 percent
18	Stomach	31 percent
11	Biliary Tract	33 percent
10	Chordoma	71 percent
69	Misc. Other Sites	23 percent

TOTAL   257

*100 percent local control after second treatment

We currently have active protocols for helium ion radiotherapy of localized carcinoma of the pancreas and localized carcinoma of the esophagus. There is an "all sites" protocol in which pilot series for several sites have been carried out, including a very interesting group of patients with tumor adjacent to critical structures. Finally, we have a very promising protocol for localized ocular melanoma. The progress to date in these protocols is detailed below and in literature.[6,7,8,9,10]

METHODS AND RESULTS

1) Carcinoma of the Pancreas

Irradiation of patients with localized, unresectable carcinoma of the pancreas has been carried on at LBL since 1976. Our initial study began as a pilot series utilizing helium ion irradiation at the 184-inch synchrocyclotron. The tumor dose was escalated fairly rapidly reaching a level of 6000 ^{60}Cobalt rad equivalent (CoRE) given in 7½ weeks at 200 equivalent rad per fraction, 4 fractions per week. This presents a minimum helium physical dose of approximately 5000 rad. The pilot study included some 35 patients who received at least 5000 CoRE tumor dose. There was approximately a 15 percent incidence of control within the irradiated area using this dose. The only morbidity has been a low incidence (∿10-15 percent) of radiation gastritis and/or duodenitis although recently it has become clear that this complication has occurred less often than thought earlier. Autopsy and surgical re-exploration have shown local failure without distant metastases to occur more frequently than originally thought and have shown that some patients initially thought to have hemorrhagic radiation gastritis have recurrent tumor invading duodenum or stomach. The percentage of patients living free of disease for greater than 6 months is ∿10 percent.

Although we made every attempt to exclude patients with hepatic metastases, a very high incidence of patients developed such metastases either during therapy or in the subsequent followup period. This incidence appears to be in excess of 75 percent of the patients.

A randomized prospective study was begun in 1978 comparing 6000 rad photon irradiation given in split course fashion with 6000 CoRE of helium irradiation. Both arms of the study received 5-Fluorouracil chemotherapy.

To date, 52 patients have been entered in this randomized study. However, there have been 8 patients who have been unevaluable for various reasons. Therefore, 44 patients are evaluable to date. There has been no difference between the two arms with respect to time to failure, time to local recurrence, or overall survival. Failure within the irradiation field in both arms has been very high with or without distant metastases (Figure 1). In the helium arm, the incidence of normal tissue morbidity is small and comparable to that in the pilot study. We will therefore increase the dose in this arm to 6600 CoRE.

We are currently planning to continue this protocol until approximately 40 patients per arm have been accrued. At the current rate of patient entry, this should be reached by late 1982. At that time we hope to expand this protocol by adding a third arm utilizing one of the heavy particles, probably neon.

FIGURE 1

TIME TO LOCAL FAILURE ONLY
(August 31, 1978 - December 31, 1980)

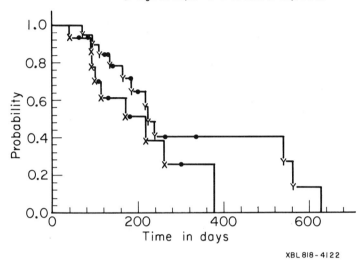

XBL 818-4122

Fig. 1. Randomized trial for carcinoma of the pancreas: time to local recurrence. Treatment corresponding to curves X and Y known only by statistician. No significant difference between curves.

2) Carcinoma of the Esophagus

Twenty-two patients have now been accrued in a Phase II nonrandomized prospective study for helium ion irradiation of localized carcinoma of the esophagus. Since this protocol was activated in December of 1978, the dose has been gradually escalated. The current dose level is 6525 CoRE given at 225 CoRE per fraction, in 4 fractions per week. As summarized in Table 2, the local failure rate remains high. Seven patients have had local control of their tumor, with followup ranging from 3 to 16 months. Two of these patients have had distant metastases; however, thirteen of the patients had local failure with or without distant metastases. An additional two patients have just recently completed treatment.

TABLE 2

3E81 CARCINOMA OF THE ESOPHAGUS

Number of Patients	Status
5	NED
7	LF only
6	LF and DM
2	DM only
2	Followup too short

NED = No Evidence of Disease
LF = Local Failure
DM = Distant Metastases

In summary, two-thirds of the patients in this protocol have failed in the treatment field. Escalating the tumor dose to 6525 CoRE at 225 CoRE per fraction has not appreciably altered this. We therefore intend to begin a pilot trial for carcinoma of the esophagus using heavier ions, such as neon. We hope that the superior OER and RBE values of these beams will be reflected in higher local control rates. The heavier ions will not be available for several months each year. During those periods, patients will be treated with helium. The tumor dose will be increased since the morbidity rate has been small.

3) Dose Localization Studies

A heterogeneous group of 92 patients with a variety of tumors has been entered into Phase I protocols to evaluate normal tissue, acute effects, and to develop charged particle treatment techniques as well as investigate possible clinical benefits of superior dose distributions with the helium ion beam. Our general impression is that for tumors adjacent to critical organs such as the spinal cord, we are able to deliver a higher dose to the tumor than could be delivered with photons, while keeping the doses to normal tissues at acceptable levels. Tumor control in this group of patients has been excellent, and normal tissue damage minimal.

This is perhaps best illustrated by a subgroup of these patients with chordomas or low grade chondrosarcomas of the base of skull, high cervical spine, or sacrum. Most of these tumors can be controlled if a photon dose $\geq$ 7000 rad can be delivered to the tumor. However, this is often impossible to accomplish with photons because of unavoidable irradiation of nearby spinal cord, brain, or gut. We have treated 10 such patients to date. Five have had the tumor in the bones in the base of the skull, three had sacral tumors, and in two the second cervical vertebra was involved. Seven patients in this group have had followup of greater than 1 year, ranging from 12 to 43 months. Four of them are alive and well with no evidence of disease, 2 had persistence of their tumor and expired, and 1 is alive with local control but has an apparent metastasis to the mandible (Table 3).

TABLE 3

Chordoma or Low Grade Chondrosarcoma

Number of Patients	Status
4	No evidence of disease
1	Local control, distant metastasis
2	Local persistence of tumor
3	Followup too short
TOTAL 10	

Some of these patients had part of their treatment with photons. Total tumor dose has ranged from 6500 CoRE to 7500 CoRE, except for 1 patient whose treatment was not completed and who received only 3600 CoRE. Interestingly, this patient is alive with no evidence of disease 45 months following treatment.

The 2 patients with involvement of the C2 vertebra are of particular interest even though their followup is too short to assess tumor control or complications. Coincidentally, both of these patients had tumor in the body and pedicles of C2, forming a "U" shaped lesion around the spinal cord. It would be extremely difficult, if not impossible, to achieve a sufficient tumor dose with photon irradiation while keeping the spinal cord dose at an acceptable level.

The treatment plan for one of those patients is presented in Figure 2. The patient is a 65 year old previously healthy male who consulted his physician because of neck pain. Plain x-rays of the neck revealed a lytic lesion in the body of the C2 vertebra. Tomograms, a myelogram, and a CT scan of the area showed involvement of the body, odontoid process, and pedicles of C2. The patient then had a surgical procedure to biopsy the tumor and to stabilize his neck by wiring the spinous processes of C1, C2, and C3 together and by applying a quick setting plastic to the area. After recovering from the surgery, the patient was referred for consideration of helium ion radiotherapy. Since the high dose region is adjacent to the spinal cord, precise verification of treatment delivery is essential. We are presently unable to verify the stopping point of the beam in vivo, so we elected to avoid the spinal cord by precisely

FIGURE 2

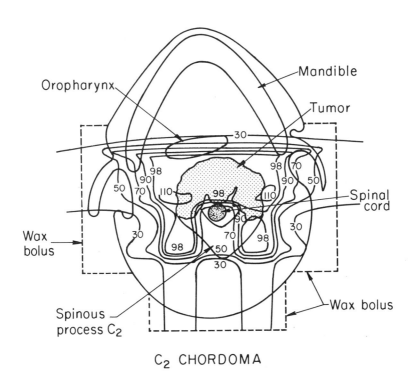

C₂ CHORDOMA

100% = 7000 Cobalt equivalent rads

XBL818-4121

FIGURE 2. Treatment plan for helium ion irradiation of a
chordoma involving the body and pedicles of the second
cervical vertebrae.

positioning the edge of the beam to include the tumor and exclude the spinal
cord. This position can be verified with a routine portal film.

The patient was treated to a tumor dose of 4000 CoRE with opposed lateral
fields which included the tumor volume and the spinal cord. The posterior portion of this field was then blocked off so that the tumor in the vertebral body
was in the treatment field, but the spinal cord and the tumor in the pedicles
were not irradiated. This portion of the tumor was treated with a direct posterior field with a midline spinal cord block. The beam was stopped abutting the
edge of the lateral conedown field. The lateral conedown fields and the posterior field were treated until the whole tumor volume received 7000 CoRE. At
this dose level, there is a very good chance of curing the tumor.

In our opinion, there is no other potentially curative treatment available
for this patient. If charged particle radiotherapy had not been available, he
would likely have been treated with photon radiotherapy. Because of the position of the spinal cord, some or all of the tumor would have been treated with a
palliative dose only, with the expectation of a tumor recurrence in the future.

In addition to the above mentioned sites where dose localization has proven
of value with helium ion irradiation, there have been several patients with
localized soft tissue sarcoma, metastatic disease in paraaortic lymph nodes, and
localized carcinoma of the biliary tract in whom the ability to deliver 6000
equivalent rad with helium ions without exceeding the tolerance of adjacent
normal tissues has clearly been of value. Several of these patients have had
long term control of their local disease. This tends to confirm the observation
although not statistically proven in a prospective randomized trial that the
improved dose localization with charged particle radiotherapy will clearly be of
value in selected clinical situations.

4) Ocular Melanoma

The clinical trial which most strongly supports the postulate that the
improved dose localization with the helium ion beam will be reflected clinically
in improved rates of tumor control and decreased normal tissue damage is the
trial investigating the treatment of ocular melanomas.

Ocular melanomas are malignant tumors of the pigmented layer of the eye.
This tumor seems nearly ideal for testing the possible benefits of helium ion
irradiation. When discovered, these tumors are generally small and have not
metastasized. They are therefore potentially curable by a localized treatment
such as surgery or irradiation. This tumor can be precisely localized for
radiotherapy by noninvasive tests such as ultrasound, CT, fluorescein angiogram,

clinical examination, and by a minor surgical procedure which involves suturing radio-opaque markers around the base of the tumor. As well, the results of therapy can readily be followed by the same noninvasive tests.

The standard therapy for this tumor in most parts of North America is enucleation of the eye. Various types of radiotherapy have been attempted in order to both control the tumor and spare the useful vision in the eye. The most widely used technique involves the application of [60]Cobalt plaques to the base of the tumor. Experience at the University of California, San Francisco with that technique resulted in 40 percent of the eyes having subsequently to be enucleated either for tumor recurrence or for radiation damage to the eye, although others have had better results with this modality[11,12]. We therefore elected to initiate treatment with helium ion radiotherapy for this tumor, thinking that by placing the Bragg peak over the tumor and sharply collimating the beam, a high uniform dose could be delivered to the tumor with a small dose to nearby critical structures in the eye. We are using a technique pioneered at the Harvard Cyclotron by the Massachusetts General Hospital Department of Radiation Medicine. By precisely positioning the Bragg peak over the tumor with a 3 mm margin proximally and distally along the beam, and a 2 mm margin laterally, a high uniform dose can be delivered to the tumor, while nearby critical structures such as optic disc and macula can be spared if the tumor is a few millimeters away from them. We are currently delivering a dose of 8000 CoRE (6150 physical rad) in 5 fractions over 8 days with a very high rate of tumor control, a low rate of normal tissue damage, and preservation of useful vision in a large number of these patients.

We have now completed treatment of 42 patients. Thirty-seven patients have followup ranging from 2 to 35 months. Five patients have had local recurrence of their tumor. Two of these are from among the first few patients treated by us. It is now apparent that these represent marginal misses of the tumor. A third patient has recurred on the side of the eye opposite to that treated and is thought to have a "ring melanoma" of the ciliary body. The other two local failures have no discernable technical problems in their treatment, and are thought to represent two examples of radioresistent tumors (Tables 4 and 5). One patient has a biopsy proven lung metastasis, with local control of the primary tumor.

TABLE 4

Ocular Melanoma - Results

(37 Patients Evaluable)

Number of Patients	Status
31	No evidence of active disease
1	Local control, distant metastasis
5	Local failure (all salvaged)
TOTAL 37	

TABLE 5

Ocular Melanoma - Local Failures

(37 Patients Evaluable)

5 Local Failures:

    2 - Marginal Misses
    1 - "Ring Melanoma"
    2 - Apparently Radioresistent Tumors

Normal tissue morbidity has been very mild, most commonly consisting of epitheliitis of the eyelid and loss of lashes in those cases where the lid could not be retracted out of the radiation field. Two patients have cataracts which are not affecting their vision significantly. About two-thirds of the patients have vision greater than 20/50 in the treated eye. One patient, with a very large tumor, had shrinkage of the tumor, but severe pain secondary to glaucoma in the eye and a retinal detachment requiring enucleation.

The patients with tumor recurrence have all been successfully salvaged. Four by enucleation of the eye and one by re-irradiation of the eye.

In summary, we have had excellent local control of these tumors with minimal normal tissue morbidity. Thus, we are preserving useful vision in most patients.

CONCLUSION

Preliminary clinical results of helium ion radiotherapy are very promising in situations where the excellent dose localization properties of that beam can be used optimally, such as treating ocular melanomas or a small tumor abutting the spinal cord. Our local control rates for pancreatic and esophageal carcinomas have been low; however, there has been little damage to normal tissues. We therefore plan to escalate the tumor dose until either local control rates are acceptable or morbidity is unacceptable.

REFERENCES

1. Suit HD (1969) Statement of the problem pertaining to the effect of dose fractionation and total treatment time on response of tissue to x-irradiation. Time and Dose Relationships in Radiation Biology as Applied to Radiotherapy. Carmel Conference, Brookhaven National Laboratory Report BNL-5023 (C-57) p vii-x.
2. Kaplan HS (1976) Hodgkin's disease and other human malignant lymphomas: advances and prospects. Cancer Research 36:3863-3878.
3. Suit HD and Goitein M (1974) Dose limiting tissues in relation to type and location of tumor. Implications for efforts to improve radiation dose distributions. European J. Cancer 10:217-224.
4. Chapman JD, Blakely EA, Smith KC, and Urtasun RC (1977) Radiobiological characteristics of the inactivating events produced in mammalian cells by helium and heavy ions. Int J Radiation Oncology Biol and Phys 3:97-102.
5. Phillips TL, Fu KK, and Curtis SB (1977) Tumor biology of helium and heavy ions. Int J. Radiation Oncology Biol and Phys 3:103-113.
6. Castro JR, Tobias CA, Quivey JM, Chen GTY, Lyman JT, Phillips TL, Alpen EL, and Sing RP (1979) Results of tumor treatments with alpha particles and heavy ions at Lawrence Berkeley Laboratory. European J of Cancer, Barendsen Broerse and Breur (eds) Pergamon Press, New York.
7. Castro JR, Quivey JM, Lyman JT, Chen GTY, Phillips TL, and Tobias CA (1980) Radiotherapy with heavy charged particles at Lawrence Berkeley Laboratory. J of the Can Assoc of Rad 31:30-34.
8. Char DH, Castro JR, Quivey JM, Chen GTY, Stone RD, Irvine AE, Barricks M, Crawford JB, Hilton GS, Lonn LI, and Schwartz A (1980) Helium ion charged particle therapy for choroidal melanoma. Ophthalmology 87:105-110.
9. Castro JR, Quivey JM, Lyman JT, Chen GTY, Tobias CA, and Phillips TL (1980) Current status of heavy charged particle radiotherapy at Lawrence Berkeley Laboratory. Cancer 46:633-641.
10. Chen GTY, Castro JR, and Quivey JM (1981) Heavy charged particle radiotherapy. Annual Review of Biophysics and Bioengineering 10:499-529.
11. Char DH, Lonn LI, and Margolis LW (1977) Complications of cobalt plaque therapy of choroidal melanomas. Am J Ophthal 84:536-541.
12. Stallard HB (1966) Radiotherapy for malignant melanoma of the choroid. Br J Ophthal 50:147-155.

Supported by the NIH/NCI Grant #5P01CA19183,

#2 R10 21744-05, and DOE Contract #W7405-ENG-48

CLINICAL EXPERIENCE WITH HEAVY ION BEAMS
AT LAWRENCE BERKELEY LABORATORY

Joseph R. Castro, William M. Saunders, Cornelius A. Tobias, George T.Y. Chen,
J. Michael Collier, Samuel Pitluck, John T. Lyman, Kay H. Woodruff, Eleanor A.
Blakely, Theodore L. Phillips and Edward L. Alpen

University of California Lawrence Berkeley Laboratory
Division of Biology and Medicine
University of California School of Medicine, San Francisco
Department of Radiation Oncology

Supported in part by NIH/NCI CA19138, CA15184, CA21744, and DOE W740ENG-48

Helium and heavier particles such as carbon, neon, silicon and argon ions are
under investigation in the irradiation of human cancers at the University of
California Lawrence Berkeley Laboratory in a systematic study of the role of
such particles in clinical practice (1-7).

Study of the biological and physical parameters of these beams have also been
carried out in cell, tissue and tumor systems in order to focus on the properties desirable for radiation therapy (8-12,16,17).

Molecular and cellular studies have been carried out by Tobias and associates
(10,11,13,14,15,18) to include the effects of heavy ions on survival of mammalian cells in tissue culture and the modification of these effects by oxygen.
These studies include the nature of sublethal and potentially lethal lesions and
the repair capabilities of such damage. Tissue radiobiological studies have
included the effects of heavy ions on normal mammalian tissues such as skin,
lung, spinal cord and gut (9,12,18). Other studies include genetic effects and
chronic effects of heavy ion irradiation (13).

These studies have been utilized by Tobias to formulate a new model, the
repair-misrepair model (18), to explain the fundamental radiobiological
phenomena associated with heavy ion radiotherapy.

These heavy charged particles have physical and biological advantages for
delivery of therapy to many cancers. In addition to improved dose localization,

silicon and argon beams significantly depress the oxygen effect to OER values
between 1.4 and 1.6 in the extended parallel opposed Bragg peak.

Heavy ions also depress enzymatic repair mechanisms, decrease variations of
radiosensitivity during the cell division cycle, cause greater than expected
delay in cell division and decrease the protective effects of neighbouring cells
in organized systems (9).

Potential therapeutic advantage may result from these effects if a significant differential in the above parameters can be found between normal and tumor
cells and if hypoxia is a critical factor in failure of radiation to control
some tumors.

The effectiveness at depth of argon ions is limited because of particle
fragmentation and greater biological effectiveness in the entrance region than
in the spread peak.

However, silicon, intermediate between neon and argon in the periodic table,
offers an attractive combination of enhanced biological effect, low OER and
reasonable depth dose characteristics.

Neon ions, at 670 MeV/amu, while not offering as great a reduction in the
OER, have a range in tissue up to 23 cm with a field size of 20 cm diameter.

Carbon ions, while offering the best physical dose distribution, do not
appear to have sufficiently high LET to significantly depress the OER or offer
evidence in limited clinical practice of improved tumor control over helium or
photon irradiation.

The goal of the clinical program at Lawrence Berkeley Laboratory (LBL) has
been to systematically investigate the potential advantage of improved dose
localization through irradiation of selected tumor targets with helium ions, and
to study the combined potential of enhanced biologic effect and dose localization by irradiation with one of the heavier particles.

Carbon and argon ions do not appear optimal for the above stated reasons.
Therefore, during the next 18-24 months we plan to focus on neon and/or silicon
ions in order to determine their suitability for phase III prospective testing
in the treatment of selected human cancers.

MATERIALS AND METHODS

From July 1975 through December 1981, 378 patients have been irradiated with
particles and 27 patients irradiated as controls (Table 1). Of the 378 heavy
charged particle patients, 298 have been treated with helium ions, either solely

or in combination with photon irradiation, and 80 have received all or part of their irradiation with one of the heavier particles, either carbon, neon or argon ions.

Table 1

Heavy Particle Clinical Trial Patients

(7/75-12/81)

ANATOMIC REGION	HELIUM	HEAVY PARTICLE
Head/Neck	26	15
Intracranial	17	20
Ocular	56	--
Thoracic	41	11
Abdomen	128	25
Retroperitoneal	11	3
Pelvis	18	1
Skin & Subcutaneous	1	5
	298	80

Low LET Photon Control Patients
(randomized pancreas trial)   27

TOTAL   405

In order to complete the phase I-II studies for helium and heavier particles and implement prospective phase III controlled clinical studies, we envision the following overall plan:

Phase I:

Establish maximum tolerable heavy charged particle dose using dose fractions of 2.0-3.0 Gray equivalents. Establish parameters and levels of toxicity.

Helium:

Dose localization studies:

Chordoma, juxtaspinal tumors

Ocular melanoma

Other localized tumors such as localized soft tissue sarcomata

> Localized carcinoma of the biliary tract
> Localized carcinoma of the pancreas

Heavy ions:

> RBE and toxicity studies:
>> Skin, subcutaneous nodules
>> Metastatic lymph nodes
>> Ca pancreas
>> Ca head/neck
>> Ca stomach

Phase II:

> Establish levels of local control in specific tumors
> using maximum tolerable dose as determined in Phase I.

Helium:

>> Chordoma
>> Juxtaspinal tumors
>> Ocular melanoma

Heavy ions:

>> Ca pancreas
>> Advanced tumors head/neck
>> Brain tumors
>> Ca esophagus

Phase III:

> Establish definite superiority of modality
> (randomized or single arm)
> To be selected from:
>> Ca pancreas
>> Advanced tumors head/neck
>> Brain tumors
>> Ca esophagus

Considerable progress has been made on completing the phase I and II studies for helium, carbon and neon ions.

Phase I studies for silicon ions are scheduled to begin this year and should lead to phase II studies by next year.

Selection of particle(s) and tumor sites for phase III studies should be completed in order to implement such studies by 1984 at which time improvements in beam delivery at the Bevalac will facilitate the heavy particle clinical trial. These will include upgrading of the local injector to the Bevatron (instead of the Super HiLac) to permit ions as heavy as neon or silicon to be accelerated and design of a new beam spreading system to permit large field irradiation with heavier ions.

A phase III study of helium ion therapy in carcinoma of the pancreas is underway and almost completed.

CURRENT TREATMENT PROTOCOLS

The following protocol studies have been developed with the assistance of interested radiotherapists, biologists, physicists and others through the Northern California Oncology Group (NCOG) and the Radiation Therapy Oncology Group (RTOG):

1. LBL-NCOG 3P81/RTOG 79-10   Randomized Trial of Localized, Unresectable Carcinoma of the Pancreas. (Helium)

2. LBL-NCOG 3E81/RTOG 79-09   Localized Squamous Cell Carcinoma of the Esophagus, Nonrandomized. (Neon)

3. LBL-NCOG 7081/RTOG 79-08   Localized Ocular Melanoma, Nonrandomized. (Helium)

4. LBL-NCOG 3S91/RTOG 81-14   Localized, Unresectable Adenocarcinoma of the Stomach, Nonrandomized. (Neon)

5. LBL-NCOG OR81/RTOG 79-11   Phase I-Phase II Study of Locally Advanced Tumors:
   - Head/Neck--Neon, Silicon
   - Brain--Neon, Silicon
   - Pancreas--Neon
   - Esophagus--Neon
   - Stomach--Neon

6. LBL-Veterans Administration Surgical Oncology Group   Localized, Unresectable Carcinoma of the Pancreas, Nonrandomized. (Helium and Heavy Ions)

PRELIMINARY CLINICAL STUDIES WITH HEAVY PARTICLES

Carcinoma of the Pancreas

Irradiation of patients with localized, unresectable carcinoma of the pancreas has been carried on at Lawrence Berkeley Laboratory since 1976. Our interest was directed at this disease site because of the increasing incidence of this disease within the United States and the potential for local control in patients with localized disease provided a high dose could be delivered without injury to adjacent normal structures.

A pilot study was accomplished in which 35 patients received helium ion irradiation to a minimum of 50 (usually 60) Gray equivalents given at 2.0 GyE per fraction, 4 fractions per week in a period of 7-8 weeks.

The most common dose prescription utilized was 60 GyE (6000 rad equivalents) given at 2.0 GyE per fraction, 4 fractions per week over a time course of 7.5-9 weeks. The total dose has gradually been escalated reaching a current level of 66 GyE in 8 weeks.

With this dose we have achieved local and regional control in about 15% of patients with several patients surviving for long periods without recurrence of disease.

A randomized trial between helium therapy and photon therapy was begun in 1978. In this study patients in both arms also received 5-FU chemotherapy. Although the study is not completed, we have seen no significant difference between the two arms, with perhaps a small trend to a longer time to local failure in the helium arm. Survival is similar in both arms in part because a a 65% incidence of liver metastases has been encountered despite careful preliminary evaluation.

Morbidity in these patients has chiefly consisted of radiation gastritis and/or duodenitis in about 15% of patients, although a higher incidence of severe reactions might have been encountered if more patients survived longer (average survival was ~9 months).

This protocol will be closed shortly and we are currently continuing phase I studies of neon ion irradiation of patients with carcinoma of the pancreas.

We have already irradiated a previous group of 19 patients with advanced carcinoma of the pancreas who were not eligible for the randomized clinical trial because of extent of disease. These patients received heavy ions such as carbon or neon for only part of their therapy except for one patient who was treated entirely with heavy particles (neon). Eleven other patients were treated with neon irradiation following helium or photon irradiation: 7 patients received carbon boost irradiation following helium or photon treatment. The total doses ranged from 40 to 65 GyE. Dose per fraction ranged from 2.0-2.25 GyE.

Four of these patients have local control of their tumor with three remaining without evidence of disease for 10 to 26 months.

Addition of low dose whole liver irradiation and/or multi-drug chemotherapy such as FAM could offer an improved chance of control of occult metastases within the liver, as well as improved local and regional control. Such studies will be considered for piloting within our own facility.

A continued search for better chemotherapeutic agents is needed in view of the prevalence of this disease and its high rate of liver metastases.

Carcinoma of the Esophagus

Twenty-five patients have now been accrued in a phase II nonrandomized prospective study for helium ion irradiation of localized carcinoma of the esophagus. Since this protocol was activated in December 1978, the dose has been gradually escalated from 60 GyE at 2.0 GyE per fraction. Only seven patients have had local control of their tumor, with followup ranging from 5 to 14 months. Eighteen of the patients have had local failure, with or without distant metastases.

We therefore have begun a phase I trial of carcinoma of the esophagus using a heavier ion (neon). The dose to be employed will be 69.75 GyE at 2.25 GyE per fraction or 54 GyE at 3.0 GyE per fraction. We hope that the superior OER and RBE of these beams will be reflected in a higher local and regional control rate.

Advanced Head and Neck Tumors

A small group of 15 patients with far advanced head and neck tumors were treated with carbon or neon ions. Most of these patients had only a portion of their treatment given with heavy particles. The total dose was low, because of use of a conservative RBE and particle dose. These patients were irradiated as part of the phase I study to evaluate toxicity. In most instances therefore tumor persistence was seen in the radiation field. Further dose escalation is required with a larger number of patients treated entirely with heavy particles. Initially, neon ions will be utilized to be followed by pilot silicon irradiations. Subsequently one of these ions will be selected for phase II (and possibly phase III) head and neck trials. Analysis of normal tissue effects and tumor response should be facilitated in this group of accessible neoplasms.

Glioblastoma Multiforme

Since 1975, fifteen patients have received irradiation for primary malignant glioma of the brain with carbon or neon ions. Most of these patients have received boost therapy following photon irradiation. More recently a small group of 8 patients received treatment entirely with neon ions. The results in these patients as yet have not been different from historical results with photon irradiation. Five already have tumor recurrence and the followup period in the other patients is short. One patient appears to have died without tumor

but with an exact cause of death not being determined as yet. Her clinical
course was marked by gradual deterioration and inanition; whether from radiation
caused brain injury or other causes is still under investigation.

The tumor dose utilized in these patients may have been too low (48 GyE in
16 fractions over 4 weeks) and will be gradually raised. We expect to deliver
52.8 GyE in 16 fractions in the next group of patients to be treated with neon
ions. Subsequently we also plan to investigate the use of silicon ions in
patients with glioblastoma.

Carefully integrated studies with the Brain Tumor Research Center at UCSF
will be done including followup CT scanning to detect both effects on normal
brain as well as the tumor. Nuclear magnetic resonance scanning and positron
emission scanning will also be accomplished on selected patients through collaboration with the UCSF Diagnostic Radiology Department and the Research
Medicine Group at LBL.

Miscellaneous

A number of patients with miscellaneous locally advanced and/or metastatic
tumors in various sites have been irradiated. Treatment tolerance has been
generally good in these patients without unduly severe skin, mucosal or intestinal reactions.

The treatment techniques utilized in these patients have been similar to
those developed at the 184-inch synchrocyclotron using helium ions. Experience
has shown it possible to treat virtually any anatomic site although dosimetric
problems remain to be solved, particularly in the thorax.

Our goals in the phase I-II studies of heavy particles remain as follows:

1. Evaluation of acute and subacute response of normal tissues
   such as mucosa, skin and intestine.
2. Initial evaluation of tumor response.
3. Development of effective treatment techniques using carbon,
   neon, and argon ions based on experience obtained with helium ions.
4. Clinical evaluation of the physical and biological dose
   distributions available with carbon, neon, silicon and argon ions.
5. Design and implementation of phase III studies.

Since silicon appears to have a more favorable dose distribution than argon
as well as a low OER, it may prove to be the optimal heavy ion for irradiation
of such tumors as carcinoma of the pancreas, advanced head and neck tumors and
malignant gliomata of the brain.

Neon ions will be tested for more deeply seated tumors such as carcinoma of the esophagus, pancreas and stomach, at least until beam delivery improvements permit deeper penetration with large field silicon beams.

REFERENCES

1. Woodruff, K.H., Castro, J.R., Quivey, J.M., Saunders, W.M., Chen, G.T.Y, Lyman, J.T., Tobias, C.A., Walton, R.E., and Peters, T.C.: Postmortem Examination of Twenty Pancreatic Carcinoma Patients Treated with Helium Ion Irradiation. Presented in part at the National Pancreatic Association, Chicago, IL, November, 1981.

2. Debelbower, Jr., R.R.: Current Radiotherapeutic Approaches to Pancreatic Cancer. Cancer, 47:1729-1733, 1981.

3. Castro, J.R., Quivey, J.M., Lyman, J.T., Chen, G.T.Y., Phillips, T.L., and Tobias, C.A.: Radiotherapy with Heavy Charged Particles at Lawrence Berkeley Laboratory. J. Canadian Assoc of Radiol, 31:30-34, 1980.

4. Castro, J.R., Quivey, J.M., Lyman, J.T., Chen, G.T.Y., Phillips, T.L., Tobias, C.A., and Alpen, E.L.: Current Status of Clinical Particle Radiotherapy at Lawrence Berkeley Laboratory. Cancer, 46:633-641, 1980.

5. Quivey, J.M., Castro, J.R.,Chen, G.T.Y., Moss, A.A., and Marks, W.M.: Computerized Tomography in the Quantitative Assessment of Tumor Response. British J. Cancer, 41:31-34, Supple. IV, 1980.

6. Castro, J.R.: Particle Therapy: The First Forty Years. Seminars in Oncology, Vol 8, No 1, March, 1981.

7. Castro, J.R., Hendrickson, C., Quivey, J.M., Saunders, W.M., Hannigan, J.F., Silverberg, I.J., and Torti, F.M.: Heavy Charged Particle Radiotherapy for Localized Esophageal Squamous Cell Carcinoma. Proceedings of Am Soc Clin Oncol, 22:450, 1981.

8. Chen, G.T.Y., Castro, J.R., and Quivey, J.M.: Heavy Charged Particle Radiotherapy. Ann Rev of Biophysics and Bioengineering, 10:419-429, 1981.

9. Tobias, C.A., Blakely, E.A., Alpen, E.L., Castro, J.R., Ainsworth, E.J., Curtis, S.B., Ngo, F.Q.H., Rodriguez, A., Roots, R.J., Tenforde, T., and Yang, T.C.H.: Molecular and Cellular Radiobiology of Heavy Ions. Presented at the CROS/RTOG PART III International Particle Workshop, Houston, TX, February, 1982.

394

10. Tobias, C.A.: Pretherapeutic Investigations with Accelerated Heavy Ions. Radiobiology, 108:145-158, 1973.

11. Blakely, E.A., Tobias, C.A., Ngo, F.Q.H., Yang, T.C.H., Smith, K.C., and Lyman, J.T.: Inactivation of Human Kidney Cells by High Energy Monoenergetic Heavy Ion Beams. Radiation Research, 80:122-160, 1979.

12. Goldstein, L.S., Phillips, T.L., Fu, K.K., Ross, G.Y., and Kane, L.J.: Biological Effects of Accelerated Heavy Ions: Single Doses in Normal Tissues, Tumors and Cell in Vitro. Radiation Research, 86:529-554, 1981.

13. Roots, R., Yang, T.C.H., Craise, L., Blakely, E.A., and Tobias, C.A.: Rate of Rejoining of DNA Breaks Induced by Accelerated Carbon and Neon Ions in Spread Bragg Peak. Int. J. Rad. Res., 38:203-210, 1980.

14. Blakely, E.A., Ngo, F.Q.H., Chang, P.Y., Lommel, L., and Tobias, C.A.: Silicon: Radiobiological Cellular Survival and the Oxygen Effect. Lawrence Berkeley Laboratory Report LBL-11220:119-124, 1980.

15. Ngo, F.Q.H., Blakely, E.A., and Tobias, C.A.: Sequential Exposures of Mammalian Cells to Low and High-LET Radiations: Lethal Effects Following X-ray and Neon Ion Irradiation. Radiation Research, 87:59-78, 1981.

16. Raju, M.R., Bain, E., Carpenter, S.G., Cox, R.A., and Robertson, J.B.: A Heavy Particle Comparative Study. Part II: Cell Survival Versus Depth. British J. Radiology, 51:704-711, 1978.

17. Rodrigues, A. and Alpen, E.L.: Cell Survival in Spheroids Irradiated with Heavy Ion Beams. Radiation Research, 85:24-37, 1981.

18. Tobias, C.A., Blakely, E.A., Ngo, F.Q.H., and Yang, T.C.H.: The Repair-Misrepair Model of Cell Survival. Radiation Biology in Cancer Research (R. Meyn and H.R. Withers) pp. 195-230, Raven Press, New York, 1980.

CLINICAL STUDIES -- PIONS

CURRENT STATUS OF PION RADIOTHERAPY AT LAMPF

STEVEN E. BUSH AND ALFRED R. SMITH
Cancer Research and Treatment Center, The University of New Mexico, and the
Department of Radiology, The University of New Mexico, School of Medicine

INTRODUCTION

The theoretical advantages of negative pi meson (pion) radiotherapy were reviewed by Fowler and Perkins in 1961[1], however, it was not until 1974 that the first cancer patients were treated with pions using the Biomedical Channel at the Los Alamos Meson Physics Facilty (LAMPF). One hundred seventy-three patients have now been treated at the facility under the auspices of the Cancer Research and Treatment Center of The University of New Mexico and have been followed for periods of six to fifty months. This experience has led to the standardization of treatment planning and therapeutic technique. At the same time increasing knowledge of the clinical effects of pions has led to refinement of treatment volumes and dosage schedules. Ninety-six patients with 97 large, deep seated neoplasms have been treated with curative intent since 1977 and followed for a minimum of one year. Preliminary results of treatment of these patients have previously been reported.[2,3] Additional observations in this group and a subsequently treated group of 33 patients with less than one year follow-up form the basis of this report.

MATERIAL AND METHODS

LAMPF is a one-kilometer-long proton linear accelerator which produces an 800 MeV proton beam with an average current of approximately 650 microamperes. Pions are collected for biomedical application in a fixed vertical channel which produces approximately 5 rad per minute in treatment volumes up to 2 liters. Characteristics of the channel as well as immobilization, treatment planning, and simulation techniques have previously been reported.[4,5,6,7] One hundred seventy-three patients with locally advanced neoplasms were treated between 1974 and 1980. All but six patients were treated under Phase I and II trials intended to determine tumor response and normal tissue reaction for a variety of anatomic sites. Ninety-six patients without metastatic disease were treated with curative intent and have been followed for a minimum of one year. Five of

these patients received doses in the range of 1500 pion rad to cone-down volumes
in the planned combined management of malignant gliomas using conventional whole
brain irradiation with subsequent pion boosting therapy. The remaining patients
all received a minimum prescribed dose of 2700 pion rad, that dose at which
complete tumor regression was first noted. The minimum tumor dose was 80% of
the prescribed dose in most cases. Sixty-seven patients received pion
irradiation alone while 19 received supplemental conventional irradiation and
ten underwent pion radiotherapy in combination with surgery. Such supplemental
therapy was used primarily in those patients treated to low dose with pion
irradiation during early trials designed to determine normal tissue tolerance.
Table 1 shows the reasons for exclusion of 77 patients from that group
considered for curative potential. Thirty-three patients have been followed for
less than one year while 9 patients were excluded because of treatment of
metastatic skin nodules in early Phase I trials. An additional 15 patients
were excluded because of the presence of known distant metastases at the time
of treatment. Twenty patients received less than 2700 pion rad because of the
planned low dose pilot studies or because of beam malfunction or medical
problems during the course of therapy.

TABLE 1

PION PATIENTS 1974-1980

Total Cases	173
Exclusion:	
Follow-Up < 1 year	33
Skin Metastases	9
Distant Metastases	15
Low Dose Pilot	7
Low Dose Beam	10
Low Dose Medical	3
Total Exclusions	77
Total Curative Cases	96

The group of patients treated with curative intent included 36 patients with
advanced neoplasms of the head and neck. Three of these patients had minor
salivary gland tumors and one had an anaplastic carcinoma of the nasopharynx.
The remaining patients had stage T3 and T4 squamous carcinomas with or without
regional adenopathy but with no known metastases. Twenty-three patients had
malignant glioma with astrocytomas grade III diagnosed in eight cases and glio-
blastomas multiforme in fifteen. Fifteen patients had stage T3 or T4 adeno-

carcinoma of the prostate and 11 had unresectable adenocarcinoma of the pancreas.
Among 12 patients with locally advanced lesions of other miscellaneous sites,
there were 3 with transitional cell carcinoma of the bladder, two each with
carcinoma of the esophagus, lung and rectum and single patients with carcinoma
of the stomach, uterine cervix and skin.

RESULTS

Tables 2 and 3 show crude survival and local control statistics related to
dose range and site of disease in a group of patients followed from 12 to 50
months. The survival rate was lowest for patients treated for adenocarcinoma
of the pancreas with none of the 11 patients surviving. All 11 expired with
clinical or autopsy proof of locally persistent disease, although only four had
received a dose of 4000 pion rad and only one received 4500 pion rad. Nine of
11 patients had distant metastases and the liver was involved as the sole site
of distant disease in 7 of these cases. Fourteen of 36 patients treated for
tumors of the head and neck survived from 15 to 40 months. The 14 survivors
have no evidence of disease and an additional three patients expired with intercurrent or metastatic disease but local control.

TABLE 2

SURVIVAL OF PION PATIENTS TREATED WITH CURATIVE INTENT BY SITE AND DOSE

	$\leq$2000	< 4000	> 4000	Total	
Head & Neck	-	6/12	8/24	14/36	(39%)
Brain	3/5	2/12	1/6	6/23	(26%)
Prostate	-	3/4	10/11	13/15	(87%)
Pancreas	-	0/6	0/5	0/11	(0%)
Other	-	4/8	0/4	4/12	(33%)

TABLE 3

LOCAL CONTROL IN PION PATIENTS TREATED WITH CURATIVE INTENT BY SITE AND DOSE

	< 2000	$\leq$4000	> 4000	Total	
Head & Neck	-	6/12	11/24	17/36	(47%)
Brain	1/5	1/12	1/6	3/23	(13%)
Prostate	-	3/4	10/11	13/15	(87%)
Pancreas	-	0/6	0/5	0/11	(0%)
Other	-	5/8	2/4	7/12	(58%)

Six of 23 patients treated for malignant gliomas survived from 13 to 28 months following therapy. Four of 8 patients with grade III glioma survived while only 2 of 15 patients treated for glioblastoma multiforme or combined grade III and grade IV astrocytomas survived more than one year. The median survival of that group of patients with grade III astrocytomas treated more than 12 months ago is 16 months; that for patients with grade IV lesions is 12 months. Three patients, all of whom were treated for grade III astrocytomas survived without evidence of disease. The criteria for local control are stable neurological symptoms, absence of steroid dependence and absence of contrast enhancement or mass effect on CT scan.

Thirteen of 15 patients treated for advanced carcinoma of the prostate survived from 15 to 44 months. One patient expired seven months following therapy with hepatic metastases and widespread nodal involvement. The second patient expired as a consequence of chronic obstructive pulmonary disease 20 months following prostate irradiation and had evidence of persistent carcinoma as well as gross involvement of para-aortic and mediastinal lymph nodes at autopsy. A third patient had confirmation of locally persistent disease 13 months following 4300 pion rad for a T4 prostatic carcinoma.

Twelve patients were treated for lesions of miscellaneous sites including three with advanced transitional cell carcinoma of the urinary bladder. Two of these three patients had local control, although one expired of intercurrent gastrointestinal bleeding unrelated to disease or treatment. Two patients were treated for carcinoma of the lung, one of whom survives without evidence of disease at three years. The second expired with local recurrence and metastases two years following therapy. Those two patients treated for esophageal carcinoma have expired although one was free of tumor at autopsy, having died as a consequence of chronic alcoholism. Both patients treated for rectal carcinoma died with metastatic disease, although one who had been treated for a locally recurrent lesion following abdominoperineal resection had no evidence of disease at autopsy. The patient with gastric carcinoma died with local recurrence and the single patient treated for the stage III B carcinoma of the cervix died with lung metastases and small bowel necrosis one year following combined pion and interstitial template irradiation. This complication is believed to be therapy related. One patient with a large squamous cell carcinoma of the face invading the malar bone remains free of disease two years following therapy. Crude survival rates of 87, 39, 26 and 0% for patients with neoplasms of the prostate, head and neck, brain and pancreas respectively

were recorded at a minimum follow-up of one year following therapy.
Corresponding local control rates were 87, 47, 13 and 0%. Table 4 shows local
control statistics for 67 patients, including one patient with simultaneous
carcinomas of the prostate and bladder, treated for cure with pions alone.
Nine of 31 patients (29%) receiving less than 4000 pion rad had no evidence of
local disease at last follow-up or death, while 17 of 37 (46%) receiving greater
than 4000 pion rad had local control.

TABLE 4

LOCAL CONTROL AFTER PION IRRADIATION ALONE BY SITE AND DOSE

	<4000	> 4000	Total
Brain	1/10	1/6	2/16
Head & Neck	1/4	4/12	5/16
Prostate	3/4	10/11	13/15
Pancreas	0/5	0/5	0/10
Other	4/8	2/3	6/11

Table 5 shows crude survival and local control statistics for a group of 33
patients followed for periods less than one year. Eight of 13 patients in this
group treated for glioma are surviving. Two patients expired during therapy
as a result of intercurrent disease. One of 2 patients treated for carcinomas
of the head and neck and all six treated for advanced prostatic cancer survive
without evidence of active disease. Five patients with pancreatic carcinoma
survive, however, there has been no evidence of regression of mass disease on
serial CT scans. Three patients have shown no evidence of progression of local
disease while one developed hepatic metastases and another a gradually enlarging
mass in the central abdomen. Two patients were treated for rectal cancer
including one with an inoperable lesion which was found to be sterilized at the
time of AP resection after 3000 pion rad. A second patient had a persistent
presacral mass on CT scan following pion irradiation for a locally recurrent
lesion. Two patients treated for stage III B carcinoma of the cervix survived
although both had persistence of disease at the conclusion of therapy. One
patient with recurrent anal carcinoma presented with a large pelvic mass
invading the acetabulum but had no evidence of tumor at the time of laparotomy
for small bowel obstruction 10 months later. The operative specimen in this
case showed evidence of radiation injury to the small bowel. One patient each
with esthesioneuroblastoma and T3 transitional cell carcinoma of the bladder

survive without evidence of disease.

TABLE 5

PION PATIENTS TREATED JULY 1980 TO OCTOBER 1980

	Crude Survival		Local Control	
Brain	8/13	(62%)	3/13	(23%)
Head & Neck	2/2	(100%)	2/2	(100%)
Pancreas	5/5	(100%)	0/5	(0%)
Prostate	6/6	(100%)	6/6	(100%)
Other	6/7	(86%)	3/7	(43%)

Acute reactions to pion radiotherapy have been systematically recorded on a
scale of 0 to 4 as follows: 0-nil; 1-skin erythema, mucosal injection, mild
dysuria or diarrhea, etc.; 2-dry desquamation, patchy mucositis, moderate dysuria, diarrhea with mucous, etc.; 3-moist desquamation, confluent mucositis,
severe dysuria with bladder spasms, diarrhea with blood, etc.; 4-acute necrosis.
Average sums of acute reactions were obtained by summing severities of all reactions for individual anatomic sites in an attempt to quantify the overall acute
morbidity related to treatment. Those structures scored by sites are as follows:
head and neck-mucosa, skin, salivary glands; pelvis-skin, rectum, bladder;
thorax-skin, dysphagia; abdomen-nausea, diarrhea; brain-skin. Table 6 demonstrates a trend to more severe acute reactions in all sites except the brain in
the dose range above 4000 pion rad as compared to the lower dose range although
these data do not include analysis of other potentially contributory factors
including fraction size, treatment volume, and hyperfractionation. The average
sum of acute reactions for ten patients treated for carcinomas of the head and
neck and receiving greater than 5000 pion rad was 6.2.

TABLE 6

ACUTE INJURY RELATED TO PION IRRADIATION IN DOSES > 2700 PION RAD BY SITE AND
DOSE RANGE*

Dose Range	Site	Number of Patients	Average Sum of Acute Reactions
< 4000	Head & Neck	13	5.1
	Pelvis	8	4.6
	Thorax	3	2.3
	Abdomen	6	1.8
	Brain	6	1.2
> 4000	Head & Neck	24	5.8
	Pelvis	12	4.9
	Thorax	1	3.0
	Abdomen	6	2.2
	Brain	12	1.2

* See text for explanation of scoring system.

Chronic reactions following pion irradiation had been tabulated according to the scoring system of EORTC/RTOG. Five patients have had severe chronic normal tissue reactions related to pion irradiation alone. A 75 year old female had severe laryngeal edema following 5000 pion rad for a T4 carcinoma of the larynx. Another patient developed chronically symptomatic pulmonary fibrosis following 4000 pion rad for a large adenocarcinoma of the left lower lobe of the lung. A 71 year old man required a colostomy for rectal ulceration 1½ years following 4500 pion rad for a T3 adenocarcinoma of the prostate. This patient had numerous post-operative complications necessitating reoperation for small bowel obstruction and expired as a result. A 51 year old male treated for a T3 N2b squamous carcinoma of the base of the tongue developed a pharyngeal wall necrosis approximately four months following 4600 pion rad to the primary lesion and underwent attempted resection of the lesion. He developed chronic infection and ultimately expired of pneumonia. The fifth patient with pion – related chronic injury was a 49 year old male with recurrent cloacogenic carcinoma of the anus involving left pelvic nodes and the acetabulum. He received 4900 pion rad in 150 pion rad fractions and developed severe small bowel injury necessitating ileostomy approximately 10 months later. Three patients had chronic reactions co-existent with persistent disease and one patient, with a history of previous surgeries for a large squamous carcinoma of the face, developed skin atrophy following pion irradiation to a dose of 3800 pion rad. Three patients developed mucosal necrosis following combined pion and implant or surgical therapy for head and neck tumors, however, healing occurred in each case. Two other patients are presumed to have expired from treatment related complications. The first exsanguinated from a tracheal-inominate artery fistula two weeks following salvage composite resection for tonsillar carcinoma which persisted following 5000 pion rad. The second patient received 4500 pion rad and 2500 rad by a template implant for a stage III B carcinoma of the cervix and expired with small bowel obstruction and necrosis at one year. Fourteen patients with glioma have been autopsied and all but one had gross or microscopic evidence of residual tumor. One patient who received 3800 pion rad for a grade III astrocytoma died with local recurrence at 17 months and showed histological evidence of radiation injury with reactive gliosis.

Table 7 shows a comparison of the average sums of chronic reactions for various treatment sites and dose ranges of less than 4000 pion rad and greater than 4000 pion rad. All patients received pions alone with curative intent.

Average summed reactions were obtained in a manner analagous to that for acute reactions. The average summed reactions for head and neck patients increased from 2.1 to 2.8 in comparison of low and high dose groups with a corresponding increase of 1.4 to 2.8 for patients with pelvic primaries. Twenty-six of 31 patients in the other category were treated for glioma or pancreatic carcinoma and had minimal late effects, usually grade I radiation dermatitis.

TABLE 7

CHRONIC INJURY RELATED TO PION IRRADIATION ALONE IN DOSES > 2700 PION RAD BY SITE AND DOSE*

Dose Range	Site	Number of Patients	Average Sum of Chronic Reactions
< 4000	Head & Neck	4	2.1
	Pelvis	7	1.4
	Other	19	0.9
> 4000	Head & Neck	12	2.8
	Pelvis	13	2.8
	Other	12	0.9

* See text for explanation of scoring system

DISCUSSION

One hundred seventy-three patients have completed pi meson radiotherapy for large and deep seated lesions since 1974. A subpopulation of 96 patients have been treated with curative intent and followed for a minimum of one year. This group of patients includes those with a variety of disease sites, histological types, and combination of conventional therapy with pion irradiation. The heterogeneity of this clinical material and the relatively short follow-up of these cases precludes a meaningful comparison with historical series.

These data demonstrate that pion irradiation will eradicate locally advanced lesions in a variety of sites and provide local control of such lesions for periods of two to four years. Acute normal tissue reactions have generally been mild to moderate with abbreviation of a planned course of therapy in less than 5% of cases. Chronic reactions have generally been acceptable. The pattern of acute normal tissue reactions shows that most epithelial tissues will tolerate doses of approximately 4500 pion rad in 125 rad fractions over seven weeks to clinically relevant volumes. Severity of acute reactions begins to increase rapidly at doses greater than 4500 pion rad. The incidence of chronic injury appears to increase disproportionately in patients treated to doses in excess of 4000 pion rad. While average summed acute reactions for head and neck sites increased from 5.1 to 5.8 in that group of patients receiving greater than 4000 pion rad, a 14% increase, chronic reactions increased from 2.1 to 2.8 (33%).

The average summed acute reactions for patients treated for pelvic primaries increased from 4.6 to 4.9 (7%) in that group receiving greater than 4000 pion rad as compared to those receiving less than this dose, although the average summed chronic reactions increased by 100% from 1.4 to 2.8. These injuries have manifested primarily as subcutaneous fibrosis, chronic edema, mucosal and cutaneous damage. Chronic injury to oral and pharyngeal mucosa is comparable to that of rectal mucosa for similar dose and fractionation schemes. Chronic injury including small bowel damage, fibrosis and mucosal injury may not manifest for periods of nine to twelve months following therapy. Data from the population of patients treated for cure provide promising anecdotal results for a variety of sites including the head and neck, brain and prostate. The initial experience in treatment of pancreatic carcinoma has been disappointing, however, a new pilot study combining a maximum dose of 3840 pion rad over 5 weeks to the radiographically demonstrable disease with subsequent conventional irradiation of the entire upper abdomen including pancreas, liver and regional nodes to a dose of 2400 rad in 3½ weeks, appears more promising. The first five patients in this group survived for eight to twelve months from diagnosis. Other non-randomized trials continue for treatment of malignant gliomas, advanced carcinomas of the uterine cervix, esophageal carcinoma and squamous cancer of the lung confined to the chest. Phase III trials have been activated for stage III and IV carcinoma of the oral cavity and pharynx as well as for inoperable and locally recurrent adenocarcinoma of the rectum in order to compare best conventional irradiation and pion radiotherapy in a prospective fashion. Continued accession of patients with various locally advanced lesions and additional follow-up of previously treated patients will certainly provide necessary information in the guidance of future clinical trials of pion radiotherapy.

ACKNOWLEDGMENTS

These investigations were supported in part by U.S. Public Health Service Grant No. CA-16127 from the National Cancer Institute and by the U.S. Department of Energy.

REFERENCES

1. Fowler PH, Perkins DH (1961) The possibility of therapeutic applications of beams of negative pi mesons. Nature 189: 524-528.
2. Kligerman, M., Tsujii, H., Bagshaw, M., Wilson, S., Black, W., Mettler, F., and Hogstrom, K. (1979) Current observations of pion radiation therapy at LAMPF, in Abe, M., Sakamoto, K., Phillips, T.L., Treatment of Radioresistant Cancers, Elseveir/North-Holland Biomedical Press, Amsterdam, 145-157.
3. Kligerman, M.M., Bush, S.E., Kondo, M., Wilson, S. and Smith, A., Results of Phase I-II Trials of Pion Radiotherapy, Proceedings of the Second Annual Rome International Symposium of Biological Bases and Clinical Implications of Tumor Radioresistance, in press.
4. Paciotti, M., Bradbury, J., Hutson, R., Knapp, E., and Rivera, O. (1977) Tuning the beam shaping section at the LAMPF biomedical channel IEEE Trans. Nuc. Sci. NS-24, 1058.
5. Kligerman, M.M., Hogstrom, K.R., Lane, R.G. and Somers, J. (1977a) Prior immobilization and positioning for more efficient radiotherapy, Int. J. Radiat. Oncol. Biol. Phys. 2, 1141-1144.
6. Hogstrom, K.R., Smith, A.R., Kelsey, C.A., Simon, S.L., Somers, J.W., Lane, R.G., Rosen, I.I., Von Essen, C.F., Kligerman, M.M., Berardo, P.A. and Zink, S.M. (1979) Static pion beam treatment planning of deep seated tumors using computerized tomographic scans at LAMPF, Int. J. Radiat. Oncol. Biol. Phys. 5, 875-886.
7. Tsujii, H., Bagshaw, M., Smith, A., Von Essen, C., Mettler, F. and Kligerman, M. (1980) Localization of structures for pion radiotherapy by computerized tomography and orthodiagraphic projection, Int. J. Radiat. Oncol. Biol. Phys. 6, 319-325.

THE PION THERAPY PROGRAMME AT TRIUMF

G.B. GOODMAN, B.G. DOUGLAS, S.M. JACKSON AND C.M. LUDGATE
A. Maxwell Evans Clinic, Cancer Control Agency of B.C., 2656 Heather Street,
Vancouver, B.C. V5Z 3J3, Canada

INTRODUCTION

In vivo skin studies in experimental animals were designed to determine the RBE for various dose parameters before the reaction of human skin to pion therapy was assessed at TRIUMF.

It was found that mouse foot skin RBE for 10 fractions ($\sim$ 500 rad x-rays) was about 1.5 and for 3 fractions ($\sim$ 900 rad x-ray) about 1.3.[1] The pig skin RBE for 10 fractions was 1.4 for the early (epithelial) acute reaction and possibly as high as 1.6 for the medium term reaction (dermal) for 330 pion rad; it was also observed that the RBE of 1.6 was not evident for 290 pi-rads or less. The control radiation used was 270 KV X-rays.[2] These data agreed reasonably with Kligerman's reports of an RBE of 1.4 for 13 - 15 fractions for human skin.[3]

Eight patients have now completed courses of treatment at TRIUMF to subcutaneous metastases from a variety of malignancies. Each patient had one nodule at least, treated by pions and 3 or more other nodules treated by 280 KV X-rays. The doses of x-rays spanned the expected RBE for pions.

Skin reactions and tumour responses were observed for 1 - 20 months up to June, 1981.

This paper describes our experience of acute skin reactions in humans treated with pion therapy and describes short term plans in relation to present technological and clinical constraints. The ultimate objective being pursued is the long term conduct of randomized comparative Phase 3 clinical trials.

I ACUTE SKIN REACTION STUDY IN HUMANS TREATED BY PI-MESON THERAPY

The object was to study the effects of pions on human skin to determine RBE values relative to 280 KV x-rays. The assessment of acute skin reaction used objective methods.

Patient Selection

The patient population included those with four or more discrete subcutaneous deposits, each nodule was capable of being subtended by an area equivalent to that of a 4 cm circle.

Additional requirements were biopsy proof of malignancy, a life expectancy of

3 months or more and informed consent that the treatment was essentially experimental.

Treatment Protocols

The physical depth dose profiles for the 280 KV and pion beams were matched at 0, 1 and 2 cm depth in the pion peak stopping region. The portal used was a 4 cm circular area and the 90% isodose subscribed a 3.6 cm circle. Pions were delivered at a dose rate of 18 rads/minute and 280 KV x-rays at 50 rads/minute. The dose fractionation schedules varied (see Table 1) while estimates of human skin tolerance were determined from clinical experience. Skin tolerance was assessed to be close to 5400 rads for 10 fractions for 280 KV[4] while 3 fraction data were based on our own experience of 100 KV irradiation of skin cancer.

TABLE 1

PION STUDY - DOSE SCHEDULES

	3 f/4d	9 f/11d	10 f/11-12d
No. Patients	1*	2	6*
Pion Dose (rads)	1900	2925	2700-3300
X-rays (rads)	2470-2850	3825-4275	4000-5250
Assumed RBE Range	1.3 - 1.5	1.3 - 1.46	1.48 - 1.76

Dose Rates: Pions   18 rads/min   280 KV = 50 rads/min
Dose Profiles matched for 280 KV and Pions
* One patient received 2 different treatment protocols for 2 separate tumour
  sites treated on different occasions: 10 f/11-12d and 3 f/4d.

10 fractions in 11 - 12 days (6 patients)

While initially the dose delivered was 90% of tolerance some later patients received doses closer to full tolerance. Initially, the pion dose used was 2700 rads and x-ray doses were so chosen as to encompass a possible RBE range of 1.48 - 1.76. The early reactions from these patients suggested an RBE for pions of about 1.5.

This led us to increase the x-ray dose and narrow the RBE range from 1.4 - 1.6 using x-ray doses of 4500 - 5250 rads with a pion dose of 3300 rads.

9 fractions in 11 days (2 patients)

Patients who failed to complete a 10-fraction course because of cyclotron breakdown received x-ray doses of 3825 - 4275 rads and a pion dose of 2925 rads, spanning an RBE range of 1.3 - 1.46. Their follow-up is only one month.

<u>3 fractions in 4 days</u> (1 patient)

This fractionation was used for a patient who presented towards the end of a scheduled beam run. X-ray doses of 2470 - 2850 rads spanned an RBE range of 1.3 - 1.5 with a pion dose of 1900 rads.

<u>Skin Reaction Assessment</u>

Reaction assessments were clinical and photographic. Clinical assessments were made by two or more clinicians (up to four) at each visit, usually weekly during the active phase but less frequently during the healing phase, up to intervals of one month. A clinical narrative followed simple guideline levels of reaction intensity from erythema through dry and moist desquamation to ulceration. Coloured photographs were taken under standard conditions at each visit. In assessing results all data have been taken into account.

TABLE 2

PION STUDY - CLINICAL SCORING OF ACUTE REACTIONS [*] [+]

0 = No reaction
1 = Erythema
2 = Dry desquamation
3 = Moist desquamation
4 = Ulceration

[*] Various subcategories of these levels exist.
[+] Narrative descriptions of reactions as well.

<u>Results</u>

Table 3 shows the various types of cancer treated. Only 8 of 9 patients are included for on-going analyses since one refused to continue after the first irradiation. Currently only 5 patients have adequate follow-up suitable for RBE estimates. Totals of 11 nodules were treated with pions and 28 with x-rays with follow-up for 1 - 20 months.

TABLE 3

PION STUDY - DISEASE, NODULES TREATED AND FOLLOW-UP

Disease	Fields Treated		Status
	Pions	X-rays	
Lymphocytic Lymphoma	2	6	A 20 mos
Mesothelioma	1	3	D 16 mos
M. Melanoma	2	4	D 12 mos
Breast Cancer	1	3	D 7 mos
Breast Cancer	1	3	A 19 mos
Breast Cancer	1	3	D 1 mo
Lung Cancer	2	3	A 1 mo
Breast Cancer	1	3	A 1 mo
Breast Cancer*			(excluded)

* Patient refused treatment

Acute Reactions - Time Courses

Clinical and photographic data indicated that the onset of reactions took place in 1 - 3 weeks for 10 fractions and 2 weeks for 3 fractions. The duration of peak intensities from these differing fractionations were respectively 3 - 6 weeks and 2 - 8 weeks. Healing occurred during the period from 8 or 9 to 14 weeks, with the exception of one patient where healing was delayed due to confluence of reactions.

TABLE 4

PION STUDY - ACUTE SKIN REACTION ASSESSMENTS

	Clinical	
	10 f	3 f
Onset	1 - 3 weeks	2 weeks
Peak Duration	3 - 6 weeks	2 - 8 weeks
Healing	9 - 14 weeks	8 - 14 weeks

Reaction time courses were similar for pions and x-rays and for different fraction schedules, although as shown in the graphs (Fig. 1) pion reactions sometimes developed more quickly and healed more rapidly.

ACUTE REACTION – CLINICAL SCORES

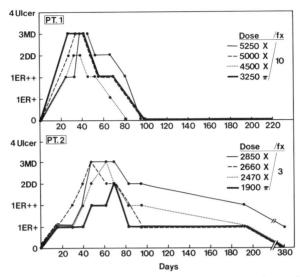

Fig. 1. Skin reaction time courses from fractionated pion and x-ray exposures. Upper frame 10 fraction treatment; lower frame 3 fraction treatment. ER: erythema, DD: Dry Desquamation, MD: Moist Desquamation, Ulcer: Ulceration.

Other Reaction Effects

Field shape differences between the pion and x-irradiated skin reactions were observed with less reaction at the edge of the pion field. Because disparity of reaction at field margins could have resulted from electron build-up from the use of lead cut-outs with 280 KV x-rays a beam shaping filter was made to match the dose distribution across the pion field.

Confluent reactions between adjacent fields resulted in reactions corresponding to a larger total area and vitiated assessment of individual dose effects.

We now feel 1 cm unirradiated skin should exist between adjacent areas.

RBE Estimations

Estimations of acute reaction RBE's were made in 5 patients combining clinical assessments and photographic material, bearing in mind possible different time scales for reaction. The biological end point used was usually moist desquamation, sometimes dry desquamation.

<u>10-fraction data</u>: for 2 patients (1 lymphoma, 1 mesothelioma) the acute skin

reactions from 2700 pion rads exceeded that of 4000 x-ray rads but were less than 4500 x-ray rads. For another patient (malignant melanoma) the 2700 pion rads skin reaction was greater than 4250 x-ray rads but less than 4500 x-ray rads. In one patient (breast cancer) the 3300 pion rads reaction was less than 5250 x-ray rads but indistinguishable from 5000 or 4500 x-ray rads.

Another patient (breast cancer) had a dose of 3250 pion rads and the skin reaction was clearly greater than 4500 x-ray rads but really indistinguishable from 5000 - 5250 x-ray rads.

3-fraction data: in one patient (lymphoma) 1900 pion rads produced a less intense skin reaction than 2470 x-ray rads.

The RBE for acute skin reactions in humans ranged from 1.43 - 1.67 for 10 fractions with a mean value of about 1.5. For 3 fractions, data suggests an RBE of 1.3 maximum.

Tumour Response

In 5 of 8 assessable patients it could be determined by clinical palpation that for those treated with pi-mesons there was a total of 6/7 complete responses compared with 12/19 complete responses for x-rays. Duration of responses ranged from 3 - 20 months. None of the nodules has shown evidence of regrowth.

II PREREQUISITES FOR CLINICAL TREATMENT OF DEEPSEATED TUMOURS

A CT whole body scanner and treatment planning unit have recently been installed in the Vancouver clinic. At TRIUMF, requirements include adequacy of pion flux, beam access and beam direction. The final prerequisite is a sufficiently large population of patients for clinical trials.

The pion beam at TRIUMF is horizontal and stationary so a special treatment couch was designed and constructed to make large field therapy possible. The couch movements provide for treatment of patients in a number of different positions relative to the beam (X, Y, Z translations and table tilting around the patient axis). Provision was made for scanning under computer control, the couch motion correlated to the pion dose rate. A laser alignment system is used and additional structures on the couch for patient immobilization and for fastening of collimators were also required. Installation of this system at TRIUMF is almost complete, and high proton beam currents of approximately 160 microamps will be available in 1982.

Short Term Plans

Phase 1-2 feasibility studies of pelvic malignancies are planned for 1982 and a conjoint study for glioblastoma with our colleagues at LAMPF and SIN will be implemented.

Patients with symptomatic advanced pelvic cancer will be treated to doses of 2000 pion rads in 10 fractions in 2 weeks to a 1 litre volume. This corresponds to an estimated 75% of "tissue tolerance". The criteria for patient selection and end-points for assessment are shown in Table 5.

TABLE 5

PION THERAPY IN SYMPTOMATIC ADVANCED PELVIC CANCER - PHASE 1-2 STUDY

Patients	Endpoints
Inoperable pelvic primary ± metastases	Tumour regression
Biopsy +ve	Survival rates
Age less than 75 years	Palliation relief
Performance Status Karnofsky higher than 60	Complication early/late
No previous radiation	

Patients with glioblastoma are being treated at LAMPF with pions only, or with whole brain photon irradiation and a pion boost. The latter treatment should be practical at TRIUMF and at SIN in the near future. Photon doses of the order of 4400 rads are delivered to the whole brain in 200 rad fractions over 4 - 5 weeks. A pion boost to the primary tumour area delivers an additional dose of about 1500 pion rads at 125 rads per fraction in about 2½ weeks. Criteria for patient selection and endpoints used at LAMPF are shown in Table 6.[5]

TABLE 6

GLIOBLASTOMA STUDY - LAMPF

Eligible	Endpoints
± primary resection	Tumour response
Biopsy +ve	Time to recurrence
Grade 3-4 Astrocytoma	Median and disease-free survival
Age 18-75 years	Complications early/late
Karnofsky higher than 60	

Constraints to Clinical Operations at TRIUMF

Only 40% of the total pion flux originally expected at TRIUMF can be realized.[6] As a result, the dose rate to a 1 litre volume for a 100 microamp proton beam is reduced from an expected 10 rads/minute to only 3 - 4 rads/minute; this would correspond to a treatment time of 25 - 35 minutes to deliver a dose of 100 rads at a beam current of 100 microamps.

Improvements can result from the use of higher proton beam currents and modification to the biomedical beamline.[6] Operation at 160 microamps proton beam could increase the dose rate to 5 - 7 rads/minute to the same volume with treatment times of 15 - 20 minutes for doses of 100 rads. The installation of another quadrupole in the biomedical beamline could augment the pion dose rate still further to within the range of 10 - 14 rads/minute with treatment times of 7.5 - 10 minutes for a dose of 100 rads.[6] These modifications are under development at TRIUMF.

Despite this, major conflicts will continue to exist with basic programmes such that we can only expect high intensity beams (i.e. greater than 100 microamp proton beam) for a maximum of 20 - 24 weeks/year.

The Availability of Patients

Registration data for the year 1980 for pelvic and brain malignancies in the Vancouver Clinic show that approximately 200 patients would be available in 24 weeks operation (Table 7).

TABLE 7

PION THERAPY - PATIENT AVAILABILITY - A.M. Evans Clinic 1980

Site	Total Nos/ Annum	% Suitable for Trials	Estimated Nos/ 24 weeks*
Prostate	253	60	70
Bladder	114	50	26
Rectum	91	50	21
Cervix	112	26	13
Ovary	90	45	19
Endometrium	170	10	8
Brain	84	80	31

* The amount of high current operation at TRIUMF will vary somewhat; a range of 18 to 24 weeks per annum is expected.

Estimates can be made of the number of treatment courses assuming a 10-hour hour day and 5.5 days weekly treatment operation (Table 8).

This evidence clearly indicates that our patient load is capable of filling the available beam time.

TABLE 8

PION THERAPY - POTENTIAL TREATMENT COURSES/YR.*

No. of Fractions	Treatment Courses/Yr.
10	158
15	105
20	79

* Assumes dose-rate of 5 - 7 rads/litre/min
  Assumes 1.5 treatments/hour (average)
  Assumes 24 weeks of 160 microamp beam current/year
  Assumes 80% efficiency in patient accrual and treatment delivery

DISCUSSION AND CONCLUSION

There is a sense of urgency abroad that "pion therapy for cancer" should justify its continuing financial support. This is legitimate because people want to know whether pions are any good or not and finally, whether pions are better than supervoltage photon irradiation.

The need for understanding and cooperation between basic scientists and medical groups is essential while international cooperation in clinical studies is required to provide answers to these questions.

ACKNOWLEDGMENTS

We wish to acknowledge the assistance of Drs. G.K.Y. Lam, R.O. Kornelsen and L.D. Skarsgard in the conduct and planning of these patient treatments.

REFERENCES

1. Skarsgard LD (1979) The biological properties of pions. In Okada S et al (ed.) Proceedings of the Sixth International Congress of Radiation Research, Tokyo, May 13-19 1979. Tokyo: Japanese Association for Radiation Research: 788-801.
2. Douglas BG, Jackson SM, Goodman GB, Ludgate CM (1980) Clinical status of TRIUMF; Maria Design Symposium, Vol II, Radiation Oncology, October, 1980 Medical Accelerator Res Inst in Alberta, Edmonton.
3. Kligerman MM, Sala JM, Wilson S, Yuhas JM (1978) Investigation of pion-treated human skin nodules for therapeutic gain. Int J Radiat Oncol Biol Phys 4:263-265.
4. Paterson R (1948) Influence of tolerance on choice of dose; The treatment of malignant disease by radium & x-rays. In Arnel (ed.), London, England, 39.
5. Bush S. Personal communication.
6. Lam GKY, Skarsgard LD (1982) Physical aspects of the pion beam at TRIUMF. In Skarsgard LD (ed.) Pion and Heavy Ion Radiotherapy: Pre-clinical and Clinical Studies. New York: Elsevier/North-Holland (these proceedings).

INITIAL CLINICAL EXPERIENCE WITH THE PIOTRON

C.F. VON ESSEN[1] , H. BLATTMANN[1] , A. BLEHER[2] , I. CORDT[3] ,
J. CRAWFORD[1] , A. ERDMAN[1] , P. FESSENDEN[4] , A. GEIGER[1] , C. GERBER[1] ,
E. HUGENTOBLER[5] , E. PEDRONI[1] , C. PERRET[1] , P. POERSCHKE[1] ,
M. SALZMANN[1] , K. SCHAEPPI[2] , K. SHORTT[6] , B. STADELMANN[1]
[1]Swiss Institute for Nuclear Research, 5234 Villigen, Switzerland
[2]Dept. of Radiotherapy, Inselspital, 3010 Bern, Switzerland
[3]Radiobiological Institute of the University of Zürich,
 8029 Zürich, Switzerland
[4]Dept. of Radiology, Stanford University, School of Medicine,
 Stanford, CA 94305, USA
[5]Dept. of Radiotherapy, Stadtspital Triemli, 8063 Zürich,
 Switzerland
[6]National Physics Laboratory, Ottawa, Ontario, Canada K1A OR6

The Piotron, a large solid acceptance angle superconducting
negative pi-meson (pion) channel, has been built at SIN for cancer
therapy. Its design, construction and performance is described
at this Workshop by G. Vécsey[1]. The design concept, originated
by Boyd, Schwettman and Simpson[2] permits simultaneous multiportal
therapy by means of the 60 converging beams. Considerable advantages may thus be provided for high dose-rate delivery and con-
formation of treatment to target volumes. However, in order to
fully exploit these advantages, new or improved approaches in
radiation therapy techniques are needed, e.g., dynamic scanning
of the target volume, meticulous patient positioning and target
localization, and accurate compensation of overlying tissue
inhomogeneities. Dosimetry aspects are reported by M. Salzmann[3]
and H. Blattmann[4] at this Workshop. The development of a 3-dimen-
sional optimization treatment planning system has been described
by E. Pedroni[5], and a positioning system by C. Perret[6].

The Piotron is designed for the treatment of larger deep-
lying malignant neoplasms. However, because of the extreme
technical complexity inherent in its design it is necessary to
proceed toward that goal by means of cautious steps, evaluating
at every level the results and problems encountered. At the same
time it is necessary to compare the effectiveness of treatment
by the Piotron with the best currently available methods since

418

the expense and complexity of Piotron therapy is not justified
if such treatment does not constitute a significant improvement.

In addition to a carefully phased clinical investigation
the biological effects of pions have been and continue to be
evaluated. Some of these studies are reported by Fritz-Niggli at
this Workshop[7].

CLINICAL PROGRAM

The clinical investigations are divided into 3 major phases,
with substeps where indicated (Table I).

TABLE I

Phase	Clinical Status	Primary Goal	Secondary Goal	Treatment Mode
Ia	Multiple small skin metastases	Palliation	RBE for acute epidermitis	Static - 15 beams
Ia'	Single skin or lymphatic nodules	Palliation	Mould techno-logy-Positioning	Static - 30 beams
Ib	Larger meta-static or surgically recurrent masses	Palliation	Confirm dose distributions	Dynamic raster scan or ring scan
II	Advanced regionally localized tumors at various sites	Curative	Seek optimum dosage. Explore "boost" therapy and radiation adjuncts	Dynamic
III	Primary tu-mors - randomized trials	Curative	Compare with "best avai-lable" treat-ments	Dynamic

Phase Ia is designed to determine the RBE (relative biological effectiveness when compared to conventional photons) of
pions for acute epithelial reactions with small treatment volumes
upon the skin of patients with metastatic skin nodules.

Phase Ia' is a transitional step from the simple, small dose
distribution achieved with the Phase Ia beam geometry to the more
complex method of Phase Ib. It has been used to treat somewhat
larger metastatic or surgically recurrent nodules on or near
the body surface. The intricate steps of creating an individually
moulded couch, performing a localizing and planning CT-scan,
"cylindrizing" the patient in the region of the treatment volume,
and, finally treating through the water bolus ring, are necessary.

Phase Ib carries this approach one step further by incorporating movement of the patient during treatment so that the isocenter of the multiple beams will scan the treatment volume
(raster scan). However, the selection of tumor sites is based
on the lack of overlying tissue inhomogeneities that would require
compensation by specially constructed absorbing materials.
Patients with larger metastatic or surgically recurrent tumors
would be treated in this phase. At one stage exploration of
the ring scan (pion momentum changing during treatment) will be
initiated.

Phase II finally will employ the technical development of
the previous steps for the radical (with curative intent) treatment of locally and regionally advanced primary neoplasms. At
this point, treatment planning based on CT scans will include
compensation for tissue inhomogeneities. Sites that are under
consideration, initially, include bladder, uterus, prostate,
and rectum in the pelvis region; pancreas, biliary tract, and
liver in the abdomen. Head and neck cancer and brain tumor will
also be treated. At this stage studies of "boost" therapy and
combination therapy with radiation adjunctive agents will be
initiated.

Phase III will consist of randomized clinical trials of
Piotron therapy and the "best available" forms of radiotherapy

and/or surgery for the curative treatment of tumors in sites where, from Phase II, pions appear promising.

INITIAL CLINICAL METHODS AND RESULTS

The Phase Ia and Ia' clinical investigations herein reported were initiated in November 1980 and terminated in April 1981.

PHASE Ia

Although the Piotron is not designed to treat small superficial nodules in a static mode, it is necessary to quickly and safely test and hopefully confirm the expected relative effectiveness of pions on the normal skin surrounding metastatic nodules while simultaneously providing palliative treatment to the metastases. Inasmuch as the RBE of pion beams changes with fraction number, dose, various tissues and reaction end-points, such an RBE determination can only be considered a relative value to be used as a guide for subsequent treatment of other volumes, tissues, reaction end points, and dosage schemes. The Phase I evaluations have been carried out by the pion therapy facilities at Los Alamos[8] and Vancouver[9] for the acute reaction of the skin and accordingly the SIN Phase I studies were designed to be comparable but also attempted to establish RBE values for a variety of fractionation schemes. The reference radiations were 250 KVp x-rays generated by a Philips x-ray unit located at the Triemli Hospital in Zurich. The desired level of comparison was the acute desquamative reaction of the skin interpreted by serial color photography and clinical observation.

Technique: A dose distribution was selected in order to treat a circle of about 5 cm to a 1 cm depth of the skin. This was accomplished by selecting a sector of 15 pion beams and designing a semi-cylindrical bolus of about 19 cm thickness to allow the stopping region to reach the desired skin depth. The pion momentum was then determined (180 MeV/c) and the dose distribution confirmed by 3-dimensional ion chamber dosimetry in a water phantom.

A collimator was selected to approximate the dose distribution of x-rays from a 250 kVp therapy unit with the dose distribution of pions in the special 15 beam configuration. The sur-
faces irradiated could not be precisely matched but approximated
5 cm in diameter. The fall-off was greater with pions, therefore
a pion isodose level of 90 % was selected to compare to the 100 %
dose level of x-rays.

The reactions were read and scored according to a scale
developed by L. Cohen[10] which involves 8 steps of visible acute
skin reactions.

Doses were calculated to give an advanced dry desquamative
reaction (level 5 in the Cohen scale) with x-rays and reduced for
pions by a factor of $\frac{1}{1.5}$ or 0.67 in accordance with the expected
RBE value.

Wherever possible comparable or bilaterally symmetric skin
areas bearing metastases were selected for comparison between
x-rays and pions. In all cases treatments with pions and x-rays
were given on the same day.

DOSAGE SCHEME

It was hoped that sufficient lesions would be available to
permit RBE's to be determined for differing numbers of fractions. Fraction numbers ranging from 1, 4, 12, to 20 were used
to calculate equivalent doses based on an empirical formula
derived from experience with x-ray therapy of skin cancer[11].
However, because of technical factors leading to interruption
of pion therapy it was possible only to compare reactions for
fraction numbers of 3, 4, and 10.

RESULTS OF PHASE Ia

Seven patients were referred for this study, four from Switzerland, and one each from Austria, France and Holland. Six of these
patients could be treated but due to technical failure of
the helium cooling plant it was possible to complete pion therapy
in only 2 patients. These will be reported in detail. However,
the general experience with treatment of patients was as follows:

Psychological factors: All patients adapted quickly to
the potentially disquieting technical array of equipment in
the treatment room and to the confining aspects of the treatment
couch and chamber. With careful introduction to the treatment
situation any apprehensions appeared to be relieved. Continuous
audio-visual monitoring and patient-to-nurse communication contributed to the patient's feelings of security.

Logistic factors: Since SIN does not have a clinical base,
it must rely on referral from a number of medical institutions
and individual physicians. A structure for referral from within
Switzerland has been established through collaboration with
the Swiss Group for Clinical Cancer Research (SAKK). Another
group, termed the International Pion Users' Group, has been established. It includes oncologists from Sweden, Great Britain,
Netherlands, France, Germany, Austria, Italy, Israel, and Kuwait.
Patients for pion treatment were referred from both of these
groups. Accomodations for stay were arranged either at nearby
hotels (3 patients), the local hospital (1 patient) or the patients
travelled from their homes for each treatment (2 patients). Local
transportation was provided by SIN vehicles.

Radiation background: The principal source of background radiation is neutrons from interactions within the Piotron system.
The second source is neutrons emitted from within the treated
volume of the patient. This source becomes more important as
the treatment volume increases[12]. Whole body dosimetry will be
reported in detail later. For treatment in the approximate center
of the body, e.g., the abdomen, the central body dose, as measured
in phantoms, ranged from about 10 mrad per rad of the maximum
skin dose to 0.6 mrad per rad along the body axis with neutron
components of 3.4 to 1 mrem per rad respectively. Thus for
a maximum cumulative dose of 2500 rads to the skin the central
body axis dose ranged from 25 rads under the beam (8.5 REM of
neutrons) to 1.5 rads (2.5 REM) in the head region. Surface doses,
measured in vivo by TLD dosimetry, varied with distance from
the treatment bolus. Particular attention was given to the ocular
dose for treatments on the thorax.

These were generally in the region of 0.2 % of the total
skin treatment dose. Serial complete blood counts were performed
on a weekly basis in all patients during and immediately following
pion therapy. No alterations in blood elements were noticed in
any patient with one exception, a patient who received concomitant Co^{60} fields to the sternum, anterior mediastinum, and
x-ray therapy to right supraclavicular and left chest wall
lesions for metastatic mammary carcinoma. This patient experienced
a leukopenia and erythrocytopenia which gradually returned to pre-
treatment levels.

SKIN AND TUMOR RESPONSES

The two patients completing planned courses of treatment serve
as the basis for calculation of RBE values. However, important
confirmatory observations were made on the other patients who
received pions and supplementary x-ray therapy. The following
briefly describes the two definitive patients.

Patient 81-1. A 52 year old female social worker had a malignant melanoma excised from the left calf 5 years previously.
Inguinal metastases were resected 4 months later but recurrence
and skin metastases developed 1 year later. Following local BCG
injection (Prof. H.J. Senn) there was a generalized remission for
approximately 2 years. Multiple skin metastases then progressed
despite further systemic therapy and at the time of referral for
pion therapy there were 31 pigmented subcuticular to subdermal
metastases ranging from 3 to 22 mm in diameter scattered over
the entire torso, head and upper proximal extremities. There
was apparent left iliac lymphatic involvement producing a moderate left lower extremity lymphedema. During the 2 weeks before
therapy could be initiated 12 more metastases were counted and an
estimation of mean volume doubling time of untreated metastases
was 20 days. Pion therapy and x-ray therapy were initiated to
5 and 10 comparable lesions respectively. Because of increasing
weakness and discomfort, however, the fractionation program was
altered so that ultimately 4 pion treated areas and 4 x-ray
treated areas could be compared. All treated areas demonstrated

424

partial tumor regression while untreated lesions relentlessly
increased. Visual inspection and color photography under constant
exposure conditions were made and the rate and magnitude of
development of skin reactions were plotted. Figure 1 demonstrates
such a plot for 2 pion and 2 x-ray fields receiving 10 fractions
in 19 days.

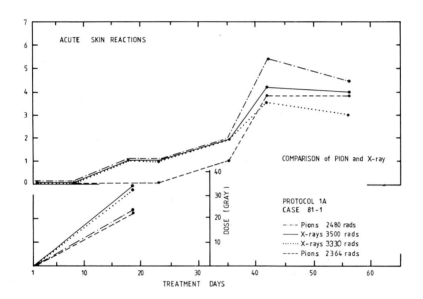

Fig. 1. Comparison of levels of acute skin reactions from pions
and 250 kVp x-rays in case 81-1. Each of 4 sites received
10 treatment fractions over 19 days of pions (2 sites) or x-rays
(2 sites). The RBE is calculated from the time of maximum reaction
(day 43).

Because of the patient's deteriorating status no further observations could be made beyond the 57th day from beginning of
treatment and she expired on the 64th day of widespread metastases.

Patient 81-2. A 56 year old farmer had a malignant melanoma
excised from the left calf 3½2 years previously. A left inguinal
lymphadenectomy for metastatic melanoma was followed by recurrence
and multiple skin metastases in the left thigh 2 years later.
Despite systemic therapy, disease progressed and the patient was
referred for pion therapy. Twelve pigmented subcuticular to subdermal metastases were noted, confined to the left adductor,
medial quadriceps and inguinal regions. They ranged in
size from 7 to 20 mm diameter. Because of the close proximity
only 3 lesions sufficiently separated were selected, one for pion
therapy and 2 for x-ray therapy. Subsequently 2 other lesions
were treated in the Phase Ia' study. Figure 2 shows the progression of skin reactions plotted for a schedule of 3 fractions
in 4 days.

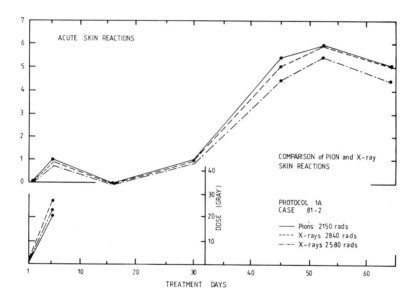

Fig. 2. Comparison of acute skin reactions for case 81-2.

Table II summarizes the data from both patients and gives the RBE values and ranges. It was not possible to accurately score rates of tumor regression, which occured in all treated sites.

TABLE II: Phase Ia skin reactions

No. Fractions	Doses for Equivalent Acute Reactions			RBE
	x-ray		Pions	
10	3500	>	2364	< 1.48
	3330	<	2364	> 1.41
4	2840	<	2150	> 1.32
3	2115	>	1577	< 1.34

PHASE Ia'

Patient 81-2 received subsequent pion therapy to a larger metastatic nodule in the left adductor region with a configuration of 30 contiguous pion beams. At this stage a specially moulded treatment couch with gelatine filled bolus was used and the patient and couch were positioned for treatment inside a water-bolus ring with an outside diameter of 61 cm. The target volume was localized by the specially designed positioning device and, by coordinate positioning, the target volume was adjusted to the isocenter of the 30 converging beams. A minimum (80 % of maximum) dose of 2040 rads was delivered in 4 fractions over 6 days. TLD dosimetry confirmed the dose distribution in vivo. The skin reaction progressed to a dry desquamative level and the nodule began slowly to regress. A mass of recurrent nodes in the left groin measuring 5 x 4 x 3 cm were similarly treated, but at this stage with 2 overlapping "spots" of the 30 converging beams. This proceedure represents the first step toward dynamic raster scanning. The reaction and response were similar and the patient continues to be followed.

DISCUSSION AND CONCLUSION

The first measurements of the acute skin reaction to peak pions giving an RBE value between 1.41 and 1.48 for 10 fractions in 19 days is in good agreement with values from Los Alamos of 1.43 for 13 fractions in 13 days, and from Vancouver of 1.5 for 10 fractions in 10 days. The RBE values for 3 and 4 fractions of about 1.3 are in good agreement with radiobiological evidence from the mouse foot experiment[13] and with expected lower values as the fraction number is reduced and the fraction size increased[14]. The ongoing clinical experience at Los Alamos, based on observations of acute skin and mucosal reactions is in the range of 1.6 to 1.8[15,16] for 24 to over 30 daily fractions. It is interesting to note that it has not been possible clinically to note quantitative RBE differences for various treatment volumes in the latter experience. Thus the first simple step has been made to confirm the biological effectiveness of pions emitted from the unique configuration of the SIN Piotron. The first advance has likewise been accomplished for dynamic therapy involving the complexity of treating a patient surrounded by a water-bolus ring.

ACKNOWLEDGEMENT

The initiation and progress of this project is due to the dynamic stimulus of Professor J.P. Blaser, Director of SIN. The design and construction of the Piotron has been accomplished by G. Vécsey and colleagues. We are indebted to the following oncologists for referral of patients and for ongoing supportive care:

Dr. P. Forrer, Chur

Prof. J.C. Horiot, Dijon

Prof. K.H. Kärcher, Vienna

Prof. G. Martz, Zürich

Prof. B. van der Werf-Messing, Rotterdam

Prof. H.J. Senn, St. Gallen

Dr. B. Späti, St. Gallen

Prof. P. Veraguth, Bern.

428

We are especially indepted to Dr. F. Heinzel, Director of
Radiotherapy of the City Hospital of Zürich, for enthusiastic
support and use of his facility for control treatments.

REFERENCES

1 Vécsey G (1982) The piotron channel at SIN. Pion and Heavy Ion
   Radiotherapy: Pre-clinical and clinical studies. Elsevier North
   Holland, New York (these proceedings)
2 Boyd D, Schwettman HA, Simpson J (1973) A large acceptance pion
   channel for cancer therapy. Nucl Instr Methods 111:315-331
3 Salzmann M (1982) The pion dosimetry program at SIN. Pion and
   Heavy Ion Radiotherapy: Pre-clinical and clinical studies.
   Elsevier North Holland, New York (these proceedings)
4 Blattmann H (1982) Treatment planning for dynamic therapy at
   SIN. Pion and Heavy Ion Radiotherapy: Pre-clinical and clinical
   studies. Elsevier North Holland, New York (these proceedings)
5 Pedroni E (1979) Development of the therapy planning programs
   for the 60 beam SIN pion applicator. Radiat Environ Biophys
   16:211-218
6 Perret C (1978) Einrichtungen für die Patientenbehandlung. SIN
   Jahresbericht E12-E13
7 Fritz-Niggli H (1982) Biological properties of single- and
   multiport pion beams: Studies on repair, RBE and OER with
   drosophila, mouse foot and mammalian cells. Pion and Heavy Ion
   Radiotherapy: Pre-clinical and clinical studies. Elsevier North
   Holland, New York (these proceedings)
8 Kligerman MM, Smith A, Yuhas JM, Wilson S, Sternhagen CJ,
   Helland JA, Sala JM (1977) The relative biological effectiveness of pions in the acute response of human skin. Int J Radiat
   Oncol Biol Phys 3:335-339
9 Goodman G (1982) The pion therapy program at TRIUMF. Pion and
   Heavy Ion Radiotherapy: Pre-clinical and clinical studies.
   Elsevier North Holland, New York (these proceedings)
10 Cohen L (1978) Personal communication
11 von Essen CF (1969) A practical time-dose formula for x-ray
   therapy of skin cancer. Br J Radiol 42:474 (letter)
12 Shillaci ME, Roeder DL (1973) Dose distribution due to neutrons
   and photons resulting from negative pion capture in tissue.
   Phys Med Biol 18:821-829
13 Fröhlich E, Binz P, Blattmann H, Fritz-Niggli H, von Essen CF,
   Josuran F, Schärer U, Zehnder J (1980) Fraktionierte Hautbestrahlungen bei der Albinomaus mit Peak-Pionen. SIN-Jahresbe-
   richt 74-75
14 Elkind MM (1970) Damage and repair processes relative to neutron (and charged particle) irradiation. In Current Topics in
   Radiation Research. North Holland, Amsterdam
15 von Essen C (1978) Personal observations
16 Kligerman MM (1980) Tissue reaction and tumor response with
   negative pi-mesons. J Can Ass Radiol 31/1:13-18

WORKSHOP SUMMARY

Gordon WHITMORE

Ontario Cancer Institute, 500 Sherbourne Street, Toronto, Ontario, Can.

While my presentation is listed on the program as a summary it
seems presumptuous to attempt such a thing. I would prefer to think
of this as a statement of one person's impressions, questions and
concerns.

In the first session we were treated to several presentations
dealing with one existing and two proposed types of facilities for
either pion or heavy ion radiotherapy. Those of us who remember 400
Kev x-ray machines and electromechanical calculators cannot help but
be impressed by the tremendous technical advances which have taken
place and must certainly express admiration to those who can describe
a 134 meter, computer-controlled, proton linac with a facility cost of
$25 x 10^6 as a PIGMI. While I make this comment somewhat facetiously,
such costs must cast a sobering influence on any discussion of the
clinical future of pions and heavy ions and serve to emphasize the
quality of data and the impact of results which will be required if
these modalities are ever to achieve wide acceptance. It must,
however, be born in mind that properly utilized, such a facility
would be capable of treating a great many patients, many on an
outpatient basis, and therefore the prorated cost per patient might
not be as formidable as one might initially expect. Furthermore, the
costs of treatment failure greatly exceed the cost of success.
However, because of the manpower and expertise requirements of such
machines it is likely that they will only be affiliated with very
major treatment centers. In this respect, Canada, because of its
centralized approach to radiation oncology may be in a position to
lead the way, and may already be doing so with one existing and one
proposed facility.

The first session raised several questions in my mind. It has
been pointed out that PIGMI is an attractive source of protons and
pions and with the addition of an appropriate but perhaps
problematical electron beam ion source could become HIGMI, an
attractive source of heavy ions. The question then arises as to
whether the PIGMI/HIGMI approach was considered and rejected for the

MARIA project in Edmonton? If so was the reasoning correct? I would have enjoyed a fuller discussion of the rationale which should now govern the choice between major particle modalities and the means of particle acceleration. Is the situation still so confused that we must build machines capable of covering every possible alternative? If it is then how long can the situation continue?

I am also concerned by the fact that while the clinical community continues to propound the merits of clinically dedicated machines that the current MARIA approach appears to be a multifacetted one with responsibilities for clinical practice, isotope production and physics research. It is my impression that such approaches often lead to difficulties; I believe that the Bevelac has faced these problems and TRIUMF is now facing just such difficulties and partly as a result is considering the acquisition of a SIN type pion collector.

Finally, with respect to this session, I must reiterate that PIGMI is proposed to operate with a 100 μAmp beam current, the beam current which is considered unacceptable at TRIUMF. This means that for pion therapy PIGMI would have to be equipped with something like a SIN type collector. These potential future demands for SIN type collectors reinforce the need for a rapid evaluation and resolution of some of the perceived problems of electron contamination and magnet heating seen in the current prototype.

Moving on from the discussion of facilities we then heard discussions of some of the problems faced by physicists doing dosimetry and treatment planning with existing machines.

My overall impression is that while the problems of absolute dosimetry are formidable for both heavy ion and pion beams and are further complicated by variations of RBE with LET, the sophistication required for practical therapy considerations may not be as difficult to achieve as originally imagined - at least in the case of particle beams used in simple parallel opposed geometries. With pions the contribution of the relatively long range neutrons produced in the stars tends to reduce the RBE variation from the proximal to distal portions of the peak. For parallel opposed fields the RBE variations will be further reduced by the averaging effect of the two fields. In the case of the heavy ions it seems reasonable to expect that the averaging phenomenon will occur with parallel opposed fields but there is likely to be greater variation with beam spread and a greater variety of filter designs will be required to produce beam uniformity and to give the therapist greater choice in determination of daily fraction sizes. The greatest uncertainty in the process is the determination of the appropriate radiobiological parameters to use to design filters for human situations and we have seen examples of filters which produced a flat response across the peak region for one cell line but certainly not for another.

Returning to the subject of pion dosimetry it must be pointed out that the presence of the high energy neutrons is not an unmixed blessing since it would appear that the pion beams will have relatively large penumbras and because of the high RBE values for neutrons the "equivalent dose penumbra" will be higher than the physical dose penumbra. With heavy ions presumably the penumbra will be much sharper. However, with heavy ions the sharper penumbra will of course be bought at the price of a greater dependence of dose distribution on tissue inhomogeneities and a greater need for the type of information which can be derived from CT scanners. This latter information includes not only the location of tumor and critical normal tissues but also measures of electron density obtained either by the use of calibration techniques such as were described or by dual wavelength or split filter CT scanning. I also feel compelled to ask whether once allowances have been made for uncertainties about tumor margins, patient inhomogeneities, uncertainties of localization, patient movement, etc., how precise will heavy ion therapy be and will precision only be possible for a very limited number of disease sites.

Precision therapy not only requires precise tumor detection and planning but also requires precision patient localization and immobilization, problems which were alluded to here but for which I believe adequate solutions are not yet available. Perhaps the Medusa device or the use of radioactive beams can be used to check the localization of patients in the heavy ion beam prior to and during each treatment and similar devices might be devised for pions. However, whatever the nature of such diagnostic devices it is my belief that after the first treatment they should only be considered as check procedures and not as primary patient set-up and immobilization devices because they will utilize the time of very costly treatment facilities.

We now come to the biological aspects of pion and heavy ion

radiation therapy. What is clear is that over the last few years
there has been a wealth of experimental data obtained on RBE's and
OER's both in vitro and in small animal systems and we have had an
opportunity to hear from a number of individuals who have been in the
forefront of this data acquisition. However, it is likely that there
will be few surprises forthcoming in this area and it is my own belief
that continued in vitro measurements are unlikely to yield information
of great significance except in one or two areas. The first and most
accessible of these areas will be information on RBE and OER as a
function of physical parameters such as, location within a beam, LET,
Y , fraction of "stars", etc. Such studies must, I believe, be aimed at
establishing general principles and not merely on the acquisition of
more values of RBE and OER. As examples of this kind of general
information we have seen indications that the biological effectiveness
of a pion beam may be dependent upon its dimensions at right angles to
the beam direction as well as along the beam axis. This would appear
to reflect a contribution from the star neutrons although some of the
physical measurements of neutron doses near the edge of pion beams
would appear to cast some doubt on this assumption. Whatever the
cause it is fortunate since, as was pointed out, it may increase the
homogeneity of biological effect across large field volumes.

A second area where we need additional information concerns the
response of mammalian cells and tissues to fractionated doses of
radiation for both γ-rays and the various particles. One thing
which seems certain is that with heavy ions there is likely to be a
much smaller effect of fractionation than is seen with γ-rays. Under
certain circumstances with heavy ions fractionation rather than
producing protection may in fact produce sensitization. However, one
would expect to see such sensitization only for closely spaced
fractions and I would always expect that pions would show increased
survival following fractionated exposures.

If we are to make the most appropriate use of particles and γ-rays
then the effects of fractionation for both modalities must be
determined in a variety of normal tissues. This is true because while
it is likely that the improved dose distributions and lower OER's of
high LET particles will always produce some therapeutic gain this may
not always be so for the shoulder removal effect of high LET particles.
The removal of the repair capacity of critical normal tissues through

the use of heavy particles may more than counteract any benefit of increased physical dose in the peak region. The determination of dose-effect curves for normal tissues as functions of fractionation regimes will be time consuming and costly and once again the emphasis in the design of the experiments should be to develop principles which will hopefully allow extrapolation to the human situation.

Much more importantly, as was pointed out, we need to understand the cellular origins or mechanisms of early (acute) and late damage in critical normal tissues. We have seen evidence that early (acute) effects may not be adequate predictors of the severity of late effects. Do late effects arise from destruction of the vascular system or from the destruction of cell renewal systems in each organ? On the answer to this may depend our ability to develop predictors of damage to other tissues. While on the subject of late effects we need to develop better information on the carcinogenic properties of high LET particles. It would appear that high LET particles have a high RBE for carcinogenesis at low doses - at least as measured in the Harderian gland. The situation with respect to lung and mammary tissue is less clear. We need to know the carcinogenic hazards of these beams and also if there are major variations from tissue to tissue and if so why?

One fact which seems to come out of all of the data and discussions to date is that there may be no ideal particle for all tumors. While ions such as silicon and argon have very low OER's they tend to have less favorable dose distributions than carbon and neon ions or pions. Pion beams are less likely to suffer major disturbances from inhomogeneities because of greater scattering and the range of the star neutrons. On the other hand these same factors produce larger penumbra effects for pions so that beam edges will never be as sharp as with heavy ions. In conclusion, it would appear the properties of the particle beam should be matched to the anatomy and biological properties of the tumor and critical normal tissues whether inside or outside the target volume. Therefore we need to develop rapid methods to assess the biological status of a tumor with respect to the level of hypoxia, potential for repair, reoxygenation and repopulation, likelihood of tumor spread, etc. All of these factors will enter into the choice of the most appropriate beam for the treatment of a particular tumor in a given site. Only at such a time when the assumptions can be clearly stated would I be willing to develop figures of merit except as a possible method for guiding experimentation. Inappropriate use of figures of merit could lead to unfortunate conclusions. I recognize that it may be a very long time before we develop such abilities and therefore in the meantime we may have to be content with less rigorous predictions based on correlations with other biological or histological characteristics. While it would be desirable to have this information it is unlikely that the funding agencies will long continue to support research on particle therapy in the absence of clinical evidence indicating a high likelihood of ultimate usefulness. This brings me to a discussion of the currently available clinical information.

I must confess that my overall impression is one of disappointment that we still know so little about the therapeutic efficacy of any of the particles. It is my understanding that proton therapy had its beginnings about 1961 and still the data while encouraging for certain very specific sites cannot be extrapolated to major disease sites. Neutron therapy in its reincarnated form is of course a newer modality but here again the clinical data, while encouraging with respect to some sites, is still relatively controversial. Given what appears to be the fragmented approach of the radiation community to the whole evaluation of particle therapy it would appear that this is likely to be the situation for a very considerable period.

If we look at the neutron trials then it seems apparent that in several trials the neutron patients have demonstrated higher levels of local control but it is usually true that such improved control has been "associated with" higher levels of complication. I have been careful here to use the phrase "associated with" because I do not know to what extent the complications are treatment induced and to what extent they are a consequence of damage done by the disease and simply manifested as a result of increased survival time. I must, however, reiterate the concern that if the sigmoidal curve of complications versus dose lies slightly to the right of local control versus dose, then major improvements in local control might be achieved with modest increases in complications but this might also be true with γ-ray treatment regimens. I realize that there are those who will state that these are only the vestigial arguments of the non believer. However, given the high personal costs of complications and

the high financial costs of particle therapy I believe such arguments
will have to be answered before neutron therapy can be adequately
assessed by the community, not only in terms of its role as a treatment
modality but what if anything the results tell us about tumor biology
and aid in the choice of future therapeutic modalities.

In the case of heavy ions and pions we must first mention the
helium ion experience although I would immediately accept the
statement that neither protons nor helium ions fall in the class of
major heavy ions and in all cases the numbers of patients treated are
small. In neither pancreas nor esophagus is there evidence of
statistically significant improvement in overall survival or of
improved local control using helium ions. Because helium ions are
basically low LET particles with RBE's and OER's not very different
from x-rays the only real hope for improved local control will come
from increases in tumor dose. It is not clear to me in the trials to
date that the effective tumor doses have been increased over
conventional photon doses or that doses have been pushed to
unacceptable levels of complication. Therefore I find it difficult to
interpret the clinical findings to date and I am concerned that
helium ions and protons may be abandoned before their time. We must
be concerned that an inadequate trial could dispense with an
effective modality.

If neutrons have the advantage of low OER but the disadvantage of
poor effective dose distributions and helium ions have the advantage
of good depth dose distribution but high OER the question then arises
what can we expect from particles with good dose distribution and
lower OER values. The argument would appear to be that we might
expect a great deal but unfortunately the supporting data from pions
and heavy ions is still not available and I am concerned that given
the rate of progress to date the question will remain open for a
very long time with a resulting decrease in the enthusiasm of the
oncology community for the support of these programs.

To circumvent these kinds of problems I believe we need concerted
approaches amongst the relatively small number of charged particle
users, both scientific and clinical. Would it not be possible to
agree on a limited number of disease sites for major efforts. In
fact if one lists the tumors of interest to the various groups there
is very considerable overlap especially in brain, head and neck and

pelvis. Even though it is too early for phase III randomized trials in these areas it would appear that there might be great merit in preliminary discussions concerning data to be acquired, types of patients, results of phase I and II trials, definitions of complications, etc. It would also be useful to have clear definitions of the questions to be answered by each trial. Are we comparing particle vs particle or particle vs photons? Are results to be compared on the basis of survival at some given level of complication or on the basis of some other cost versus benefit consideration? What will success or failure of the trial tell us about how we should proceed in the future? Since one major emphasis of such trials must be to convince other radiation oncologists of the advantages or disadvantages of particle therapy it would be useful if other institutions using the highest quality of photon therapy could be included in the evaluation scheme hopefully in the form of a friendly competition. To make these decisions and establish protocols prior to the trials will be difficult but not to do so seems likely to lead to trials the results of which will be less than convincing.

While talking about trials perhaps I could make one other point. This is that as a community we often seem to adopt approaches which are like the search for the holy grail, either we find it or we don't. In reality there is unlikely to be a holy grail in terms of a major breakthrough. What we must be concerned with is that our efforts lead to the development of the maximum amount of useful information. Much of what we can hope to learn from the study of particles and their application to radiation oncology is of relevance to the use of more conventional radiation modalities and to the nature of the disease. Much of what can be learned from conventional therapies is of relevance to particle therapy. As one example we have heard eloquent pleas for the use of isoeffect rather than isodose lines but the same plea could well be made for the case of conventional photon therapy yet it is seldom if ever done. Many of the problems of tumor localization, the causes of early and late complications, the need for measures of severity of complications, the importance of hypoxic cells, etc., are problems for us all.

In closing I would say that basic physics and biology considerations suggest that heavy ions and pions may well have a major role to play in the development of clinical oncology. If they are to play that role then the rate of clinical achievement must be markedly accelerated and I hope that the major result of this workshop will be such an acceleration and I thank the organizers for their efforts and support.

INDEX